Is That Fried Chicken Wing Worth It?

A Practical and Real Approach to Weight Loss and Healthy Living

Sharon D. Allison-Ottey, MD
(a.k.a. Dr. Sharon)

Published by Carlden Media, Marketing & Publishing, Inc.
www.carldenpublishing.com

Carlden Media, Marketing & Publishing, Inc.
Lanham, MD

Direct all correspondence to:
Carlden Media, Marketing & Publishing, Inc.
10104 Senate Drive, Suite 228
Lanham, MD 20706
301.731.8890
www.carldenpublishing.com
info@carldenpublishing.com

Library of Congress Control Number: 2009912713

ISBN-10 1-4196-6984-2 paperback
ISBN-13 978-1-4196-6984-2

Carlden books may be purchased for business or promotional use or for special sales. For information, please write to:
Carlden Media, Marketing & Publishing, Inc.
10104 Senate Drive, Suite 228
Lanham, MD 20706
info@carldenpublishing.com

Printed and Bound in the United States of America.

Table of Contents

Dedication

This book is dedicated to every woman, man, boy and girl who ever struggled with their weight, health and self-esteem. It is dedicated to everyone who so desperately wants to get a handle on the battle of the bulge and desires to be healthy. This book is dedicated to every parent that wants to model a healthy lifestyle for their children. It is dedicated to every spouse, partner and friend that desires their own personal best health but also that of their loved ones. Finally, this book is dedicated to YOU, the reader that had the courage to pick it up and take a small step toward a healthier life because you know deep in your soul that **YOU ARE WORTH IT!**

On a personal note, this book is dedicated to the next generation of the Allison family, my nephews and nieces. I love you all dearly *(Krenisha (Dee), Jeremy, Ray, Kia, Rayneshia and Darren)* and hope that as young adults you value your health/wellness and pass it on. For the younger ones, my beloved nephew, Christofferson Isaiah, my energetic and brilliant niece, Dayana, I so want you to continue to grow as the extraordinary, intelligent and remarkable people that you are becoming. I still have hope that in one of you there is a desire to become a medical doctor. Finally, this book is dedicated to my two new little princesses *(the Denises)* whose parents honored me in a way that has continued to astonish me by allowing them to share my middle name. I dedicate this book to Daila *Denise* Timberlake Allison and Kristin *Denise* Allison, may your lives be blessed with safety, health and wellness beyond measure. Your Auntie Sharon will do all that she can to stay committed and be a role model as you crawl, walk and run through the wonderful life that God has planned for you.

Acknowledgements

This book has been a labor of self-searching, love, commitment and certainly research. I've pulled this book from production three times. It has been revised in my attempt to make sure that I serve my readers well and I hope this has been accomplished. Thank you for having the patience to wait. Although it is written by Sharon Allison-Ottey, MD *(a.k.a. Dr. Sharon)*, it is a project that has required lots of helping hands, insight and assistance. I really hate naming individuals and to protect myself I say THANK YOU to all of the invaluable people that touch my life, whether on a daily basis or randomly with your emails, Facebook, Twitter, at events/conferences or in other venues.

As this is a book about nutrition and fitness, I must thank the great personal trainers that I've worked with in my own struggle over the last few years. Jennifer Boozer gave me the inspiration, during a grueling workout, for the title and premise of this book *(see Introduction)*. Jennifer is the epitome of excellence as a personal trainer and motivator. She was instrumental in my journey through the pounds and trying to find my balance between my life, health and career. Thank you Jennifer for being such a committed professional, our paths will forever cross and intersect. I would like to acknowledge and thank my current trainer, MacArthur *(Mac)* James, Jr. of Athletic Dominance. Although Mac fails to realize that I'm the client and thus should be the boss, he is nonetheless a trainer par excellence. Thanks Mac for not listening to my complaints or excuses and pushing me forward. Thank you to the management, staff and workout buddies of Bally's Total Fitness on Central Avenue in Capitol Heights, Maryland and at Sportfit Bowie on White Marsh Road in Bowie, Maryland.

I would like to acknowledge the following people for their contribution to this valuable work and my life. I'm grateful for my Executive and Personal Assistant, Sherri Warren who is my right hand and often forgets that she is not my mother. Sherri you are invaluable to me and such a blessing. I would like to also thank Sherri's predecessor, Cassandra Denise Smith, who remains an invaluable part of the *Dr. Sharon Team* and is an essential part of my life. Thanks to Sharon Silk, Alexander Maxey and Alonso Villegas, Jr. who have worked as part of my research team and are now gurus in their own right as it relates to health/ wellness. You guys have been great and I appreciate your time, energy and spirit of excellence. I would like to also thank Maria Boeding, my new editor for all aspects of my writing including the books, my website, articles and the *Cards by Dr. Sharon* greeting card line. Maria you are excellent and I thank you for assuring that my thoughts and words are grammatically correct. I also thank Sherry Buchman for her continued editorial assistance and support.

It truly does take a village, in my case, to raise Dr. Sharon. I'm grateful for the baddest photographer on the planet, Jacqueline Hicks of Fond Memories who never fails to make me look better than I could imagine. Thank you to Christian *(Chris)* Foster, my Public Relations guy for years and for those that work with you on my behalf. I would like to thank Granville Woodson and Ronda Quillen for their work on this book's layout and with my other projects. A special thanks to Juliana Doan, a graphic artist who is simply phenomenal and essential to my work. There would be no way that I could fail to acknowledge the talented, creative and innovative webmaster and graphic artist, Rachelle Harris, of *Designs by Rachelle*. Thank you Rachelle for developing my websites, book covers, advertisements and tons of other things for years. You never fail to provide a fresh look and to capture the essence of my work.

As always, I must acknowledge and thank my family and dear friends who remain so supportive of me and all that I do. Specifically Colin C. Ottey, MD, Thomas E. Allison and Guerleane W. Allison, as well as, my biological and extended family. I thank you from the bottom of my heart for being the greatest cheerleaders in the world.

Introduction

(Where in the World Did You Get the Title of this Book?)

"**Five More!**," Jennifer barked as I lie on my back in an unnatural position with my legs over an exercise ball, hands behind my head and doing my THIRD set of abdominal crunches. At this moment my devoted personal trainer had no idea that I planned on strangling her with my bare hands. I could see it, feel it and if she made me do one more set of crunches, as God was my witness, I would do it. That act would be worth the electric chair.

Then as if some supernatural voice came out of the heavens; I heard, *"Was it worth it?"* In my exercise haze, mid-crunch and with Jennifer's voice in the distance…I heard again, *"Was it worth it?"* Surely I had totally lost my mind, the abdominal crunches had cut the oxygen to my brain and I had to be passed out and hallucinating. Then the voice asked plainly, *"Was that fried chicken wing worth it?"*

"No, it wasn't worth this," I said aloud as Jennifer continued to bark at me.

"What? It's worth it—just think about the six pack abs that you'll have." She responded.

"Huh?"

"You asked if this is worth it—right?" Jennifer asked inquisitively.

"No, I was just talking aloud." I felt my abdominal muscles quivering, it was as if they were trying to escape from under the layers of fat from the countless innocent chicken wings, potato chips and chocolate that had been sacrificed to my taste buds and gluttony, and now were part of the landscape of my body.

"Ok, Dr. Sharon take a rest." Jennifer now said, almost sympathetically. Finally; she succumbed to her humanness and was giving me a break. I moved to get off the floor swiftly. *"Where are you going?"* She responded *"we have another set of 20 to do—take a 10 second REST 10-9-8."*

"Please tell me that I'm finished, I have a meeting." I responded with a little white lie. I did have to meet myself in my car on my way home. There was no way that I was going to torture myself for another minute.

"Hmmm ok, I'm going to have to get your schedule from your assistant. What did you have for dinner last night?" She asked with her hands on hips and lips tight, we both knew that the meeting was bogus.

"Why? I do have my own life; I don't have to tell you everything." I said with a quick check around me to see if she had her jump rope of torture in the room. There was no way that I was going to confess to Jennifer that I had partaken of the forbidden fruit—fried chicken wings the night before. After all, that would be fuel to her sadistic mind that thought of ways to torture me in my quest for better health and a size 8. I could not tell her that I ate the deep fried wing, meaty with crisp skin, grease dripping off of my lips and with taste buds experiencing heaven on earth. I had to pat myself on the back, I did manage to exert some control—I just ate one, well maybe one and a half—what harm could that do?

"WHAT did you have to EAT last NIGHT?" She asked again, totally unmoved by my comments, as if she was reading my mind.

"A fried chicken wing, I was hungry and couldn't find a place with a salad. Ok, you said one more set let's do this." I said quickly and pretended to be energized; maybe if I did the last set she'd let me go. The nerve of her, and I was paying for this.

"To burn off just one chicken wing we'll have to do hundreds of sit ups. Let's start NOW!" Jennifer was back in her zone and my mind was racing. Surely she was exaggerating, I have an MD—I know about this stuff, which didn't sound right, and it was just a little wing *(and a half)*. Why did I have to devour it? Was it really worth it—the wing was tasty with that meaty, juicy flesh covered in crisp skin. I'm from North Carolina so I KNOW fried chicken.. It only took about 2.9 minutes for me to INHALE the savory wing but now I would have to sweat and grunt for countless minutes to burn it off. Not to mention the millions of wings long ago devoured that were converted to fat on my body, which I was desperately trying to lose.

My hands instinctually began to contract and I restrained myself from strangling her. Instead I blurted it out, *"It is NOT WORTH IT!"*

"What are you talking about? Your health, your…" Jennifer began her motivational pep talk that I was all too familiar with. She was right, but with my abs in a knot from those darned sit-ups, I didn't care.

"The fried chicken wings, I mean WING, that I ate last night is not worth this!" I said as I got back into position to begin another set of crunches.

Jennifer finally let me escape and as I limped to my car trying to nurse my aching abs, her words would not leave me. Was it true? Would I have to do hundreds of sit-ups to burn off a measly but tasty chicken wing? Whoever just ate one chicken wing anyway—that's against the rules of chicken wing etiquette. This sparked something in my belly that I now use daily in making decisions about what I eat, if I will exercise and the WORTH of it all.

Well, the scientist in me immediately began to go to work and investigate Jennifer's statement. I REALLY wondered what I'd have to do to burn off the wings. First I looked up the calories in two fried chicken wings, and then I looked up how many calories were burned during various activities based on my weight.

Did you know that to burn off **two fried chicken wings** *(approximately 280 calories)* you would have to:

Activity	150 lbs	170 lbs	190 lbs	220 lbs	250 lbs
Aerobics, Low Impact	41 mins.	39 mins.	33 mins.	28 mins.	25 mins.
Bicycle, Stationary	35 mins.	31 mins.	28 mins.	24 mins.	21 mins.
Cleaning House	82 mins.	78 mins.	65 mins.	56 mins.	50 mins.
Sex	165 mins.	145 mins.	130 mins.	112 mins.	99 mins.
Sit Ups	31 mins.	27 mins.	24 mins.	21 mins.	19 mins.
Treadmill	27 mins.	24 mins.	22 mins.	19 mins.	17 mins.
Volleyball	62 mins.	55 mins.	49 mins.	42 mins.	37 mins.
Washing Dishes	107 mins.	95 mins.	85 mins.	73 mins.	65 mins.

Lo and behold, my life has NEVER been the same and the *Is It Worth It* Philosophy was born. All that for some dog gone chicken wings. And they weren't even that great. After all, they were not my Mama's; who by the way makes the best fried chicken wings in the world and YES they are worth it—but I've gotten off track. My research, REALLY made me think long and hard about putting the wings in my mouth. That doesn't mean I won't ever have another fried chicken wing, Mrs. Guerleane Allison's *(a.k.a. my Mama's)* chicken is worth two hours of exercise on any given day. However, when I do give in to the temptation, I have to be ready to burn it off. So, I choose the method; treadmill, cleaning the house *(NOT)*, aerobics and while sex might sound good, it is impossible to find another human to help you reach the minutes required to burn off the chicken wings. Truth be told, you will get tired even if you opted for *"self love."*

What if you aren't a wing person, what about a chicken breast?

Fried Chicken Breast

To burn off **one Fried Chicken Breast** *(approx. 510 calories)* you would have to:

Activity	130 lbs	150 lbs	170 lbs	190 lbs	220 lbs	250 lbs	270 lbs
Aerobics, General	80 mins.	69 mins.	61 mins.	55 mins.	47 mins.	42 mins.	39 mins.
Bicycle, Stationary	74 mins.	64 mins.	57 mins.	51 mins.	44 mins.	39 mins.	36 mins.
Calisthenics *(push-ups, sit-ups, pull-ups, jumping jacks)*	65 mins.	56 mins.	50 mins.	44 mins.	38 mins.	34 mins.	72 mins.
Food Shopping	225 mins.	196 mins.	173 mins.	155 mins.	133 mins.	118 mins.	109 mins.
Gardening, General	130 mins.	112 mins.	99 mins.	89 mins.	76 mins.	68 mins.	63 mins.
Raking Lawn	121 mins.	105 mins.	92 mins.	83 mins.	71 mins.	63 mins.	58 mins.
Sex, General, Moderate	399 mins.	346 mins.	306 mins.	274 mins.	235 mins.	208 mins.	193 mins.
Shoveling Snow	86 mins.	75 mins.	66 mins.	59 mins.	51 mins.	45 mins.	42 mins.
Sweeping Floors	157 mins.	136 mins.	120 mins.	108 mins.	93 mins.	82 mins.	76 mins.
Treadmill	58 mins.	50 mins.	44 mins.	40 mins.	34 mins.	30 mins.	28 mins.
Vacuuming	148 mins.	129 mins.	114 mins.	102 mins.	87 mins.	77 mins.	72 mins.
Volleyball	130 mins.	112 mins.	99 mins.	89 mins.	76 mins.	68 mins.	63 mins.
Washing Dishes	225 mins.	196 mins.	173 mins.	155 mins.	133 mins.	118 mins.	109 mins.
Weight Lifting	173 mins.	150 mins.	132 mins.	119 mins.	102 mins.	90 mins.	84 mins.

This philosophy is not just limited to chicken. I wouldn't want the poultry industry coming after me. I'm an equal opportunity "fat attacker." What about those jelly beans that you have on your desk at work? They can't harm you; after all you only eat a few a day.

Jelly Beans

To burn off **25 Jelly Beans** *(approx. 140 calories)* you would have to:

Activity	130 lbs	150 lbs	170 lbs	190 lbs	220 lbs	250 lbs	270 lbs
Aerobics, General	22 mins.	19 mins.	17 mins.	15 mins.	13 mins.	11 mins.	11 mins.
Bicycle, Stationary	20 mins.	18 mins.	16 mins.	14 mins.	12 mins.	11 mins.	10 mins.
Calisthenics *(push-ups, sit-ups, pull-ups, jumping jacks)*	15 mins.	15 mins.	14 mins.	12 mins.	10 mins.	9 mins.	9 mins.
Food Shopping	62 mins.	54 mins.	47 mins.	42 mins.	37 mins.	32 mins.	30 mins.
Gardening, General	36 mins.	31 mins.	27 mins.	24 mins.	21 mins.	19 mins.	17 mins.
Raking Lawn	33 mins.	29 mins.	25 mins.	23 mins.	20 mins.	17 mins.	16 mins.
Sex, General, Moderate	110 mins.	95 mins.	84 mins.	75 mins.	65 mins.	57 mins.	53 mins.
Shoveling Snow	24 mins.	21 mins.	18 mins.	16 mins.	14 mins.	12 mins.	11 mins.
Sweeping Floors	43 mins.	37 mins.	33 mins.	30 mins.	25 mins.	23 mins.	21 mins.
Treadmill	16 mins.	14 mins.	12 mins.	11 mins.	9 mins.	8 mins.	8 mins.
Vacuuming	41 mins.	35 mins.	31 mins.	28 mins.	24 mins.	21 mins.	20 mins.
Volleyball	36 mins.	31 mins.	27 mins.	24 mins.	21 mins.	19 mins.	17 mins.
Washing Dishes	62 mins.	54 mins.	47 mins.	42 mins.	37 mins.	32 mins.	30 mins.
Weight Lifting	47 mins.	41 mins.	36 mins.	33 mins.	28 mins.	25 mins.	23 mins.

It's not limited to just your food intake, we can rack up HUNDREDS of calories a day with what we drink and we don't really think about it. What about the cold and tasty, ever popular Frappuccino?

Frappuccino

To burn off **one Frappuccino** with whipped cream *(approx. 600 calories)* you would have to:

Activity	130 lbs	150 lbs	170 lbs	190 lbs	220 lbs	250 lbs	270 lbs
Aerobics, General	94 mins.	81 mins.	72 mins.	64 mins.	55 mins.	49 mins.	45 mins.
Bicycle, Stationary	87 mins.	76 mins.	67 mins.	60 mins.	51 mins.	46 mins.	42 mins.
Calisthenics *(push-ups, sit-ups, pull-ups, jumping jacks)*	76 mins.	66 mins.	58 mins.	52 mins.	45 mins.	40 mins.	37 mins.
Food Shopping	265 mins.	230 mins.	203 mins.	182 mins.	157 mins.	139 mins.	128 mins.
Gardening, General	153 mins.	132 mins.	117 mins.	105 mins.	90 mins.	80 mins.	74 mins.
Raking Lawn	142 mins.	123 mins.	109 mins.	97 mins.	84 mins.	74 mins.	69 mins.
Sex, General, Moderate	469 mins.	407 mins.	360 mins.	322 mins.	277 mins.	245 mins.	227 mins.
Shoveling Snow	102 mins.	88 mins.	78 mins.	70 mins.	60 mins.	53 mins.	49 mins.
Sweeping Floors	185 mins.	160 mins.	142 mins.	127 mins.	109 mins.	97 mins.	89 mins.
Treadmill	68 mins.	59 mins.	52 mins.	47 mins.	40 mins.	35 mins.	33 mins.
Vacuuming	174 mins.	151 mins.	134 mins.	120 mins.	103 mins.	91 mins.	84 mins.
Volleyball	153 mins.	132 mins.	117 mins.	105 mins.	90 mins.	80 mins.	74 mins.
Washing Dishes	244 mins.	230 mins.	203 mins.	182 mins.	157 mins.	139 mins.	128 mins.
Weight Lifting	203 mins.	176 mins.	156 mins.	140 mins.	120 mins.	106 mins.	98 mins.

What about that lunch on the run. You know the one—you're in your car and you have to grab something before you pass out. You're trying to be healthy so you opt for a chicken sandwich versus a burger.

Hardees Lunch

To burn off **one Charbroiled Chicken Club Sandwich**, Crispy Curls *(large)* and one large Coke *(approx. 1050 calories)* you would have to:

Activity	130 lbs	150 lbs	170 lbs	190 lbs	220 lbs	250 lbs	270 lbs
Aerobics, General	164 mins.	143 mins.	126 mins.	113 mins.	97 mins.	86 mins.	79 mins.
Bicycle, Stationary	153 mins.	132 mins.	117 mins.	105 mins.	90 mins.	80 mins.	74 mins.
Calisthenics *(push-ups, sit-ups, pull-ups, jumping jacks)*	133 mins.	116 mins.	102 mins.	92 mins.	79 mins.	70 mins.	65 mins.
Food Shopping	464 mins.	403 mins.	356 mins.	319 mins.	274 mins.	242 mins.	225 mins.
Gardening, General	267 mins.	232 mins.	205 mins.	183 mins.	158 mins.	139 mins.	129 mins.
Raking Lawn	248 mins.	215 mins.	190 mins.	170 mins.	147 mins.	130 mins.	120 mins.
Sex, General, Moderate	821 mins.	713 mins.	629 mins.	564 mins.	485 mins.	429 mins.	397 mins.
Shoveling Snow	178 mins.	154 mins.	136 mins.	122 mins.	105 mins.	93 mins.	86 mins.
Sweeping Floors	324 mins.	281 mins.	248 mins.	222 mins.	191 mins.	169 mins.	156 mins.
Treadmill	119 mins.	103 mins.	91 mins.	81 mins.	70 mins.	62 mins.	57 mins.
Vacuuming	305 mins.	265 mins.	234 mins.	209 mins.	180 mins.	159 mins.	148 mins.
Volleyball	267 mins.	232 mins.	205 mins.	183 mins.	158 mins.	139 mins.	129 mins.
Washing Dishes	464 mins.	403 mins.	356 mins.	319 mins.	274 mins.	242 mins.	225 mins.
Weight Lifting	356 mins.	309 mins.	273 mins.	244 mins.	210 mins.	186 mins.	172 mins.

Finally, what about our beloved holidays? The one most associated with food is THANKSGIVING. Many of us pray before this meal, *(if you're at the Allison household, my father, Thomas Allison, prays and you will burn off a lot of the calories by just standing for the hour that he takes to give his infamous Thanksgiving Day prayer)*. I would suggest that in this prayer you ask for forgivness of your gluttony and that your arteries don't jump out of your body in an attempt to not be clogged with fat. Below is just a little of a normal Thanksgiving dinner, but we all know that most of us eat TRIPLE this amount when you add in the ham, fried chicken, duck/goose, macaroni and cheese, potato salad, collard greens, chitterlings, three slices of cake, two slices of pie and the sweetened iced tea. But for the sake of making this point, here is the info on a conservative meal.

Thanksgiving Dinner

To burn off six oz. of Turkey, two cups of Mashed Potatoes, one cup of Stuffing, two cups of Cranberry Sauce, one dinner roll and one slice of Apple Pie *(approx. 1598 calories)* you would have to:

Activity	130 lbs	150 lbs	170 lbs	190 lbs	220 lbs	250 lbs	270 lbs
Aerobics, General	250 mins.	217 mins.	192 mins.	172 mins.	148 mins.	131 mins.	121 mins.
Bicycle, Stationary	232 mins.	201 mins.	178 mins.	159 mins.	137 mins.	121 mins.	112 mins.
Calisthenics *(push-ups, sit-ups, pull-ups, jumping jacks)*	203 mins.	176 mins.	156 mins.	139 mins.	120 mins.	106 mins.	98 mins.
Food Shopping	707 mins.	613 mins.	541 mins.	485 mins.	417 mins.	369 mins.	342 mins.
Gardening, General	406 mins.	352 mins.	311 mins.	279 mins.	240 mins.	212 mins.	196 mins.
Raking Lawn	378 mins.	328 mins.	290 mins.	259 mins.	223 mins.	197 mins.	183 mins.
Sex, General, Moderate	1250 mins.	1085 mins.	958 mins.	858 mins.	738 mins.	653 mins.	605 mins.
Shoveling Snow	271 mins.	235 mins.	208 mins.	186 mins.	160 mins.	141 mins.	131 mins.
Sweeping Floors	492 mins.	427 mins.	377 mins.	338 mins.	291 mins.	257 mins.	238 mins.
Treadmill	181 mins.	157 mins.	138 mins.	124 mins.	107 mins.	94 mins.	87 mins.
Vacuuming	464 mins.	403 mins.	356 mins.	319 mins.	274 mins.	242 mins.	225 mins.
Volleyball	406 mins.	352 mins.	311 mins.	279 mins.	240 mins.	212 mins.	196 mins.
Washing Dishes	707 mins.	613 mins.	541 mins.	485 mins.	417 mins.	369 mins.	342 mins.
Weight Lifting	542 mins.	470 mins.	415 mins.	372 mins.	320 mins.	283 mins.	262 mins.

Dr. Sharon's Worth It Tip:

If you are serious about really changing your life and need professional help whether you want to gain or lose weight, think about partnering with a personal trainer. Even if you can only afford one or two sessions, these experts are worth it. Keep reading and I'll give you tips on how to find a great trainer, how to afford it and easy ways to get sessions at no cost.

- Jennifer Boozer was one of my personal trainers and I got the idea for this book during one of our sessions. She is TOUGH but has a great knowledge base and is a real motivator.

- Jennifer's Advice: "No procrastination when it comes to your health, DEDICATION is the key to success!"

  - Jennifer's address: P.O. Box 5903 Takoma Park, Maryland 20913

  - Phone: 202.285.3548 or 301.779.2065

How To Use This Book

What it is NOT:

- A diet book

  - Diets don't work. I know that from personal experience, they just don't work. I'm not the expert at weight loss, but then again maybe I am because I've gained and lost several people in poundage over my lifetime.

- A coffee table book that just sits and gathers dust. This book wants to be read and used as a tool.

- A make you feel guilty and bad about being overweight/fat book. This isn't a book that is going to make you feel bad about having weight issues, I'm not here to blast anyone—except for some cellulite, I certainly am not trying to make myself feel bad.

- A book that will promise you that you will be a size six if you read it and put the tools into practice.

- Everyone will not be thin—that should never be the goal. BUT, you can be healthy and by the way what in the heck is a size 0; really? There are dangers in being too thin just as there are dangers in being too large.

What This Book Is:

This book is simply a tool for you to use in making decisions about your health which focuses on your eating and exercise habits. Again, this is NOT a diet book! It can be used no matter what your eating plan *(diet)* or strategy; whether low calorie, low carbohydrate, Jenny Craig, Weight Watchers, South Beach, Mayo Clinic, diet pills, a physician supervised program, surgical banding and even gastric bypass. The facts remain the same and the philosophy of the book is one that you can use to lose and maintain your weight. If you're looking for the next great diet book or gimmick—this is NOT the book for you! If you are looking for a tool to help you in the journey of weight loss, maintenance and even weight gain—keep reading because *It IS Worth It!*

A Dr. Sharon Sidebar:

Discuss your health issues with your private physician and/or healthcare provider—not Bubba out of the back of his car or the doctor on television late night selling you the pills that will take care of everything that ails you. We often put more thought into what we order off of a restaurant menu than we do our medical advice. I'm just saying...

This book is broken down into sections that you can understand and apply. Additionally, I invite you to go to my website, for updates and tools that you can use. I will start with the basics and build on your working knowledge of how things work. Honestly, most of us know this stuff but we don't apply it. The question is, has the information been presented in a way that we can really understand and not be bored to tears? The book is just a tool and you won't get the magical secret of how to lose 50 pounds in two hours! You will get information about nutrition, weight, your health and life lessons along the way.

"Be careful about reading health books. You may die of a misprint." Mark Twain

There are a lot of nuggets of useful information throughout that is presented in a way that we can understand. The information is presented for INFORMATIONAL purposes only and in no way should be thought of as personalized medical advice. Let me say that again; The information is presented for INFORMATIONAL purposes only and in no way should be thought of as personalized medical advice. You will need to discuss any weight or health issues with your private physician and healthcare team.

Using This Book?

1. **Buy it and Read it. It's really EASY to read.**

   a. Healthy living, why it's important to address the issue of weight.

   b. Health consequences and rewards of healthy living

   c. Facts vs. Fiction on diets, exercise and what you THINK you know.

   d. Quick reference in the back of the book.

   e. There are nuggets of information and a bit of humor thrown around.

2. **Apply the principles and the *Is It Worth It* Philosophy to your eating and exercise plan. Set REALISTIC goals.**

3. **Read it again and highlight/flag and mark the areas that you need to pay extra attention to—we all have our demons.**

4. **Learn and repeat the *Is It Worth It Affirmations* and come up with your own.**

5. **Put what you learn into action and commit to a healthier you.** The focus is NOT on your dress or pants size, you can be a cute size two but wind up in a coffin because your cholesterol was too high and you had a heart attack. Thin/slender does not always mean healthy. This is about your health and wellness, the side benefit is that healthy people actually look and feel better.

Are you ready to get started? Turn the page, push back from the wrong foods, suck in your gut and let's start burning some calories and realizing that We are WORTH it.

"Never put off till tomorrow what you can do today." Thomas Jefferson

"If you wait for tomorrow, tomorrow comes. If you don't wait for tomorrow, tomorrow comes." Senegalese Proverb

A Dr. Sharon Sidebar:

DO NOT sit and read this book inhaling potato chips, chocolate chip cookies and other stuff that you know you don't need to be eating! I've done seminars/workshops on health, nutrition, weight and during my talk people have pulled out a giant size candy bar and guzzled a slurpee. These same people stand up, laugh and push me forward with their response and applause then squeeze back into their seat. *(Thanks for the applause though).* C'mon people! Let's really get started.

OFFICIAL DISCLAIMER

The contents of this book, www.drsharononline.com, www.isthatfriedchickenworthit.com and any other media venue are for informational purposes only. The content is not intended to be a substitute for professional medical advice, diagnosis or treatment. Further, the information should be viewed as general health information and not as clinical advice or treatment from Sharon Allison-Ottey, MD or her associates. Always seek the advice of your personal physician, psychologist or other healthcare provider with any questions you may have regarding a medical or psychiatric condition. Never disregard professional medical advice or delay in seeking it because of something you have read in the writings of Sharon Allison-Ottey, MD, she encourages all people to seek personal, private care from a medical professional on a regular basis. The information in this book is in no way a substitution or extension of clinical care and Sharon Allison-Ottey, MD and associates provide the information as health educators. By reading the information, you acknowledge that you have understood the terms and conditions of use of the information. Further, Sharon Allison-Ottey, MD and associates are released from any and all liability related to the information provided.

Dr. Sharon's easy to understand translation of what the lawyers wrote: *Don't sue me!*

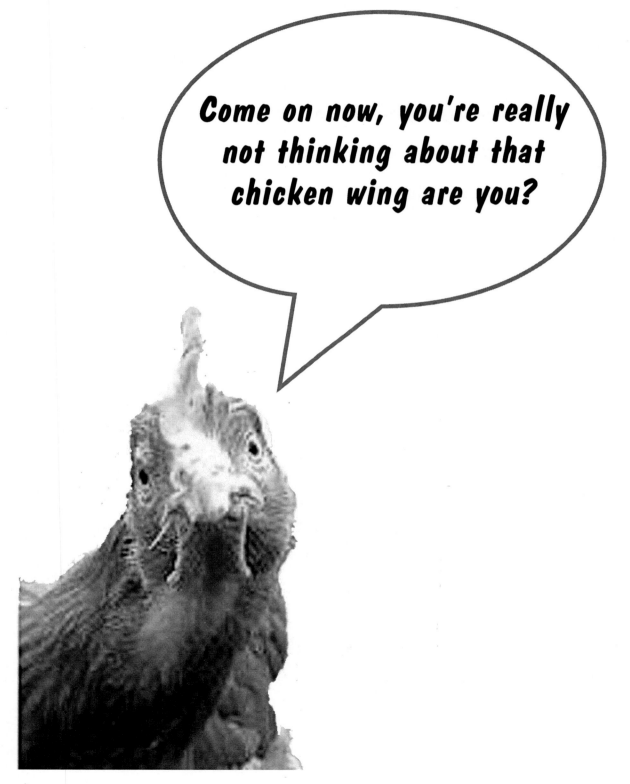

Part I: Let's Get Real and Get Down to the Basics of Nutrition

"There's no easy way out. If there were, I would have bought it. And believe me, it would be one of my favorite things!"
Oprah Winfrey, O Magazine, February 2005

Quacky Diets

I don't know about you but I've been on a diet since my preteen years. I've tried most diets/fads and even been suckered into buying miracle products that sounded too good to be true. I know that I'm not the only one who has eaten crackers and boiled eggs for two days to lose weight. A few examples of diets which most health experts **DO NOT** recommend:

- **The Grapefruit Diet**: You follow the instructions for 12 days then you take off for 2 days. There is a list of instructions, but the plan is basically below:

  - **Breakfast**
    - ½ Grapefruit or 4 oz. Grapefruit Juice *(unsweetened)*
    - 2 Eggs *(any style)*
    - 2 Slices Bacon
  - **Lunch**
    - ½ Grapefruit or 4 oz. Grapefruit Juice *(unsweetened)*
    - Meat *(any style, any amount)*
    - Salad *(any kind of dressing)*
  - **Dinner**
    - ½ Grapefruit or 4 oz. Grapefruit Juice *(unsweetened)*
    - Meat *(any style, any amount) (fish may be substituted for meat)*
    - Vegetables *(any green, yellow or red vegetables cooked in butter or any seasoning)*
  - **Bed Time Snack**
    - 1 Glass tomato juice or 1 glass Skim milk
  - **Vegetables Allowed**
    - Red onions, green onions, bell peppers, radishes, cucumbers, broccoli, spinach, lettuce, cabbage, carrots and peas.
  - **Vegetables to Avoid**
    - White onions, potatoes and celery.

- **The Apple Cider Diet**: You drink 1-3 teaspoons of an apple cider tonic before every meal.

- **The Hollywood Diet**: Basically a 48 hour liquid diet/fast with a juice/tonic/vitamin mixture.

- **The Cabbage Soup Diet**: You follow a meal plan with the main theme of a cabbage soup recipe and combinations of other foods.

- **The 3 Day Diet**: Basically 3 days of eating certain foods in combination. Here is one such version.

DAY 1		
Breakfast	**Lunch**	**Dinner**
Black coffee or tea *(Sweet & Low or Equal)* or water ½ grapefruit or juice 1 slice toast with 1 Tbsp. peanut butter	½ cup of tuna 1 slice toast Black coffee or tea *(Sweet & Low or Equal)* or water	3 oz. any lean meat 1 cup green beans 1 cup carrots 1 cup vanilla ice cream 1 medium apple Black coffee or tea *(Sweet & Low or Equal)* or water

DAY 2		
Breakfast	**Lunch**	**Dinner**
Black coffee or tea *(Sweet & Low or Equal)* or water 1 egg *(any style)* 1 slice toast 1 banana	1 cup cottage cheese or tuna 5 saltine crackers Black coffee or tea *(Sweet & Low or Equal)* or water	2 beef franks or hot dogs ½ cup carrots 1 banana 1 cup broccoli or cabbage ½ cup vanilla ice cream Black coffee or tea *(Sweet & Low or Equal)* or water

DAY 3		
Breakfast	**Lunch**	**Dinner**
Black coffee or tea *(Sweet & Low or Equal)* or water 5 regular saltine crackers 1 oz.(slice) cheddar cheese 1 apple	1 hardboiled egg 1 slice toast Black coffee or tea *(Sweet & Low or Equal)* or water	1 cup tuna 1 cup carrots 1 cup cauliflower 1 cup melon ½ cup regular vanilla ice cream Black coffee or tea *(Sweet & Low or Equal)* or water

Condiments Allowed: Lemon, a dash of salt and/or pepper, mustard and cooking spray

Substitutions: Some people use the following substitutions for the 3 day diet:

- Orange instead of Grapefruit

- Tuna instead of Cottage cheese *(and vice versa)*

- Frozen yogurt instead of Ice Cream

- Cauliflower instead of Broccoli *(and vice versa)*

- Green beans instead of Broccoli or Cauliflower

- Beets instead of Carrots

- Toast instead of five crackers *(and vice versa)*

STOP: Now, somebody has read the diets above and in their mind has decided to try one of them. I just give them as an example of what NOT to do and how silly they can be. Reread the sentence: "A few examples of diets which most health experts DO NOT recommend." This means DON'T do it.

The Truth About Fad Diets & Gimmicks

I could write an entire book on fads and gimmicks which have been used over the years. This is not to mention the use of colon cleansers and body wraps which promise to get the weight off. Many of you are saying, "She doesn't know what she's talking about; I lost weight on the XYZ diet." Guess what, you're right—you can lose weight by following these wacky diets, I'm sure that I've lost the equivalent of my three year old niece Dayanna's weight on them. The problem is I gained Dayanna, her sister *(baby Denise)*, her cousin *(baby Denise)* and a few relatives after I got off of the diet and then inhaled the refrigerator because I either starved myself or became too comfortable with the weight loss and eased up on exercise. The bottom line is if you eat fewer calories than your body uses you will lose weight; this is the fundamental basis of ALL weight loss. It's not rocket science; its physiology and basic math. The issues with crazy/quacky diets are the risks to your health and wellbeing. You can't follow such diets for the rest of your life and chances are if you follow them long term you will shorten your life.

Dr. Sharon's Let's Get REAL Moment: There is only one way to lose weight. I don't care what you do it boils down to basic math. You must eat *(consume)* fewer calories than you use *(expend)* each day to live. That's it—that's the big secret? You must find balance between the calories in and the calories burned. Further, you must create a negative balance of 3,500 calories to lose 1 pound. There are other factors like metabolism, health conditions, medications and family history which we will discuss.

Given that basic math of calories in and calories burned, fad diets do work in efforts to drop pounds. Look back at the 3 day diet; this is a very low calorie diet. If you follow this diet you will lose weight because you are eating very few calories, and much less than what your body needs to keep your heart beating, keep you walking and moving, etc. The problem with these gimmicks is that they are too hard to follow longterm, you get hungry so you get up at about 2:00 a.m. and inhale the refrigerator and gain every pound that you lost and more. You then go on to the next fad diet and become a human yo-yo up and down the scale. Further, you may not be getting the nutrients and vitamins that you need and you may be putting your health and LIFE in danger. Are the pounds that you may lose with dangerous, quacky diets Worth It?

>*"The second day of a diet is always easier than the first.*
>*By the second day you're off it."* Jackie Gleason

The DANGER of Being a Human Yo-Yo

Weight cycling *(yo-yo)* is the repeated loss and regain of body weight when the weight loss is the result of dieting it is called, yo-yo dieting. This could be a range from 5 to 10 pounds to 50 pounds or more in the cycle. This is VERY controversial; some studies have shown that there are negative effects on the heart and other organs. Other studies are less definite about the long term effects on physical health although recently there is strong evidence that there is an effect on blood pressure *(hypertension)*.

There is more evidence of the psychological effects of yo-yo dieting. Think about the real feeling of failure that you have when you regain the weight, you being your harshest critic and indeed your own worst enemy. Today you may feel great because you've finally lost that 20 pounds, then three months later when you've eased up on the exercise and slipped back into your habits, the weight has crept back on with a few additional friends—you find yourself depressed. Also, think of the money that you've spent on clothes in all the sizes that are in most of our closets: *Dream Size, Skinny, Real Me Size* and the HORRIBLE *Fat Me Sizes*.

Let's Get to the Basics

There are several factors that play a role in our weight. I like to boil it down to three basic factors that are the major players for most of us:

• **FORK**

 • **SNEAKERS**

  • **PARENTS**

Fork = Food that we take in
Sneakers = Our activity level including exercise
Parents = Family and genetics

The good news is that YOU have control over two of the big players in this equation.

The Caloric Balance Equation

- Overweight and obesity result from an energy imbalance. This involves eating too many calories and not getting enough physical activity.

- Body weight is the result of genes, metabolism, behavior, environment, culture and socioeconomic status.

- Behavior and environment play a large role causing people to be overweight and obese. These are the greatest areas for prevention and treatment actions.

Adapted from U.S. Surgeon General's Call to Action to Prevent and Decrease Overweight and Obesity, 2001. www.cdc.gov/obesity/causes/index.html.

What's the Big Deal about Calories?

A Calorie: In simple terms, think of a calorie as the gas that your body needs to move. A calorie is a measure of energy. For the more advanced, it is the amount of heat needed to raise the temperature of one liter of water.

How do calories affect our weight?

1. **Too many calories:** If you overfill your tank, you gain weight. Think of it like topping off the gas tank, what happens when the tank is full and you keep pumping? The gas spills out. Now, look down at your stomach, thighs or any area that moves when you don't want it to, or the area that hangs over your bra or over your waist. This is evidence that you've overfilled your tank, the calories have spilled over, gotten together and made some fat which is spilling over.

2. **Too few calories:** If you run out of gas what happens? You stop, can't move and need to call someone for help. If you take in too few calories you simply don't have energy to keep your body moving. I'm not only talking about moving and doing exercise or hard work. Your body needs calories to keep your heart pumping, your kidneys working, your legs moving and all of the other vital areas working in harmony. When you decrease your fuel to dangerously low levels, you could have serious health issues.

3. **What is your goal?** This will determine what you need to do. To put it simply:

   a. To maintain your weight: Eat and burn the same number of calories.

   b. To decrease your weight: Burn more calories than you eat.

   c. To increase your weight: Eat more calories than you burn.

I don't care what anybody says; the truth is that calories count! It's basic math and physiology. It is how our bodies work. Yes, there are other factors but this is the mother lode, we must balance what we take in with the fork, what we burn off with our sneakers and use every day in our activities *(i.e., keeping our heart beating, body functions, talking, breathing, etc., all burn calories)*. The other issue is that our genetics play a role but more than the actual genes, I believe that our culture, our relationship with food and other environmental factors have a major role to play. It's not so much that Big Mama was heavy and so we're destined to be heavy; what about the fact that Big Mama was the world's greatest cook and made the best fried fish, sweet potato pie, greens with ham hocks and pound cake in the world. What about the fact that you were rewarded for good behavior with food?

Weight management is all about balance; balancing the number of calories you consume *(fork)* with the number of calories your body uses *(sneakers)* or burns off. The CDC explains it like this:

- A calorie is defined as a unit of energy supplied by food. A calorie is a calorie regardless of its source. Whether you're eating carbohydrates, fats, sugars or proteins, all of them contain calories.

- Caloric balance is like a scale. To remain in balance and maintain your body weight, the calories consumed *(from foods)* must be balanced by the calories used *(in normal body functions, daily activities and exercise)*.

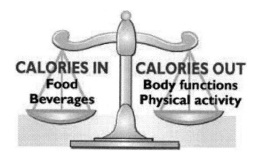

CALORIES IN
Food
Beverages

CALORIES OUT
Body functions
Physical activity

If you are...	Your caloric balance status is....
Maintaining your weight	...in balance. You are eating roughly the same number of calories that your body is using. Your weight will remain **stable**.
Gaining weight	...in caloric excess. You are eating more calories than your body is using. You will store these extra calories as fat and you'll **gain** weight.
Losing weight	...in caloric deficit. You are eating fewer calories than you are using. Your body is pulling from its fat storage cells for energy, so your weight is **decreasing**.

KEY POINT: 1 pound of body weight is equal to 3,500 calories

FOOD IS NOT THE ENEMY!

FOOD IS NOT THE ENEMY!

FOOD IS NOT THE ENEMY!

It is important for you to remember that food is not the enemy. However, too much of a good thing is bad. *"You must eat to live and not live to eat,"* as they say. Look at your goal and then develop a plan to reach it! When developing your plan, use some common sense. A diet that limits you to a certain food, food group or makes you feel deprived. I'm just going to talk about me; I'm NOT EVER going to give up Godiva chocolate. No, I'm not and I don't care what my trainer, a nutritionist or whomever has to say about it. I refuse to deprive myself of Godiva because it is worth it to me and I will do what it takes to burn off the extra calories that come with my favorite chocolate. Now, we have to be sensible; I didn't say that I was going to eat the WHOLE box of chocolates in one day. What about instead of buying 10 truffles, you buy just 2 of your favorites? Even if you must have a bite of that chocolate bar, why not buy it, take a bite and throw it away? Well, when I say this in front of audiences, inevitably someone says that you're wasting money. If that's the biggest factor, then don't buy it at all. However, if you must satisfy that craving, just take a bite or two and dump it. You're actually SAVING money. How? By throwing it away and watching your weight—you don't have to buy new clothes because your butt starts spreading more.

Dr. Sharon's Worth It Tip: 3,500 calories is a LOT of food, or is it? Ever wonder what 3,500 calories looks like on an average day? It's easy to pack on the calories without thinking AND to actually believe that you're being sensible. Let's stroll through a day.

Breakfast: You're running late so you don't have time to scramble some egg whites and have a piece of toast. You run into the nearest Dunkin' Donuts and grab something to eat, after all "breakfast is the most important meal of the day".

You decide to grab a Multigrain Bagel with light cream cheese and have a 10 oz. Vanilla Chai drink. You walk out feeling good about yourself; you've started off the day on the right foot. Or have you?

Multigrain Bagel with light cream cheese: 500 calories and 15 g fat

Vanilla Chai: 230 calories and 8 g fat

Mindless Munchies: You finally make it to work and after putting in two solid hours, you decide that you deserve a snack. You grab a Reese's Peanut Butter Cup out of the vending machine; you're brilliant! You justify it by saying that you're eating your protein (*peanut butter*) and having chocolate which is good for your heart. That's also why you have Tootsie Rolls (*midgets of course!*) on your desk which you eat throughout the day to make sure that you're eating enough chocolate for your healthy heart. Since you've been at work, you've eaten 18 (*give or take a few*).

Reese's Peanut Butter Cup (1 pack): 280 calories and 15 g fat

Tootsie Rolls (18 midgets): 420 calories and 9 g fat

Lunch: You decide to run out during lunch for some fresh air and grab something good. Panera is right on the corner and better yet, it's next to Starbucks. You decide that you will eat a Turkey sandwich and stop at Starbucks for a Grande Green Tea Frappuccino.

Sierra Turkey Sandwich: 840 calories and 40 g fat

Grande Green Tea Frappuccino with 2% milk and whipped cream: 490 calories and 14 g fat

Mid Day Meeting: You're feeling good about your healthy choices (*or so you think*) for the day as you walk into your meeting. You bring a bag of trail mix because you don't want to be tempted to eat the snacks that are out on the table. You eat only ½ of the bag and drink an energy drink that is full of antioxidants for a boost and grab a few of the Hershey's chocolate kisses that are sitting on the conference room table.

Planter's Nut & Chocolate Trail Mix (3 oz.): 480 calories and 30 g fat

Sobe Energy Essential Berry Pomegranate (16 oz.) Drink: 240 calories and 0 fat

Hershey's chocolate kisses (9 pieces): 230 calories and 13 g fat

YOUR Total BEFORE 3:00 p.m. - 3,710 calories and 144 g fat. You haven't even started to think about what you're cooking for dinner.

FOOD IS NOT THE ENEMY!

FOOD IS NOT THE ENEMY!

FOOD IS NOT THE ENEMY!

The calorie balance system reminds us that any calories that you take in and your body doesn't use for energy are going to be stored as fat. That is whether it is from a piece of grilled chicken or a greasy, fat-filled cheeseburger. A calorie is indeed a calorie, the nutritional value changes based on the food and you should make healthy choices which we will discuss, but for the sake of pure weight loss, a calorie really is a calorie.

Even though I'm making a big case for calories, we shouldn't just look at calories as the ONLY thing that contributes to weight. Unfortunately, there are factors which you cannot possibly control like your gender (*male vs. female*), your family history/genetics and your age. Remember when you were a kid (*before the video game generation)* and you actually road a bike, played hopscotch, soccer, football or another activity? You were a constant calorie burning machine, because you were growing and you were active. Unfortunately, we've begun to think ONLY of calories as they relate to the food that we put in. Just as important are the amount of calories that we burn. As we age, our activity level and calorie burn slow down and we get behind the calorie curve. How do we now go back to being active and burning through the calories? Keep reading.

Genetics/Family and Your Weight

"Call it a clan, call it a network, call it a tribe, call it a family. Whatever you call it, whoever you are, you need one." Jane Howard

"Families are like fudge—mostly sweet with a few nuts." Author Unknown

On the issue of family history, we have to spend another moment here because some of you read this and said, "That's it! I'm fat because my parents are fat." Well, I hate to burst your bubble, but the fact is that you are probably overweight because of the habits that you picked up and part of that may have come from your parents. While there is some relationship to genetics and your weight, most of it is based on lifestyle. For instance, if you grow up in a family that plays outdoor sports, took hiking vacations and was very active, you probably will love exercise and being fit. The likelihood of you carrying over those habits into your adult life is high and thus your weight may be under better control. If you grew up eating lots of green vegetables, fruits, drinking water and having balanced meals with little red meat, fried foods and sugary snacks then you probably have a better chance at being a normal weight. On the other hand, if you grew up sitting in front of the television and not participating in any outdoor activities, then exercise is foreign to you and you probably avoid it like the plague. Further, if you learned how to cook using fat back, lard, big frying pans and skillets with large amounts of country bacon drowning your poor little green beans, then you my dear probably have a weight problem. This is a lifestyle and you learn a lot about who you will be as an adult during your early childhood/adolescent life.

"You don't choose your family. They are God's gift to you, as you are to them." Desmond Tutu

Just as you may try to easily blame your family for your weight gain, are you making sure that no one is pointing a finger at you? What are we doing for our families now? Are we modeling healthy behavior with our children, spouses and extended family? Have you EVER exercised with your children? Have they seen you exercise? Do you get them off the couch? Are you the family member bringing salad to your family meal versus the 10,000 calorie-a-slice super cake that you're famous for? *Oops, did I get you on that one?*

A Dr. Sharon Sidebar:

I'm by all accounts the world's greatest auntie, just ask my nephew Christofferson. We spent time together and at the end of our week, I asked him what he learned about his favorite Auntie *(sorry other family members—I've locked up this title).* The first thing he said was; "You don't eat all your food." I laughed because I remembered that throughout the week he'd really try to clean his plate. He would actually say I don't want to waste it and I'd tell him that he could just taste it and move on. This was a hard concept for him because his father, my beloved brother, has a REAL concept of not wasting anything—even a paper clip— some people would call him a cheapskate but of course I never would. Anyway, while I do believe that you shouldn't intentionally waste food, I believe more that you shouldn't deprive yourself and that it really is okay to eat half of something and throw the rest away or save it. However, with my willpower, if I don't dump it—at right about midnight I will crawl out of bed and finish it...after all, 12:01 a.m. is a new day. You have to do whatever it takes and really be TRUE to yourself. By the way, the second thing that my nephew said: "You really can shop."

A Dr. Sharon Sidebar:

There has been A LOT of attention given to thyroid disease and weight gain in recent years. We need to make sure that we are clear about the actual AMOUNT of weight gain that you may see from thyroid disease and in health issues in general. As I've said in talks around the country—"thyroid disease may add 5-10 pounds but not 50 pounds." The 50 pounds comes from sitting on the couch eating fried chicken, cake, pies, chips and reading about your poor thyroid. GET UP and GET MOVING! Seriously, an underactive thyroid may account for 5-10 pounds—in order for you to gain massive amounts of weight from hypothyroidism you would have to have SEVERE disease. If you had severe disease there would be other symptoms that would be of great health concern. Some symptoms include: feeling very tired all the time (fatigue), weakness, coarse/dry hair, hair loss, feeling cold, constipation, depression, irritability, decreased libido (sex drive), abnormal menstrual cycles, muscle cramps and aches, weight gain or difficulty in losing weight, dry/rough skin and other symptoms. If you are experiencing any of these symptoms, call your doctor for a full evaluation—it could be a number of medical conditions. However, if your ONLY symptom of an underactive thyroid gland is weight gain, it is probably due to other factors as well such as hand to mouth syndrome (i.e., eating too much).

Medications and Disease

There are many roads leading to our increased weight, we've discussed the fork, sneakers and family. However, there are other factors which include medications and diseases/illnesses. Let's look a little further.

Other factors that affect your weight:

- Certain medications may cause weight gain based on several factors, including the way the medication works, the way it affects your metabolism (how you burn calories), the drug may increase your appetite, make you crave certain foods or cause water retention. The medication may make you feel sleepy and therefore you have decreased activity and gain weight, and many other causes that you should discuss with your doctor.

- If you believe that a medication is making you gain weight, you should talk to your doctor and really try to pinpoint the issue. There is a balance between your health, the medication benefit versus the weight gain or side effects. You may need to continue the medication but make lifestyle changes to offset the weight gain, like increasing your exercise and really decreasing your food intake. Also, it is important to ASK the doctor at the time of getting the prescription about all the side effects including weight gain.

- **A few types of medications that may cause weight gain** (limited list):
  - Birth control pills/medications
  - Allergy medications
  - Steroids (example: prednisone)
  - Some antidepressants
  - Antipsychotics
  - Insulin
  - Seizure medications
  - Some high blood pressure medications

- **Certain illnesses may cause weight gain** (limited list):
  - Genetic diseases in children (Prader-Willi syndrome, Cohen syndrome and others)
  - Polycystic ovary syndrome (PCO)
  - Cushing's syndrome
  - Depression
  - Psychiatric conditions
  - Thyroid disease (hypothyroidism)

"I saw a large woman wearing a sweatshirt with "Guess" on it. I said, "Thyroid problem?"
Arnold Schwarzenegger

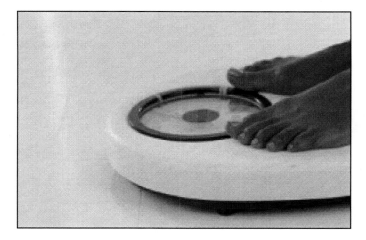

The SCALE IS NOT THE ENEMY!

The SCALE IS NOT THE ENEMY!

The SCALE IS NOT THE ENEMY!

Bathroom Scale Diet Tricks

Found at www.dietjokes.co.uk/jokes

1. Weigh yourself fully clothed after dinner and again the next morning without clothes and before breakfast, because it's nice to see how much weight you've lost overnight.

2. Never weigh yourself with wet hair.

3. When weighing, remove everything, including eyeglasses. In this case, blurred vision is an asset. Don't forget to remove jewelry as it could weigh as much as a pound.

4. Buy only cheap scales, never the medical kind. Accuracy is the enemy and high quality scales are very accurate.

5. Always go to the bathroom first.

6. Weigh yourself after a haircut, this is good for up to half a pound of hair (*hopefully*).

7. Exhale with all your might BEFORE stepping onto the scale. (*Air has weight, right?*)

8. Start out with just one foot on the scale, then holding onto a towel rod slowly edge your other foot onto the scale while slowly releasing your hold on the towel rod. Admittedly, this takes time, but it's worth it. You will weigh at least two pounds less than if you'd stepped onto the scale normally.

We're focused on weight and the factors contributing to the increased pounds, let me know how these scientific methods work for you on your scale, I'm particularly fond of #8. However, when you ask the average person on the street what their weight should be, I dare say that most do not know. As we address the weight issue, we should really focus on being healthy and fit versus getting to some magical number on a scale by any means necessary. It should be about adopting a healthier lifestyle and reaping the benefits of feeling AND looking better. You can be an ideal weight, but have too much body fat or not be toned and look horrible. You can also be a perfect weight but have bad eating habits, avoid exercising and have elevated cholesterol which leads to heart disease. There is no iron clad rule on what your ideal weight is, there are ranges and other measures *(body mass index)* that we have to consider.

What Should You Weigh? This is the billion dollar question. I've long hated these stupid tables and justified why I was off the charts! After all, I'm big boned, *WHAT on earth does that mean*?

Look at your height and then you will see a RANGE for your ideal weight. Go ahead—LOOK!

Determining Your Ideal Weight

Found at www.rush.edu

Male		Female	
Height	**Ideal Weight**	**Height**	**Ideal Weight**
4' 6"	63 - 77 lbs.	4' 6"	63 - 77 lbs.
4' 7"	68 - 84 lbs.	4' 7"	68 - 83 lbs.
4' 8"	74 - 90 lbs.	4' 8"	72 - 88 lbs.
4' 9"	79 - 97 lbs.	4' 9"	77 - 94 lbs.
4' 10"	85 - 103 lbs.	4' 10"	81 - 99 lbs.
4' 11"	90 - 110 lbs.	4' 11"	86 - 105 lbs.
5' 0"	95 - 117 lbs.	5' 0"	90 - 110 lbs.
5' 1"	101 - 123 lbs.	5' 1"	95 - 116 lbs.
5' 2"	106 - 130 lbs.	5' 2"	99 - 121 lbs.
5' 3"	112 - 136 lbs.	5' 3"	104 - 127 lbs.
5' 4"	117 - 143 lbs.	5' 4"	108 - 132 lbs.
5' 5"	122 - 150 lbs.	5' 5"	113 - 138 lbs.
5' 6"	128 - 156 lbs.	5' 6"	117 - 143 lbs.
5' 7"	133 - 163 lbs.	5' 7"	122 - 149 lbs.
5' 8"	139 - 169 lbs.	5' 8"	126 - 154 lbs.
5' 9"	144 - 176 lbs.	5' 9"	131 - 160 lbs.
5' 10"	149 - 183 lbs.	5' 10"	135 - 165 lbs.
5' 11"	155 - 189 lbs.	5' 11"	140 - 171 lbs.
6' 0"	160 - 196 lbs.	6' 0"	144 - 176 lbs.
6' 1"	166 - 202 lbs.	6' 1"	149 - 182 lbs.
6' 2"	171 - 209 lbs.	6' 2"	153 - 187 lbs.
6' 3"	176 - 216 lbs.	6' 3"	158 - 193 lbs.
6' 4"	182 - 222 lbs.	6' 4"	162 - 198 lbs.
6' 5"	187 - 229 lbs.	6' 5"	167 - 204 lbs.
6' 6"	193 - 235 lbs.	6' 6"	171 - 209 lbs.
6' 7"	198 - 242 lbs.	6' 7"	176 - 215 lbs.
6' 8"	203 - 249 lbs.	6' 8"	180 - 220 lbs.
6' 9"	209 - 255 lbs.	6' 9"	185 - 226 lbs.
6' 10"	214 - 262 lbs.	6' 10"	189 - 231 lbs.
6' 11"	220 - 268 lbs.	6' 11"	194 - 237 lbs.
7' 0"	225 - 275 lbs.	7' 0"	198 - 242 lbs.

Figuring out how much you should weigh isn't as simple as looking at a height-weight chart, but includes considering the amount of bone, muscle and fat in your body's composition. The amount of fat is a major piece to this puzzle. There are many ways to measure your body fat and muscle.

Other Tests/Guidelines:

1. **The Skin-fold tests:** Usually done in a gym or sports facility and fat calipers are used to measure body fat at various points, such as the back of the arm, abdomen and thighs.

2. **Underwater weight:** This is obviously more advanced but it is a common lab test that determines how much of a person's body is fat and how much is muscle by weighing under water.

3. **The Waist-to-hip ratio:** Measures abdominal fat by looking at the waist versus the hip and determines ratio. This is important because if you carry more weight in the middle than at the hips *(pear vs. apple shape)* you are at more risk for heart disease.

4. Body Mass Index (BMI): A good measure of how much fat you carry is the Body Mass Index *(BMI)*. This is what can be used to determine at a glance if your weight is normal, overweight or obese.

Calculate Your BMI

BMI	19	20	21	22	23	24	25	26	27	28	29	30	31	32	33	34	35
Height							Weight in Pounds										
4'10"	91	96	100	105	110	115	119	124	129	134	138	143	148	153	158	162	167
4'11"	94	99	104	109	114	119	124	128	133	138	143	148	153	158	163	168	173
5'	97	102	107	112	118	123	128	133	138	143	148	153	158	163	158	174	179
5'1"	100	106	111	116	122	127	132	137	143	148	153	158	164	169	174	180	185
5'2"	104	109	115	120	126	131	136	142	147	153	158	164	169	175	180	186	191
5'3"	107	113	118	124	130	135	141	146	152	158	163	169	175	180	186	191	197
5'4"	110	116	122	128	134	140	145	151	157	163	169	174	180	186	192	197	204
5'5"	114	120	126	132	138	144	150	156	162	168	174	180	186	192	198	204	210
5'6"	118	124	130	136	142	148	155	161	167	173	179	186	192	198	204	210	216
5'7"	121	127	134	140	146	153	159	166	172	178	185	191	198	204	211	217	223
5'8"	125	131	138	144	151	158	164	171	177	184	190	197	203	210	216	223	230
5'9"	128	135	142	149	155	162	169	176	182	189	196	203	209	216	223	230	236
5'10"	132	139	146	153	160	167	174	181	188	195	202	209	216	222	229	236	243
5'11"	136	143	150	157	165	172	179	186	193	200	208	215	222	229	236	243	250
6'	140	147	154	162	169	177	184	191	199	206	213	221	228	235	242	250	258
6'1"	144	151	159	166	174	182	189	197	204	212	219	227	235	242	250	257	265
6'2'	148	155	163	171	179	186	194	202	210	218	225	233	241	249	256	264	272
6'3'	152	160	168	176	184	192	200	208	216	224	232	240	248	256	264	272	279
	Healthy Weight						Overweight					Obese					

Body Mass Index Table: To use the table, find the appropriate height in the left-hand column and then move across to a given weight. The number at the top of the column is the BMI at that height and weight. Pounds have been rounded off.

Source: *Clinical Guidelines on Identification, Evaluation, and Treatment of Overweight and Obesity in Adults*, NHLBI, September 1998

What is BMI?

Body Mass Index *(BMI)* is a number calculated from a person's weight and height. BMI is a screening tool to identify where adults stand as it relates to their weight and gives an indication for risks of disease based on weight. BMI is a good screening tool or indicator for body fatness.

BMI = Your Weight *(kg)*/Height *(m²)*

Important Notes about BMI Charts: These charts are a general guide and provide a range for people. However, there are some exceptions:

- At the same BMI, women tend to have more body fat than men *(even thin women)*.

- At the same BMI, older people, on average, tend to have more body fat than younger adults.

- Highly trained athletes may have a high BMI because of increased muscularity rather than increased body fat.

What does your BMI score mean?

BMI	Weight Status
Below 18.5	Underweight
18.5 – 24.9	**Normal**
25.0 – 29.9	Overweight
30.0 and Above	Obese

Dr. Sharon's Let's Get REAL Moment: Denial is a very comforting blanket. Many of us will look at the height/weight charts and declare that they are somehow biased because of our race and gender. Trust me, there is no conspiracy theory and for most people these are the actual guidelines that you should follow. This is NOT about getting into your perfect size 8 and being sexy. It is about your health; the more overweight you are, the increased chance for you to have major health challenges. According to a study conducted by the National Cancer Institute *(NCI)* and the AARP, the nation's leading organization for persons 50-Plus, being overweight during midlife is associated with an increased risk of death.

According to the CDC, the BMI ranges are based on the relationship between body weight, disease and death. Overweight and obese individuals are at increased risk for many diseases and health conditions, including the following:

- Hypertension

- Arthritis

- Dyslipidemia *(for example, high LDL cholesterol, low HDL cholesterol or high levels of triglycerides)*

- Type 2 diabetes

- Coronary heart disease *(Heart Attacks/Heart Disease)*

- Stroke

- Gallbladder disease

- Osteoarthritis

- Sleep apnea and respiratory problems

- Some cancers *(endometrial, breast and colon)*

This is also not just about YOU. What about my readers who are parents and are modeling behavior and lifestyle for their children? Don't you want the best for your children? Don't you sacrifice and plan on watching them grow into the best people that they can become? Well, if you are obese, your risk of dying early is increased. Your risk of stroke, heart attack, diabetes and some cancer goes up and therefore you may not be around to see little Susie get married. Now I must ask you again, *Is that Fried Chicken Wing, REALLY, REALLY worth it?* Or is your health, your life and being there for your children worth it?

Determining Worth

This is an easy concept for us to understand because we use it every single day. I'm just proposing that we begin using it as we try to tackle longstanding weight issues. Let me give you an example of how you use the worth it philosophy:

You're walking in the mall and you see a beautiful pair of shoes. For most of us, we immediately want to know two things (*not necessarily in this order*);

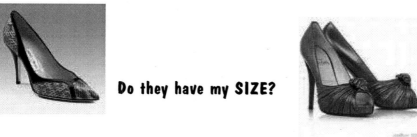

Do they have my SIZE?

How much do they COST?

The question of cost speaks to the worth that we place on the shoes. In our mind, we juggle the cost with our bank account and our obligations. We place a value on how much we want the shoes versus how much we are willing to give up to get them. It's not just shoes; I dare say we apply this principle to all of our major purchases and even in our relationships. Is starting the argument worth the risk of my spouse being mad and me having to deal with the drama? Is it worth starting the argument so that we can have great makeup sex? *Oops sorry—wrong book.*

My challenge to you is to use this thought process every day as it relates to eating and not just negatively. For instance: Is this nice, juicy apple worth it? YES—it tastes good, gives me fiber, it will cut down my risk of grabbing some junk food in a few hours and the calories are not high so it won't end up as more padding on my hips.

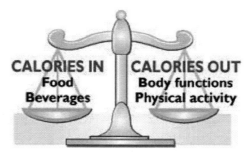

Let's look at some popular foods and you tell me if they are worth it for you? Keep in mind that 3,500 calories in excess will put an additional pound of fat on your body. Further, we will talk about how many calories the average person should be taking in every day in total, but for now let's just use 1,500-2,000 calories for the WHOLE day as our guide.

How Many Calories Does That Food Cost?

Calories In:

- Coldstone Cake Batter Ice Cream 6 oz. *Like It* size = 560 calories and 28 g fat
  - With cookie dough mixed in.
- Egg, Cheese and Sausage Croissant = 523 calories and 38g fat
- Pillsbury Grands! Flaky Supreme Cinnabon Cinnamon Rolls with Icing, 1 roll = 380 calories and 19 g fat
- Chick-fil-A Chick-n-Strips Salad with Buttermilk Dressing = 800 calories and 60 g fat
- Boston Market three piece Dark Rotisserie Chicken Meal with sweet potato casserole and market chopped side salad = 1,410 calories and 90 g fat

Calories Out: How many calories per minute do you burn doing certain activities?

Activity	130 lb	150 lb	170 lb	190 lb	220 lb	250 lb	270 lb	290 lb	320 lb
Aerobics, Step: 6" - 8" step	8	10	11	13	14	16	18	19	21
Aerobics: high impact	7	8	9	11	12	13	15	16	17
Aerobics: low impact	5	6	7	8	8	9	10	11	12
Aerobics: water	4	5	5	6	7	8	8	9	10
Basketball: playing a game	8	9	11	12	14	15	17	18	20
Basketball: shooting baskets	6	5	6	7	8	8	9	10	11
Bicycling, Stationary: moderate, 150 watts	7	8	9	11	12	13	15	16	17
Bicycling, Stationary: vigorous, 200 watts	10	12	14	16	18	20	22	24	26
Bowling	3	3	4	5	5	6	6	7	7
Boxing: punching bag	6	7	8	9	10	11	12	14	15
Calisthenics: Moderate, back exercises, going up and down from the floor	3	4	5	5	6	7	7	8	9
Child games: moderate, hop-scotch, jacks	4	5	5	6	7	8	8	9	10
Cleaning House: general	3	3	4	5	5	6	6	7	7
Cooking / Food Preparation	2	3	3	4	4	5	5	6	6
Dancing: disco, ballroom, square, line, Irish step, polka	4	5	6	7	8	8	9	10	11
Dancing: slow, waltz, foxtrot, tango	3	3	4	5	5	6	6	7	7
Food Shopping: with or without cart	2	3	3	3	4	4	5	5	6
Football or Baseball: playing catch	2	3	3	4	4	5	5	6	6
Gardening: general	4	5	5	6	7	8	8	9	10
Golf: driving range, miniature	3	3	4	5	5	6	6	7	7
Gymnastics: general	4	5	5	6	7	8	8	9	10
Ice Skating: general	7	8	9	11	12	13	15	16	17
Ironing	2	3	3	3	4	4	5	5	6
Mowing Lawn: push, power	5	6	7	8	9	10	11	12	13
Raking Lawn	4	5	6	7	7	8	9	10	11
Rock Climbing	11	12	14	16	18	21	22	24	27
Rope Jumping: general, moderate	10	11	13	15	17	19	21	23	24
Rowing, Stationery: moderate, 100 watts	7	8	9	11	12	13	15	16	17
Running: on track	10	11	13	15	17	19	21	23	24
Running: stairs, up	15	17	20	23	26	28	31	34	37
Shoveling Snow: by hand	6	7	8	9	10	11	12	14	15
Sitting: light office work, meeting	1	2	2	2	3	3	3	3	4
Skateboarding	5	6	7	8	8	9	10	11	12
Ski Machine: general	7	8	9	11	12	13	15	16	17
Skiing: cross-country, light effort, general	7	8	9	11	12	13	15	16	17
Skiing: downhill, moderate effort	6	7	8	9	10	11	12	14	15
Sleeping	1	1	1	1	2	2	2	2	2
Soccer: general	7	8	9	11	12	13	15	16	17
Stretching: Mild, Yoga	2	3	3	4	4	5	5	6	6
Swimming: butterfly	10	12	14	17	19	21	23	25	27
Swimming: general, leisurely, no laps	6	7	8	9	10	11	12	14	15
Tennis: general play	7	8	9	11	12	13	15	16	17
Trampoline	3	4	5	5	6	7	7	8	9
Typing: Computer, electric or manual	1	2	2	2	3	3	3	3	4
Vacuuming	3	4	5	5	6	7	7	8	9
Walking for Pleasure	3	4	5	5	6	7	7	8	9
Walking the Dog	3	3	4	5	5	6	6	7	7
Watching TV	1	1	1	2	2	2	2	2	2
Weight Lifting: Light, free weight, nautilus or universal	3	3	4	5	5	6	6	7	7

Dr. Sharon's Let's Get REAL Moment: Often we will do a little 30 minute workout after eating a meal and say *we've worked off our food* and then expect a pat on the back. I want to challenge us to REALLY understand what it takes to burn off those calories:

For Example: What about that Boston Market three piece Dark Rotisserie Chicken Meal with sweet potato casserole and market chopped side salad which is approximately 1,410 calories?

If you weigh 220 pounds, you would need to ride a stationary bike *(12 calories/minute)* for almost 2 hours. Are you going to do that? Additionally, if you're trying to lose weight and are following a 1,200-1,800 calorie per day program, this one meal has pretty much taken all of your calories for the day. I simply have one question: *Is It WORTH It?*

It isn't about what you cannot eat, it really is about the choices that you make and how you choose to interact with food. Is food ruling you or do you have an oz. of discipline to just say—It's NOT Worth It? Just like you can get into credit card debt by buying shoes that you can't afford; you can get into physical and emotional debt that will chase you down and stick on your hips, thighs or wherever with poor food choices. You will either pay now or pay later. How can you pay for your food choices? Let's revisit the whole concept of calories in versus calories burned. If you make the choice to eat it then you can make the choice to turn up the heat and burn it off.

How do you know when it's time to go on a diet and exercise?

Found at www.dietjokes.co.uk/jokes

- You try to do a few push-ups and discover that certain body parts refuse to leave the floor.

- Your children look through your wedding album and want to know who daddy's first wife was.

- You get winded just saying the words "six-kilometer run."

- You come to the conclusion that, if God really wanted you to touch your toes each morning, He would have put them somewhere around your knees.

- You analyze your body honestly and decide what you should develop first is your sense of humor.

- You step on a talking scale and it says, "Come back when you're alone."

- To you, *Itsy-Bitsy Teenie-Weenie Yellow Polka dot Bikini* and *To Dream the Impossible Dream* become the same song.

- You accept the fact that you can fool some of the people all of the time and all of the people some of the time, but not while you're wearing a bathing suit.

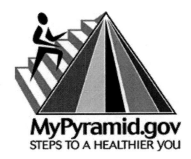

MyPyramid.gov
STEPS TO A HEALTHIER YOU

Nutrition Basics

Okay, so you have looked at your Ideal Body Weight; you've reviewed the BMI and are aware of all of the consequences of being overweight. You've begun to think more carefully about what you eat and the worth factor of food. The question becomes what is my long term weight loss and maintenance plan? Even if you don't need to LOSE weight, we all need to be HEALTHY.

In order for you to choose your method to address your weight, whether you want to lose, gain or stay the same; you must understand all that you just read in the first part of the book. Now, we have to go a little further and go over the basics of nutrition:

1. **We've discussed Calories as gas for your body**. Calories are found in foods; remember that a calorie is just that a calorie, no matter where it comes from. However, there are foods that cost more calories (*i.e., the same amount of food has more calories*); the breakdown of the calorie counts found in food is as follows:

   - 1 g of protein provides 4 calories

- 1 g of fat provides 9 calories

- 1 g of carbohydrate provides 4 calories

- 1 g of alcohol provides 7 calories

How much gas does your body need to run each day?

We've discussed calories a lot; remember that even while you sit and watch TV that you're burning calories. For your heart to beat; lungs to expand; mind to roam, eyes to blink and all of your bodily functions—it takes gas and calories are that gas. The question is often, how many calories does my body need just to exist and the answer is complicated. The basal metabolic rate *(BMR)* is simply the amount of energy that your body needs to function at rest. This must also be coupled with your activity level and what is called the thermic effect of food, which means the calories that your body needs to burn the food that you eat *(i.e., digest)*. The BMR is about 60-70% of all of the calories that you burn a day. Men generally have a higher BMR than women; this is why a man can eat more and not gain weight. *(When I get to heaven—I'm looking for EVE!)*. How do you calculate your BMR and thus get an understanding of how many calories you need to eat *(at minimum)* a day? Get out the calculators 'cause this is a brain teaser.

First Step: Estimate your BMR

This is a formula that uses your BMR and then applies an activity factor to determine your total daily calorie use.

English BMR Formula

The number of calories you would burn if you didn'thing all day; *(i.e. stayed in bed)*.

Women: BMR = 655 + *(4.35 x weight in pounds) + (4.7 x height in inches) - (4.7 x age in years)*

Men: BMR = 66 + *(6.23 x weight in pounds) + (12.7 x height in inches) - (6.8 x age in year)*

Examples:

1. A 43 year old, 5'7" female that weighs 190 pounds BMR = 1,594.3 calories.

   - What does this mean in very simple terms? If she ate 1,594.3 calories a day, she wouldn't gain or lose weight.

   - What about a man the same age/height/weight: BMR = 1,808.2 calories *(a difference of 213.90 calories)*.

   - *(I told you I'm gonna get EVE, a man can eat an extra jumbo chicken wing roasted every day vs. a woman and still not gain weight)*.

2. A 55 year old, 6'2" male that weighs 290 pounds BMR = 2,438.5 calories

3. A 30 year old, 5'9" female that weighs 210 pounds BMR = 1,751.8 calories

*The wonderful thing about living in this century is the INTERNET. You can find online calculators wherein you just put in your age, height, weight and activity levels and they do the calculations for you! I wanted to give you the background but there are plenty of sites that will calculate this for you. I recommend: www.bmi-calculator.net/bmr-calculator. Remember that weight is a factor in the calculations so as you lose or gain weight your BMR changes.

Second Step: Estimate your Activity Level

Now that you've calculated your BMR, you have to account for how active you are. This is why if you increase your activity level, you can burn more calories and lose weight. The Harris Benedict Equation is a formula that uses your BMR and then applies an activity factor to determine your total daily calories used. The only factor omitted by the Harris Benedict Equation is lean body mass. Leaner bodies need more calories than less leaner ones. Therefore, this equation will be very accurate for most people, except the very muscular *(will under-estimate calorie needs)* and the very fat *(will over-estimate calorie needs)*.

Harris Benedict Equation

Depending on your activity level, the amount of calories burned each day may be anywhere from 20 to 50 percent of your BMR. Use the Harris Benedict Equation to determine the amount of calories burned due to your activity level.

Sedentary *(little to no exercise)*: BMR x 1.2

Lightly Active *(light exercise/sports 1-3 days/week)*: BMR x 1.375

Moderately Active *(moderate exercise/sports 3-5 days/week)*: BMR x 1.55

Very Active *(hard exercise/sports 6-7 days a week)*: BMR x 1.725

Extra Active *(very hard exercise/sports & physical job)*: BMR x 1.9

Let's go back to our 30 year old, 5'9" female that weighs 210 pounds BMR = 1,751.8 calories

Her activity level now increased her calorie needs:

If she does light sports like calm, stretching yoga two times a week *(lightly active)* her calorie requirements would be:

$$1751.8 \ (BMR) \times 1.2 = 2,102.16 \text{ calories}$$

If she increased her activity and wanted to take a spin class three times a week (moderately active), her calorie requirements would be:

$$1751.8 \ (BMR) \times 1.55 = 2,715.29 \text{ calories}$$

Do you understand how exercise fits into all of this? By increasing your activity, you burn more calories and as long as you don't eat those extra calories burned, you will lose weight. Whew!!! Math class is over, go online and find the calculators.

A Dr. Sharon Sidebar: Don't even bother counting the thermic effect; let this one be a bonus because most people underestimate how much food they really eat and over estimate their calories burned. Let this one go. Plus I'm confused and I have a Medical Degree *(MD)*.

One more thing: Your body also needs calories *(fuel)* to burn the food that you eat. Opening your mouth, biting, chewing, swallowing and digesting require about 10 percent of your total caloric intake. This is called the **Thermic Effect**. For the 150-pound woman, the thermic effect would account for burning about 150 calories.

2. **Protein:** This is the building block of muscle and comes from both animals *(meat, poultry, fish, eggs and dairy products)* and plants *(nuts, grain products and legumes)*. The difference between animal protein and plant protein is the amount of fat that is found in them, with animal protein sources *(i.e., red meat)* being higher in fat. If you eat more protein than you need, it will be stored in your body as fat. Most adults in the United States get more than enough protein to meet their needs. It's rare for someone who is healthy and eating a varied diet to not get enough protein.

How much protein do you need a day? According to the CDC, in general, it's recommended that 10–35% of your daily calories come from protein. Below is the Recommended Dietary Allowance *(RDA)* for different age groups.

Recommended Dietary Allowance for Protein	
	Grams of protein needed each day
Children ages 1–3	13
Children ages 4–8	19
Children ages 9–13	34
Girls ages 14–18	46
Boys ages 14–18	52
Women ages 19–70+	46
Men ages 19–70+	56

Here are examples of amounts of protein in food:

- 1 cup of milk has 8 grams of protein

- A 3-oz. piece of meat has about 21 grams of protein

- 1 cup of dry beans has about 16 grams of protein

- An 8-oz. container of yogurt has about 11 grams of protein

3. **Fat:** Let's have a moment of reverence for fat; it's been given a lot of grief. Fat does NOT make you fat. Eating too much fat *(and protein, carbohydrates, etc.)* makes you fat. Your body must have fat to live and a calorie is just that a calorie. But you can see that when you eat fat, you eat almost twice as many calories per gram as protein so the potential to pack on the calories is there. Fat is not bad and indeed, it is essential for good skin, your digestive system and it is your body's coat so that you don't freeze to death. *(Some of us have heavier coats than we need.)*

   a. How much fat does the average person need a day
   The Dietary Guidelines for Americans 2005 recommends that Americans keep their total fat intake within certain limits. This limit is defined as a percentage of your total calorie needs.

Age Group	Total Fat Limits
Children ages 2-3	30-35% of total calories
Children and adolescents ages 4-18	25-35% of total calories
Adults, ages 19 and older	20-35% of total calories

   b. What are the different types of fats and are they all the same? All fats are not created equal. While fats are essential for normal body function, some fats are better for you than others. *Trans* fats, saturated fats and cholesterol are less healthy than polyunsaturated and monounsaturated fats.

4. **Carbohydrates (*carbs*):** This is the body's primary source of fuel/energy and includes sugars and starches. Your body uses carbs to make glucose *(sugar)*, which is the fuel that gives you energy and helps keep everything going. Your body can use glucose immediately or store it in your liver and muscles for when it is needed.

   There are two types of carbohydrates; complex and simple. The complex carbohydrates are found in grains, legumes and vegetables. These foods are rich in fiber, minerals, vitamins and other nutrients. They are nutritious and necessary for a balanced diet. The simple carbohydrates include sugar, syrup and milk.

You can find carbohydrates in the following:

- Fruits

- Vegetables

- Breads, cereals and other grains
- Milk and milk products
- Foods containing added sugars *(e.g., cakes, cookies and sugary beverages)*

How much of my diet should have carbs? This gets tricky, because of the popularity of the Atkins diet and other diets, carbs have been painted as badly as fats. Remember that food is not bad; it is how much we take in of that food and how we try to live in balance.

5. **Fiber:** Fiber is a complex carbohydrate and is found in vegetables, fruits and whole grains. Fiber is absolutely necessary for good health.

- It makes you feel fuller longer and helps keep you from overeating.
- It softens and adds bulk to your stools and makes bowel movements faster and easier.
- A high-fiber, low-fat, balanced diet helps control your cholesterol and decreases the risk of colon cancer.
- It helps regulate your blood sugar.
- You should eat about 20-35 grams of fiber every day even if you don't want to lose weight. This is a healthy lifestyle recommendation. You will need to make sure that you are drinking plenty of fluids with your fiber.

Foods High in Fiber:

Soluble Fiber

- Oatmeal
- Oat bran
- Nuts and seeds
- Most fruits *(e.g., strawberries, blueberries, pears and apples)*
- Dry beans and peas

Insoluble Fiber

- Whole wheat bread
- Barley
- Brown rice
- Couscous
- Bulgur or whole grain cereals
- Wheat bran
- Seeds
- Most vegetables

Easy Dietary Fiber Estimator	
Daily calorie needs	Daily dietary fiber needs

1000	14 grams
1200	17 grams
1400	20 grams
1600	22 grams
1800	25 grams
2000	28 grams
2200	31 grams
2400	34 grams
2600	36 grams
2800	39 grams
3000	42 grams

6. **Water:** Yes, water is an essential nutrient—we often forget this fact. You can live without food longer than you can without water. The human body is 66% water. I say all the time, *"Water is to the body like oil is to the car."* The engine will lock up if there is no oil and you will not be driving anywhere. Well, the same thing with water and you—two words DRINK IT!

I don't have to spend a lot of time telling you the merits of water. You've known since a child that you should drink more water. It keeps the kidneys flowing and the skin glowing; just to name a few of its benefits. There is the added benefit of it being filling; especially if you're eating your fiber. The controversy of how much you should drink a day continues to rage on. The truth of the matter is that very few people; except in the case of some psychological conditions, drink too much water. It is very important for you to drink when you are thirsty and actually to keep hydrated so that you do not become thirsty at all. One of the major problems with persons who desire to lose weight is that they mistake thirst for hunger. So you're really thirsty and some zero calorie water would have been gratifying but because you missed the cues of your body; you grab a candy bar *(approx. 300 calories)* wolf it down and then grab a soft drink *(16 oz. = 200 calories)* for a total of 500 calories. When you could have just had a tall glass of water first, quenched your thirst and saved those 500 calories and the additional 250-400 calories you're going to eat in about two hours when you have the sugar rush and sugar crash that will cause you to need to eat something else. Do you see the vicious cycle that a little sip of the zero calories liquid would have prevented.

Each day your body loses about two to three quarts of water that needs to be replaced. The old advice was to drink at least 64 oz. of water every day. Recent studies have It is important for you to remember that you do get water from your other beverages like teas, juices, coffee and even soft drinks. Additionally, some foods have high water content like vegetables, low-fat milk, soups, stews, etc.

What about Vitamin Water?

There is a huge marketing campaign that has been quite successful encouraging us to drink water enriched with vitamins. While it is true that this is better for you than sodas; my advice is to grab natural water. I've a rule; I don't drink calories—I'd rather chew them. That's just me but I dare say if you would take that little tip and run with it; you'd probably lose five pounds in your first month.

You make your own call on vitamin water but remember to add the calories into your daily totals and to ask the question—*Is it Worth It?* For many it is, but as for me simple zero calorie, regular H^2O will do just fine on both my lips, hips, skin and pocket book.

---

7. **Vitamins and Minerals:** Vitamins and minerals are essential to human life. We get them from food and water and they are the building blocks for our bodies. One of the major problems with starvation or fad diets is that we deprive ourselves of vitamins and minerals which could have serious health complications. Vitamins and minerals are nutrients that your body needs to grow and develop normally.

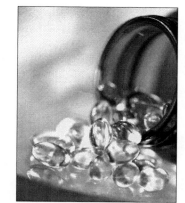

The question is always asked regarding the need to take vitamins, minerals and other supplements. Ideally, you should get your vitamins and minerals from your food and that's why it is important to eat plenty of fresh fruits, vegetables, drink water and milk every day. However, if you are not eating diets which are rich in the essential vitamins and minerals; taking a supplement would be beneficial.

Remember that too much of a good thing is bad. Well, this is no different with vitamins and supplements. You don't need to take 20 pills three times a day. A single multivitamin and calcium—especially for women in conjunction with a healthy, well balanced diet is all that you need. Discuss your vitamins, minerals, supplements and herbal products with your doctor.

Visit www.cdc.gov for more information on protein, fat, carbs, water, vitamins and minerals.

****

Ok, Dr. Sharon—I got it but how do I know how many calories, fat grams, proteins, nutrients, etc. are in the foods that I eat?

Reading is Fundamental! Learn to read nutrition labels, purchase a good calorie/nutrition counter and keep it nearby. There are also GREAT websites with lots of information; one of my personal favorites: www.sparkpeople.com. I've included information from the Food and Drug Administration's website *(www.fda.gov/Food/LabelingNutrition/ConsumerInformation/ucm078889.htm)*; I caution you—get ready for class, because this is detailed info.

The Nutrition Facts Label—An Overview: from FDA.gov

The information in the main or top section *(see #1-4 and #6 on the sample nutrition label below)*, can vary with each food product; it contains product-specific information *(serving size, calories and nutrient information)*. The bottom part *(see #5 on the sample label below)* contains a footnote with Daily Values *(DVs)* for 2,000 and 2,500 calorie diets. This footnote provides recommended dietary information for important nutrients, including fats, sodium and fiber. The footnote is found only on larger packages and does not change from product to product.

The Serving Size

The first place to start when you look at the Nutrition Facts label is the serving size and the number of servings in the package. Serving sizes are standardized to make it easier to

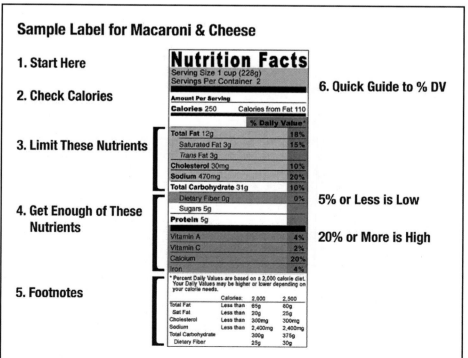

compare similar foods. They are provided in familiar units, such as cups or pieces, followed by the metric amount, e.g., the number of grams.

The size of the serving on the food package influences the number of calories and all the nutrient amounts listed on the top part of the label. **Pay attention to the serving size, especially how many servings there are in the food package. Then ask yourself, "How many servings am I consuming?"** *(e.g., ½ serving, 1 serving or more.)* In the sample label, one serving of macaroni and cheese equals one cup. If you ate the whole package, you would eat **two** cups. That doubles the calories and other nutrient numbers, including the % Daily Values as shown in the sample label.

Example				
	Single Serving	% DV	Double Serving	% DV
Serving Size	1 cup *(228g)*		2 cups *(456g)*	
Calories	250		500	
Calories from Fat	110		220	
Total Fat	12g	18%	24g	36%
Trans Fat	1.5g		3g	
Saturated Fat	3g	15%	6g	30%
Cholesterol	30mg	10%	60mg	20%
Sodium	470mg	20%	940mg	40%
Total Carbohydrate	31g	10%	62g	20%
Dietary Fiber	0g	0%	0g	0%
Sugars	5g		10g	
Protein	5g		10g	
Vitamin A		4%		8%
Vitamin C		2%		4%
Calcium		20%		40%
Iron		4%		8%

② Calories *(and Calories from Fat)*

Calories provide a measure of how much energy you get from a serving of this food. Many Americans consume more calories than they need without meeting recommended intakes for a number of nutrients. The

Amount Per Serving

Calories 250   Calories from Fat 110

calorie section of the label can help you manage your weight *(i.e., gain, lose or maintain.)* **Remember: the number of servings you consume determines the number of calories you actually eat (your portion amount).**

In the example, there are 250 calories in one serving of this macaroni and cheese. How many calories from fat are there in ONE serving? Answer: 110 calories, which means almost half the calories in a single serving, come from fat. What if you ate the whole package? Then, you would consume two servings or 500 calories, and 220 would come from fat.

General Guide to Calories

- 40 calories is low

- 100 calories is moderate

- 400 calories or more is high

The *General Guide to Calories* provides a general reference for calories when you look at a Nutrition Facts label. This guide is based on a 2,000 calorie diet.

Eating too many calories per day is linked to being overweight and obese.

③④ The Nutrients: How Much?

Look at the top of the nutrient section in the sample label. It shows you some key nutrients that have an impact on your health and separates them into two main groups:

Limit These Nutrients

The nutrients listed first are the ones Americans generally eat in adequate amounts, or even too much. They are identified in yellow as **Limit these Nutrients.** Eating too much fat, saturated fat, *trans* fat, cholesterol or sodium may increase your risk of certain chronic diseases, like heart disease, some cancers or high blood pressure.

Total Fat 12g		**18%**
Saturated Fat 3g		**15%**
Trans Fat 3g		
Cholesterol 30mg		**10%**
Sodium 470mg		**20%**

Important: *Health experts recommend that you keep your intake of saturated fat, trans fat and cholesterol as low as possible as part of a nutritionally balanced diet.*

Get Enough of These

Most Americans don't get enough dietary fiber, vitamin A, vitamin C, calcium and iron in their diets. They are identified in blue as **Get Enough of these Nutrients**. Eating enough of these nutrients can improve your health and help reduce the risk of some diseases and conditions. For example, getting enough calcium may reduce the risk of osteoporosis, a condition that results in brittle bones as one ages. Eating a diet high in dietary fiber promotes healthy bowel function. Additionally, a diet rich in fruits, vegetables and grain products that contain dietary fiber, particularly soluble fiber, and low in saturated fat and cholesterol may reduce the risk of heart disease.

Dietary Fiber 0g	**0%**
Vitamin A	**4%**
Vitamin C	**2%**
Calcium	**20%**
Iron	**4%**

Remember: *You can use the Nutrition Facts label not only to help limit those nutrients you want to cut back on but also to increase those nutrients you need to consume in greater amounts.*

⑤ Understanding the Footnote on the Bottom of the Nutrition Facts Label

Note the * used after the heading "% Daily Value" on the Nutrition Facts label. It refers to the Footnote in the lower part of the nutrition label, which tells you **"% DVs are based on a 2,000 calorie diet.".** This statement must be on all food labels. But the remaining information in the full footnote may not be on the package if the size of the label is too small. When the full footnote does appear, it will always be the same. It doesn't change from product to product, because it shows recommended dietary advice for all Americans, it is not about a specific food product.

Percent Daily Values are based on a 2,000 calorie diet. Your Daily Values may be higher or lower depending on your calorie needs.

		Calories:	2,000	2,500
Total Fat	Less than		65g	80g
Sat Fat	Less than		20g	25g
Cholesterol	Less than		300mg	300mg
Sodium	Less than		2,400mg	2,400mg
Total Carbohydrate			300g	375g
Dietary Fiber			25g	30g

Look at the amounts circled in red in the footnote—these are the Daily Values *(DV)* for each nutrient listed and are based on public health experts' advice. DVs are recommended levels of intakes. DVs in the footnote are based on a 2,000 or 2,500 calorie diet. Note how the DVs for some nutrients change, while others *(for cholesterol and sodium)* remain the same for both calorie amounts.

How the Daily Values Relate to the % DVs

Look at the example below for another way to see how the Daily Values *(DVs)* relate to the % DVs and dietary guidance. For each nutrient listed there is a DV, a % DV, and dietary advice or a goal. If you follow this dietary advice, you will stay within public health experts' recommended upper or lower limits for the nutrients listed, based on a 2,000 calorie daily diet.

Examples of DVs versus % DVs
Based on a 2,000 Calorie Diet

Nutrient	DV	% DV	Goal
Total Fat	65g	= 100% DV	Less than
Sat Fat	20g	= 100% DV	Less than
Cholesterol	300mg	= 100% DV	Less than
Sodium	2400mg	= 100% DV	Less than
Total Carbohydrate	300g	= 100% DV	At least
Dietary Fiber	25g	= 100% DV	At least

Upper Limit - Eat Less than...

The nutrients that have upper daily limits are listed first on the footnote of larger labels and on the example above. This means it is recommended that you stay below, eat less than, the Daily Value nutrient amounts listed per day. For example, the DV for Saturated fat *(in the yellow section)* is 20g. This amount is 100% DV for this nutrient. What is the goal or dietary advice? To eat less than 20 g or 100% DV for the day.

Lower Limit - Eat At least...

Now look at the section in blue where dietary fiber is listed. The DV for dietary fiber is 25g, which is 100% DV. This means it is recommended that you eat *at least* this amount of dietary fiber per day.

The DV for Total Carbohydrate *(section in white)* is 300g or 100% DV. This amount is recommended for a balanced daily diet that is based on 2,000 calories, but can vary, depending on your daily intake of fat and protein.

Now let's look at the % DVs.

⑥ The Percent Daily Value *(% DV)*:

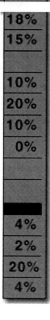

The % Daily Value *(% DVs)* is based on the Daily Value recommendations for key nutrients but only for a 2,000 calorie daily diet—not 2,500 calories. You, like most people, may not know how many calories you consume in a day. But you can still use the % DV as a frame of reference whether or not you consume more or less than 2,000 calories.

The % DV helps you determine if a serving of food is high or low in nutrients.

Note: a few nutrients, like trans fat, do not have a % DV—they will be discussed later.

Do you need to know how to calculate percentages to use the % DV? No, the label *(the % DV)* does the math for you. It helps you interpret the numbers *(grams and milligrams)* by putting them all on the same scale for the day *(0-100% DV)*. The % DV column doesn't add up vertically to 100%. Instead each nutrient is based on 100% of the daily requirements for that nutrient *(for a 2,000 calorie diet)*. This way you can tell high from low and know which nutrients contribute a lot, or a little, to your **daily** recommended allowance *(upper or lower)*.

Quick Guide to % DV: 5% DV or less is low and 20% DV or more is high

This guide tells you that **5% DV or less is low** for all nutrients, those you want to limit *(e.g., fat, saturated fat, cholesterol and sodium)*, or for those that you want to consume in greater amounts *(fiber, calcium, etc.)* As the **Quick Guide** shows, **20% DV or more is high** for all nutrients.

Example: *Look at the amount of Total Fat in one serving listed on the sample nutrition label. Is 18% DV contributing a lot or a little to your fat limit of 100% DV? Check the* **Quick Guide to % DV**. *18% DV, which is below 20% DV, is not yet high, but what if you ate the whole package (two servings)? You would double that amount, eating 36% of your daily allowance for Total Fat. Coming from just one food, that amount leaves you with 64% of your fat allowance (100%-36%=64%) for all of the other foods you eat that day, snacks and drinks included.*

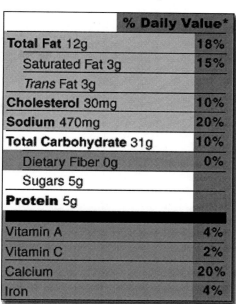

	% Daily Value*
Total Fat 12g	18%
Saturated Fat 3g	15%
Trans Fat 3g	
Cholesterol 30mg	10%
Sodium 470mg	20%
Total Carbohydrate 31g	10%
Dietary Fiber 0g	0%
Sugars 5g	
Protein 5g	
Vitamin A	4%
Vitamin C	2%
Calcium	20%
Iron	4%

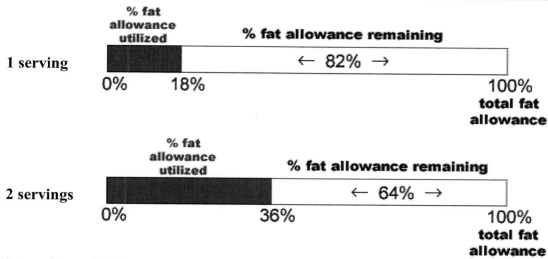

1 serving

% fat allowance utilized

% fat allowance remaining

← 82% →

0%   18%   100% total fat allowance

2 servings

% fat allowance utilized

% fat allowance remaining

← 64% →

0%   36%   100% total fat allowance

Using the % DV for:

Comparisons: The % DV also makes it easy for you to make comparisons. You can compare one product or brand to a similar product. Just make sure the serving sizes are similar, especially the weight *(e.g., gram, milligram, oz.)* of each product. It's easy to see which foods are higher or lower in nutrients because the serving sizes are generally consistent for similar types of foods, except in a few cases like cereals.

Nutrient Content Claims: Use the % DV to help you quickly distinguish one claim from another, such as reduced fat vs. light or nonfat. Just compare the % DVs for Total Fat in each food product to see which one is higher or lower in that nutrient; **there is no need to memorize definitions.** This works when comparing all nutrient content claims, e.g., less, light, low, free, more, high, etc.

Dietary Trade-Offs: You can **use the % DV to help you make dietary trade-offs** with other foods throughout the day. You don't have to give up a favorite food to eat a healthy diet. When a food you like is high in fat, balance it with foods that are low in fat at other times of the day. Also, pay attention to how much you eat so that the **total** amount of fat for the day stays below 100% DV.

Nutrition Facts

Serving Size 1 cup (228g)
Servings Per Container 2 — Start here

Amount Per Serving — Check calories

Calories 250   Calories from Fat 110

                % Daily Value* — Quick guide to % D

Total Fat 12g	**18%**
Saturated Fat 3g	**15%**
Trans Fat 3g	
Cholesterol 30mg	**10%**
Sodium 470mg	**20%**
Potassium 700mg	**20%**
Total Carbohydrate 31g	**10%**
Dietary Fiber 0g	0%
Sugars 5g	
Protein 5g	

5% or less is low
20% or more is hi

Limit these

Get enough of thes

Vitamin A	4%
Vitamin C	2%
Calcium	20%
Iron	4%

Footnote

* Percent Daily Values are based on a 2,000 calorie diet.
Your Daily Values may be higher or lower depending on
your calorie needs.

Understanding and USING the Food Label is so very vital to your health and journey to wellness that I wanted to give you another view. You can't really make good decisions about what you eat without understanding how to read the nutrition label. It is worth spending the additional time for another quick review. This information can be found at www.health.gov/dietaryguidelines/dga2005/healthieryou/html/tips_food_label.html.

Tips for Using the Food Label

Another quick look

Check servings and calories. Look at the serving size and how many servings you are actually eating.

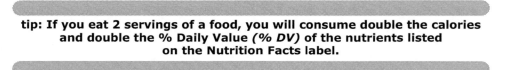

tip: If you eat 2 servings of a food, you will consume double the calories
and double the % Daily Value (*% DV*) of the nutrients listed
on the Nutrition Facts label.

Make your calories count. Look at the calories on the label and compare them with the nutrients they offer.

Eat less sugar. Foods with added sugars may provide calories, but few essential nutrients. So, look for foods and beverages low in added sugars. Read the ingredient list, and make sure added sugars are not one of the first few ingredients.

tip: Names for added sugars (*caloric sweeteners*) include sucrose,
glucose, high fructose corn syrup, corn syrup, maple syrup and fructose.

Know your fats. Look for foods low in saturated and trans fats, and cholesterol to help reduce the risk of heart disease. Most of the fats you eat should be polyunsaturated and monounsaturated fats, such as those in fish, nuts and vegetable oils.

tip: Fat should be in the range of 20-35% of the calories you eat.

Reduce sodium (salt), increase potassium. Research shows that eating less than 2,300 milligrams of sodium *(about 1 tsp of salt)* per day may reduce the risk of high blood pressure. Older adults tend to be salt-sensitive. If you are an older adult or salt-sensitive, aim to eat no more than 1,500 milligrams of sodium each day, the equivalent of about ¾ teaspoon. To meet the daily potassium recommendation of at least 4,700 milligrams, consume fruits, vegetables, fat-free and low-fat milk products that are sources of potassium including: sweet potatoes, beet greens, white potatoes, white beans, plain yogurt, prune juice and bananas. These counteract some of sodium's effects on blood pressure.

tip: Most sodium you eat is likely to come from processed foods, not from the salt shaker. Read the Nutrition Facts label and choose foods lower in sodium and higher in potassium.

Use the % Daily Value (% DV) column: 5% DV or less is low, and 20% DV or more is high.
Keep these low: saturated and trans fats, cholesterol and sodium.
Get enough of these: potassium, fiber, vitamins A, C and D, calcium and iron.
Check the calories: 400 calories or more per serving of a single food item is high.

The Reality of the Serving Size: One of the biggest mistakes that I make, as well as most humans, is underestimating my serving size. Let's take a few minutes to get a good feel for what a serving size is; I remain shocked at the amount of food that is served at restaurants and even at my kitchen table.

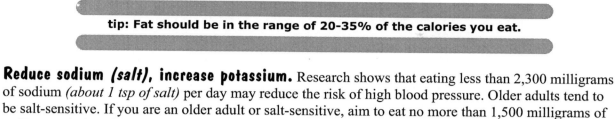

► ► ► ► Tipsheet ◄ ◄ ◄ ◄
Sizing Up Servings

Found at www.nhlbisupport.com/chd1/Tipsheets/sevenways.htm

Food Groups	One Serving Size Equals...
Breads, Cereals, Rice, Pasta and other Grains Group	• 1 slice bread or ½ bagel the size of a hockey puck • ½ cup cooked rice equals a cupcake wrapper • ½ cup pasta equals an ice cream scoop
Fruit and Vegetable Groups	• One fruit and vegetable serving is equal to one piece the size of a tennis ball or ½ cup, the size of a light bulb
Meat, Chicken, Fish, Dry Beans and Peas, Eggs and Nuts Group	• 3 oz. lean meat, chicken or fish measures up to a deck of cards or a check book.
Dairy Group	• 1 oz. cheese equals about 4 dice.
Fats, Oils and Sweets Group	• Use sparingly, for a teaspoon of fat, look to the tip of your thumb

This tipsheet is adapted from the American Dietetic Association, Eat Right Minute Nutrition Tip of the Day located at www.eatright.org.

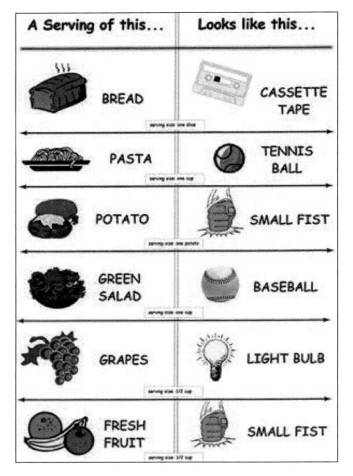

A Serving of this...	Looks like this...
BREAD	CASSETTE TAPE
PASTA	TENNIS BALL
POTATO	SMALL FIST
GREEN SALAD	BASEBALL
GRAPES	LIGHT BULB
FRESH FRUIT	SMALL FIST

"Nothing so needs reforming as other people's habits." Mark Twain

A Dr. Sharon Let's Get REAL Moment: Now look at the serving size of pasta; are you REALLY only eating one serving *(i.e., the size of a tennis ball)*? You also have to be aware that different restaurants, boxed/prepackaged foods, etc. really do have different serving sizes. Think about it, you cannot compare a slice of carrot cake out of the freezer at your local grocer to the Cheesecake Factory Restaurant which serves enough food for an entire family of six on one plate. If you lie to yourself and underestimate calories, then who do you harm?

The lies we tell: "I just had a slice of carrot cake, I looked it up and it has *(with frosting)* 385 calories, 21 g fat. That's not too bad."

Reality: You had a slice of carrot cake from the Cheesecake Factory; 1 slice equals approx: Calories: 1,010, 62 g fat.

Get into the habit of reading the label, asking the server for nutritional information or looking it up online and understanding the portion size.

BIG DIFFERENCE!

"Habits are at first cobwebs, then cables." Spanish Proverb

Name That Diet?

I've been on almost every diet that there is, again I tell you what we already know—diet's don't work. Even if you opt for the more invasive methods like gastric bypass surgery, stomach banding or wiring your mouth shut (*do they still do that?*), you are doomed for weight gain unless you modify your lifestyle. Again, the bottom line is if you eat fewer calories than you burn, you WILL lose weight; that is the fundamental basis of ALL weight loss. However, we all have different personalities, likes and dislikes and if you find a healthy weight loss or management plan that is healthy and works for you—stick to it. On the following pages, I have given you information on various diets. I have pointed out a few of my favorites and given some colorful comments along the way.

Overview of ALL Diets

Diets that generally fall into one of these categories.

Diet Type	Fast Facts	Other Information
Liquid Diets	• Liquid diets contain a reduced number of calories resulting in (*often temporary*) weight loss. • Ideally, liquid diet drinks should contain a balance of nutrients you need throughout the day, but that isn't always the case.	
Low Calorie Diets	• Very low calorie diets should be done under the supervision of a physician. • Weight loss may subside if metabolism slows to adjust to calorie intake.	
Low Carbohydrate Diets	• Factors that contribute to weight loss with this program type: loss of water weight, decreased appetite, increased feeling of fullness, and reduced calories. • Can lead to lack of nutrients.	
Low Fat Diets	• Frequent strategy for reducing the risk of heart disease. • Ideally should concentrate on eliminating bad fats rather than all fats in order to avoid missing out on important nutrients.	• *American Heart Association and the National Cholesterol Education Program recommend restricting consumption of fat to an upper limit of 30% of daily caloric intake, with no lower limit set.* • *The World Health Organization Study Group recommends that 15% of total calories be derived from fat.*

Most Popular Diets

Here is some info that we found from various sources. Remember the basics of weight loss are physics and caloric balance. There is no magic bullet!

Diet Type	Fast Facts	Other Information
Atkins Diet	• Has been around for 30 years. • High fat, low carb diet. • Reduces to carbs in an effort to reduce insulin levels that result in carbs being stored as fat.	• Promotes ketosis, an unhealthy condition that can damage kidneys.
Biggest Loser Club	• Adaptation of the popular television program. • 12 week program that includes a low-calorie diet based on 4-3-2-1 *(4 servings of fruits and veggies; 3 of lean protein; 2 of whole grains; and 1 "extra")*, along with a healthy emphasis on exercise. • Offers support and advice about nutrition, exercise, and healthy goals via online community.	
Blood Type Diet	• Claims different blood types have different nutritional needs. • Diets based on blood types developed predispositions to various illnesses.	• *What blood type likes fried chicken?*
Cabbage Soup Diet	• A seven day plan that specifically states it is not for long term weight loss. • Low fat, high fiber diet consisting of cabbage soup.	• Dieters may spend the week at home as not only are the limited food options unlikely to be found in restaurants, but large quantities of cabbage soup may also cause gas. • The weight that you lose is primarily fluids and not fat. This will more than likely return once you start eating your normal foods.
Cayenne Pepper Diet *(also known as Master Cleanse or Lemonade Diet)*	• Claims to cleanse body of toxins. • 10 day diet consisting of lemonade, cayenne pepper, and maple syrup only.	• Made popular by celebrities such as Beyoncé. • Since this plan is a liquid fast, once the user starts putting solid food into their system, the weight will come back.
Dr. Phil Diet	• Addresses the underlying causes of weight problems. • Aims to change behaviors toward and thoughts about food, weight loss and one's self. • There is a healthy emphasis on exercise. • Utilizes his book as guide and there is an online support group.	• A generally well-balanced approach to weight loss.

Diet Type	Fast Facts	Other Information
eDiets	▪ Online collection of customized diet and exercise plans. ▪ Online sessions with personal trainer and nutritionist. ▪ Online community for support and resources.	
Grapefruit Diet *(Also known as the Mayo Clinic Diet)*	▪ Low calorie, low carbohydrate, high protein 12 day diet. ▪ Based on the idea that an ingredient in grapefruits, when eaten with protein, triggers fat burning and causes weight loss. ▪ Not associated with actual Mayo Clinic hospital.	▪ The weight that you lose is primarily fluids and not fat. This will more than likely return once you start eating your normal foods.
Herbalife Weight Loss Program	▪ The program, ShapeWorks, personalizes daily protein intake for your body's individual needs, with the aim that you feel full, satisfied and energized as you lose your unwanted weight. ▪ Includes a 7 day recommended meal plan.	▪ The weight that you lose is primarily fluids and not fat. This will more than likely return once you start eating your normal foods.
Hollywood Diet	▪ Juice diet for either 24 or 48 hour cycles. ▪ Claims to detoxify and cleanse body. ▪ Promoted for rapid weight loss. ▪ Claims juice is rich in nutrients and antioxidants.	• The weight that you lose is primarily fluids and not fat. This will more than likely return once you start eating your normal foods.
Jenny Craig	▪ Franchised weight loss centers. ▪ Emphasizes portion control, nutritious food, and an active lifestyle. ▪ Personal consultants aid in motivation.	▪ Promoted by Valerie Bertinelli, Phylicia Rashad, Queen Latifah, and Kirstie Alley.
LA Weight Loss	▪ Center-based weight loss program. ▪ Private consultations and customized meal plans. ▪ Encourages portion control and healthy activity.	
Maker's Diet	▪ Biblically based 40 day lifestyle program that includes diet. ▪ Promotes eating food in as natural a state as possible, looking down on things like chemicals, preservatives and even refrigeration. ▪ Encourages clearing of toxins, exercise, and mental approaches.	
Medifast	▪ Portion controlled, nutritionally balanced, low-fat program. ▪ Utilizes shipped pre-packaged foods in various foods and flavors.	

Diet Type	Fast Facts	Other Information
Nutrisystem	<ul><li>Portion control diet with delivered pre-made food.</li><li>Promotes easy dieting as there are no calories or carbs, etc. to count.</li><li>Online community for tracking weight loss.</li></ul>	<ul><li>Promoted by Marie Osmond and Dan Marino.</li></ul>
Optifast	<ul><li>Medically monitored weight loss program aimed primarily at obese individuals.</li><li>Utilizes a mainly liquid, pre-packaged diet with nutritional bars available.</li><li>Provides support, counseling, lifestyle education and medical monitoring.</li><li>While this plan is designed to be long term, it more importantly is made to break the habits of overeating and unhealthy choices so that even after ending the diet, the user's food choices will be changed for the better.</li></ul>	<ul><li>Oprah has followed this diet plan, but regained the weight.</li><li>One component of this diet is liquid meal replacement.</li></ul>
Scarsdale Diet	<ul><li>High protein, low fat, low carb.</li><li>Contains five 14 day menu plans.</li><li>Claims to be healthier than Atkins as it is low fat and includes complex carbs like whole grain bread and fruit.</li></ul>	
Slim Fast	<ul><li>Weight loss program utilizing two meal replacements per day along with one regular meal.</li><li>Made to control hunger and reduce unhealthy food cravings.</li><li>Offers online support community.</li></ul>	
Sonoma Diet *(Also known as Mediterranean Diet)*	<ul><li>Diet based on the cuisine of the Mediterranean and portion size.</li><li>Online meal plans and recipes offered.</li></ul>	
South Beach Diet	<ul><li>Promotes a healthy balance of nutrients in food and proper portion sizes.</li><li>Recipes and food guides available online.</li><li>Temporary restrictions on certain food groups.</li></ul>	
SparkPeople	<ul><li>Online weight loss program based on high carb, low fat nutrient ratios.</li><li>Personal diet and fitness plans.</li><li>Online resources include calorie counter, exercise tracker, recipes, and support community.</li></ul>	<ul><li>A Dr. Sharon favorite!</li><li>FREE</li><li>Great online food and exercise diary</li></ul>
Subway Diet	<ul><li>A diet consisting of only low cal food options from the fast food chain, Subway.</li><li>By choosing the healthiest menu options, it is possible to follow what is essentially a low fat, low calorie diet.</li></ul>	<ul><li>Made popular by Subway spokesperson, Jared who lost 245 pounds in a year.</li><li>Though cutting calories helped to lose weight, Jared also began exercising more.</li></ul>

Diet Type	Fast Facts	Other Information
Weight Watchers	▪ Longstanding program that offers both online and in-person program options. ▪ Customized diet and fitness plans utilizing point system. ▪ Support includes motivation, weight tracking, and interactive tips and tools.	
The Zone	▪ Meals based on 40% carbs, 30% protein, 30% fat ratio. ▪ Promotes portion control, low fat and complex carb intake. ▪ Requires planning to organize and maintain meals.	▪ Followed by Jennifer Aniston.

Other Weight Loss Diets

Diet Type	Fast Facts	Other Information
3 Day Diet	▪ Low calorie diet. ▪ Claims the specific food combinations have a beneficial metabolic reaction.	
3 Hour Diet	▪ Promotes eating the right foods every three hours to control appetite. ▪ Claims to control blood sugar levels and reduce belly fat.	▪ *What if I eat a jelly donut every 3 hours?*
5 Factor Diet	▪ 5 week plan containing 5 meals a day with 5 ingredients each. ▪ Promotes exercise as part of the plan *(5 workouts for 5 minutes)*. ▪ Encourages 5 diet "cheat days" in the 5 weeks. ▪ Online support includes eating out guide, recipes, and meal planners.	▪ Site quotes Alicia Keys, Vanessa Williams Kanye West, Jessica Simpson and John Mayer in support.
7 Day Diet	▪ Promotes eating certain foods on specific days such as one day eating certain fruits, and another involves eating all kinds of vegetables. ▪ The diet claims to detoxify the body and lead to weight loss. ▪ Most of the limited calorie intake is from fruits and vegetables and, therefore, many nutrient groups are lacking.	
Abs Diet	▪ 6 week program designed to flatten stomach. ▪ Combines Abs Diet Powerfoods and The Abs Diet Workout to create a healthy body and lifestyle.	▪ *What happens if my stomach is flat but my thighs grow?*
Anne Collins Weight Loss Program	▪ 9 diets designed to be easy and healthy for long term weight loss. ▪ Online support community. ▪ Offers fitness advice and healthy motivation.	

Diet Type	Fast Facts	Other Information
Apple Cider Vinegar Diet	▪ Based on the idea that consuming a few teaspoons of apple cider vinegar prior to meals will curb the appetite and reduce cravings. ▪ Some believe it to aid the body's ability to burn fat and lower blood glucose levels.	▪ Acetic acid can damage teeth, parts of the digestive tract and the esophagus. ▪ May have a negative affect on potassium and bone density levels. ▪ May present problems with drug interactions. ▪ *Can we say DUMB?*
Bernstein Diet	▪ This medically supervised program is a combination of low calorie foods, behavior modification, education, and vitamin supplements. ▪ Aims to lose 4-5 pounds per week and involves 3 visits to the clinic each week during the program.	
Best Life Diet	▪ Promotes a lifestyle of healthy eating with an emphasis on regular physical activity. ▪ Not designed for quick or temporary weight loss ▪ Encourages healthy food choices, portion control, and physical activity.	▪ Promoted by Oprah and her personal trainer, Bob Greene.
Beverly Hills Diet	▪ Based on eating the right foods at the right time. ▪ Food groups are to be eaten only within the same group *(protein with protein, etc.)* and during certain times of day *(fruit in the morning)*.	
Body for Life	▪ Health Program based on long term wellness goals. ▪ Combination of lean protein and healthy carbohydrates every few hours throughout the day to speed up fat loss and maintain stable energy levels. ▪ Promotes exercise and a healthy lifestyle.	
British Heart Foundation Diet *(Also known as the Greenlane Diet.)*	▪ 3 day very low calorie diet. ▪ Not affiliated with the actual British Heart Foundation.	
Cambridge Diet	▪ Assortment of delivered pre-packaged foods. ▪ Designed to be nutritionally balanced meal replacements.	
Carbohydrate Addicts Diet	▪ Aims to eliminate the underlying cause of carb addiction by controlling insulin levels. ▪ Seeks to control appetite and weight by alleviating the carb addiction.	▪ *Are you an addict?* ▪ *Is there a 12 step program for carbaholics?*
Change One	▪ Promotes healthy lifestyle by encouraging the adoption of one healthy habit at a time. ▪ Online community offers support, and fitness and diet resources.	

Diet Type	Fast Facts	Other Information
DASH Diet	▪ Low-sodium diet rich in fruits and vegetables and low fat or non-fat dairy. ▪ Designed to lower blood pressure and reduce the risk of stroke and heart disease.	▪ Recommended by the National Heart, Lung and Blood Institute, the American Heart Association, and helped form the basis for the new USDA MyPyramid. ▪ A Dr. Sharon favorite for people with high blood pressure and heart disease.
Diet Smart	▪ The plan involves a series of small, healthy changes to a person's diet that result in more significant benefits over a period of time rather than drastic measures to meet a expected deadline for weight loss goals. ▪ Participants are asked to eat at least 5 times a day and stay under a daily caloric intake amount equal to 8 times their body weight to lose weight.	
Diet Watch	▪ Online program that allows users to track calories, carbs, fat, exercise, and weight. ▪ Online resources include support communities, fitness programs and meal plans.	
F-Plan	▪ A low-fat high-fiber diet based on the idea that high intake of dietary fiber fills you up quickly, providing the bulk of food without the high calories. ▪ Staples of the diet are complex carbs, such as whole grains, baked potatoes, legumes and lots of fruits and vegetables. ▪ Superseded by the F2 Diet by the same author.	
Fat Flush Diet	▪ Both a detox diet and a weight loss diet. ▪ Aims to boost metabolism, reduce water retention and promote fat loss. ▪ Promotes vegetables and lean proteins.	
FatLoss4Idiots	▪ Calorie shifting diet. ▪ Claims that by eating the right foods at the right intervals, weight will be lost by way of fat burning hormones.	▪ *What if I'm smart and fat?*
Fat Smash Diet	▪ Lifestyle approach focused on eating healthful, filling foods, and getting lots of exercise ▪ 90-day program divided into four phases: Detox, Foundation, Construction and The Temple.	▪ Method used on the television show Celebrity Fit Club.
Flat Belly Diet	▪ It is a calorie-controlled, Mediterranean-style diet plan. ▪ Based on the idea that mono-unsaturated fats work to dissolve belly fat. ▪ While the Mediterranean diet is a generally nutritious and healthy plant-based plan, it has not been proven that monounsaturated fats, though healthy, do anything to reduce body fat.	

Diet Type	Fast Facts	Other Information
Flavor Point Diet	• Proposes that by controlling flavors at a meal, dieters can turn off their appetites and eat less, and therefore, lose weight. • The way to satisfy your flavor point is by limiting the variety of flavors at a meal. Claims that an overabundance of flavors at one meal can stimulate appetite centers in the brain and cause a person to overeat. For example, eating lemon at every meal to fatigue your palate and make you less likely to overeat. • There are three phases. In phase 1, which lasts 4 weeks, dieters eat according to flavor-themed days. During phase 2, or weeks 5 through 6, these flavor themes can vary from meal to meal. Finally, by phase 3, dieters drop the flavor themes and simply search out whole foods such as whole grains, lean meats, and fresh fruits and vegetables. • There are no studies that actually look at eating according to flavor themes and how it impacts appetite, feelings of fullness, and weight loss.	• *What???* • *I'm confused , what is the EXACT flavor of a fried chicken wing?*
French Women Don't Get Fat	• Only about 7 percent of French people are obese, compared to 24 percent of Americans. • Proposes that Americans need to emphasize quality over quantity and learn to slow down so that they savor meals instead of eating on the run. • In the first phase, dieters jot down everything they eat in a food journal for a few weeks to pinpoint where they are overindulging. In the next phase, which lasts about three months, dieters gradually adjust their eating habits. For example, they may temporarily give up certain foods and cut back on portions. After dropping the pounds, dieters work to keep their weight stable. • Dieters who thrive on structure might feel lost with the strategies since they're general guidelines rather than a specific calorie-controlled weight loss plan.	• A drawback is that the author is asking dieters to behave like the French, but to do it in the United States. And that can be tough because the same environment that makes it easy to live the French lifestyle *(daily farmer's markets, less access to snack foods, exorbitant gas prices that discourage unnecessary driving)* isn't found in most areas of the United States.
Glycemic Index Diets	• Seeks to stabilize the blood sugar levels and increase energy while losing weight. • Claims that people on this diet will feel full for longer periods of time and have reduced cravings for sugar laden foods.	
Hallelujah diet	• A heavily supplemented, low calorie vegan diet, consisting of 85% raw organic foods and 15% cooked foods, is the core of the faith-based *Hallelujah Diet* program	
Hamptons Diet	• Lifestyle diet, not short term. • Encourages one to eat more vegetables, fish, and omega-3 fatty acids and consume most of one's fats in the form of monounsaturates.	

Diet Type	Fast Facts	Other Information
High Protein Diets	▪ Some studies show higher protein diets help people better control their appetites and calorie intake. ▪ People may not get enough vitamins and minerals.	▪ The American Heart Association doesn't recommend high-protein diets for weight loss, but suggest balanced nutrition.
Hilton Head Metabolism Diet	▪ The program is in two *(repeated)* stages: *The weight reduction or low calorie stage and the maintenance stage (also low fat, high carb).* ▪ Designed to increase the body's metabolism.	
Hip and Thigh Diet	▪ A low calorie and very low fat diet. ▪ Allows lean meat, unlimited vegetables and medium amounts of carbs, but avoids nuts, oils, dairy and butter. ▪ Despite the title, this diet does not provide targeted weight loss to the hip and thigh area.	▪ *Where did this name come from?*
Israeli Army Diet	▪ 8 day diet that allows only four foods: apples, cheese, chicken, salad. ▪ Every two days a new food is eaten. ▪ Very low calorie and restricted food diet. ▪ Not affiliated with the Israeli Army.	
Japanese Women Don't Get Old or Fat	▪ Describes the seven pillars of Japanese home cooking: fish, vegetables, rice, soy, noodles, tea *(particularly green tea)* and fruit. ▪ There are seven secrets of the Tokyo kitchen. First, preferred foods include fish, soy, rice, vegetables and fruit. Second, portions are small. Third, breakfast is powered by miso soup. Fourth, cooking is light and gentle. Fifth, rice replaces bread. Sixth, desserts are teeny-tiny. And seventh, Japanese women don't deprive themselves or go on diets, but eat small amounts of whatever they like. ▪ Key concepts include eating until you are 80 percent full and accruing exericse through a walking intensive lifestyle. ▪ While numerous scientific studies support the health benefits of eating Asian-style, others find college-age Japanese women are some of the most weight-conscious in the world, and older Japanese women are increasingly battling weight problems. ▪ Dieters who thrive on structure might feel lost with the strategies since they're general guidelines rather than a specific calorie controlled weight loss plan.	▪ Includes 36 family recipes and some quaint Japanese folk sayings like, "If you have a pleasant experience eating something you have never tasted before, your life will be lengthened by 75 days." ▪ Liberal use of soy sauce and vegetables preserved in salt makes most Japanese diets too high in sodium recommend that people eat brown rice instead of white in light of the beneficial effects of whole grains on cardiovascular disease and type 2 diabetes. ▪ *I wonder if shrimp tempura is on this diet?*
Ketogenic Diets	▪ A diet high in fat and protein, and virtually no carbohydrates. ▪ Moves the body into a state of **ketosis** whereby ketones are used as a fuel source rather than glucose. ▪ Some use this technique to burn as much fat as possible while retaining muscle mass.	▪ Promotes ketosis, an unhealthy condition that can damage kidneys. ▪ Can place significant strain on the body, particularly liver and kidney function.

Diet Type	Fast Facts	Other Information
Leptin Diet	▪ Leptin is a hormone that assists in regulating both appetite and metabolism. ▪ Five basic rules: ▪ Never eat after dinner. ▪ Eat three meals per day. ▪ Do not eat large meals. ▪ Eat a high-protein breakfast. ▪ Reduce the amount and glycemic index of carbohydrates consumed.	▪ *Do Leprechauns follow this diet?*
Lindora	▪ Clinically based medical weight control system. ▪ Promotes healthy eating and exercise habits to last for life. ▪ Offers additional online programs and nutritional products.	
Macrobiotic Diet	▪ Combines tenets of Zen Buddhism with a Western-style vegetarian diet to form a natural, organic, plant-based diet eaten in a natural state or prepared in traditional manners. ▪ So that foods attain a balance of yin and yang, they are paired based on their sour, sharp, salty, sweet, or bitter characteristics. ▪ Excluded foods are considered to be extreme, over-stimulating, or too concentrated and therefore not capable of achieving balance.	▪ Also promotes practices such as eating slowly and chewing thoroughly. ▪ *Is a fried chicken wing balanced?*
Mayo Clinic Plan	▪ The official recommendation of the prestigious hospital is a lifestyle aimed to maintain a healthy weight for a lifetime, not the grapefruit diet that often goes by the same name. ▪ Incorporates nutrition plans and exercise sustainable for long-term use.	
Morning Banana Diet	▪ Each breakfast consists of only bananas and room-temperature water. For lunch, dinner and snacks, you can eat whatever you like as long as you don't eat after 8 p.m. ▪ The only restrictions: No ice cream, dairy products, alcohol or dessert after dinner, and the only beverage you may have with meals is room-temperature water. One sweet snack is allowed midafternoon. ▪ One of the most popular aspects of the plan is the lack of emphasis on exercise.	▪ According to *The Japan Times* online, ever since former opera singer Kumiko Mori announced she had lost 15 pounds on the "Morning Banana" diet, there has been a shortage of bananas in Japan.
Neanderthin	▪ Promotes the consumption of food which is *edible in its raw state* and which was available in the Paleolithic age. ▪ The exclusion of grains and dairy as products of agricultural society makes it low carb.	▪ FYI: average life expectancy for a Neanderthal was between 30 and 35 years. ▪ *Duhhh?*

Diet Type	Fast Facts	Other Information

Naturally Thin Diet	• Provides 10 golden rules for being naturally thin:
	  • Your diet is a bank account *(you need to balance your calories for the day)*.
	  • Taste everything, eat nothing *(share food, eat small bites)*.
	  • Pay attention *(say no to mindless eating)*.
	  • Downsize your portions.
	  • Cancel your membership in the Clean Plate Club.
	  • Check yourself before you wreck yourself *(stop emotional and binge eating)*.
	  • Know thyself *(know your trigger foods)*.
	  • Get real *(eat more whole foods and fewer processed ones)*.
	  • Good for you *(make peace with food)*.
	  • You can have it all—just not all at once.
	• Promotes eating lots of low calorie veggies, small amounts of fruits, whole grains and meat, and moderate amounts of protein.
		• Some health experts have stated that this diet plan does not provide enough daily calories to support extended practice. Concern was also expressed about the advice that meals should be skipped, to allow for more indulgences like alcohol.
		• I like the 10 golden rules. I think that they can be a part of any well balanced nutritional program.

Negative Calorie Diet	• Strives for the negative caloric effect, in which the number of calories the body expends to chew, digest, metabolize and eliminate the food is more than it gains from the food itself. • Mostly fibrous vegetables and fruits. • Can lack in many essential nutrients.	• *Lookout, bathroom.*
Ornish Diet *(Also known as Eat More, Weigh Less)*	• High-fiber, low fat vegetarian diet • Encourages avoiding sugars, meats, oils, most dairy and additional food groups with the goal of maintaining less than 10% calories from fat in one's diet.	• Dr. Ornish is well known in the medical community because of his success in reversing blockages to the heart, once thought impossible without surgery or drugs.
Park Avenue Diet	• The six week program is more than a low calorie diet. It includes a lifestyle makeover encompassing beauty, etiquette, poise, fitness and fashion, designed to give you the look of the rich and famous. • Also addresses seven fundamental components of lifestyle to have a better chance of physical and mental self-improvement, including: weight, physique, hair, skin, clothing, self confidence and interpersonal skills. • Two behavior modifications work on self-confidence and interpersonal skills, and the other sections focus on appearance, which is designed to capture more than just weight and enhance what everyone notices when you walk into a room.	• *Do I get new Manolo Blahniks or Jimmy Choos if I do this diet?*

Diet Type	Fast Facts	Other Information
Peanut Butter Diet	• Moderate calorie restriction. • Regular aerobic exercise every day. • Regular small meals and snacks throughout the day that encourage fat burning and discourage binge-eating. • Less demanding restrictions may make it an easier diet for many to follow.	• One can expect to eat between 4-6 tablespoons of peanut butter a day.
Personality Type Diet	• Asks users to answer 66 questions about their habits and attitudes toward eating, exercise, and coping. Offers specific advice to change the behaviors and attitudes with which a person self-identifies. Method points you to the areas where diet and lifestyle change will do you the most good. • Based on the scores, a person falls into one or more categories. • Emphasizes "super foods." These are all plant-based foods: Fruits, vegetables, grains, nuts, seeds, dried beans, lentils and soy products. All are low or moderate fat foods rich in vitamins and other important nutrients. Not a vegetarian diet, but there is a focus on vegetarian dishes. Fish and poultry are on the menu. Lean red meat is OK, but not encouraged.	• *What personality craves Godiva chocolate?*
Pritikin Diet	• A low fat diet, not vegetarian, but largely based on vegetables, grains and fruits.	
Protein Power	• Low carb, high protein diet.	
Raw Food Diet	• Consists of consuming unprocessed, organic and plant based foods. • Seeks to benefit from the enzymes and chemicals contained in foods in the raw form since cooking foods at high temperatures usually destroys these beneficial compounds. • Promise of efficient digestion, enhanced energy levels, better skin and flushing of toxins from the body.	• *Can we say flush?*
Rice Diet	• Consists of a very low calorie, high-complex carbohydrate, low sodium, low fat, low sugar, low protein, whole foods diet designed to detoxify, cause and prevent or reverse chronic diseases.	
Rosedale Diet	• High fat, very low carb, low protein diet. • Places emphasis on eating a lot more healthy fats. • Based on controlling the hormone *leptin*.	
Sacred Heart Diet	• A soup-based diet that resembles the cabbage soup diet. • Claims that you will lose 10-17 pounds in the first week.	• The American Heart Association have claimed that the diet is phony. • *10-17 pounds in a week? Is that even OK? C'mon people this is NOT SACRED, this is SATANIC.*

Diet Type	Fast Facts	Other Information
Seattle Sutton	• A calorie and fat controlled plan. • Pre-made meals available for order and delivery.	
Six Week Body Makeover	• A customized process of learning your own reaction to particular foods, then combining them in your diet so that your unique metabolism burns more fat. • The package includes a starting up video, a body 'blueprinting' kit, exercise bands & training video, custom eating & body shaping plans, a guide for dining out, a 'Living Lean' program & audio cassette and a recipe guide/menu planner.	
The Shangri-La Diet	• Advertised as the ''no hunger, eat anything weight loss plan,'' it proposes to curb your appetite and lower your body's set point *(the weight at which it naturally wants to settle)* with concoctions of sugar water or extra-light olive oil consumed between meals which teaches your body to stop associating taste with calories. So you'll want less of whatever foods you're eating. • The diet is based on the premise of taste association. The theory: If you eat a variety of familiar foods that are rich in flavor, the brain stimulates hunger, raising the set point and causing weight gain. But if you consume foods with little taste, or that taste unfamiliar, the brain thinks the body must be starving thus lowering the set point and causing weight loss. • Dieters can eat whatever foods they like, but are advised to stay away from processed foods, refined grains, and foods containing high-fructose corn syrup, and to choose more wholesome foods such as fruits, vegetables, whole grains, and foods high in fiber.	• *Drink olive oil? Not!* • *I'm sorry but I LIKE the taste of food.*
Slim4Life	• Combines individual supervision with a well-balanced food program that is based on regular everyday food purchased from the supermarket.	
Somersizing	• Food combining to not only help you burn fat more efficiently, but also balance your hormones and improve your metabolism.	• Promoted by Suzanne Somers.
Sugar Busters	• Promotes reducing the sugar in one's daily menu through easy-to-follow recipes and meal plans. • Determines the glycemic levels of various foods with a accessible glycemic index.	
Ultra Metabolism Plan	• Designed to control appetite and inflammation. • Aims to prevent cellular "rust" that interferes. with metabolism and turn calories into energy. • Seeks to make sure the thyroid, the master metabolism hormone, is working optimally. • Claims to detoxify the liver and subdue stress.	

Diet Type	Fast Facts	Other Information
Ultra Simple Diet	- Designed to provide your body with foods and activities that help fight the inflammation, food insensitivities, and environmental toxins that an unhealthy diet creates. - Promoted Foods: fish, especially small, non-predatory species such as sardines, herring, wild salmon, black cod or sable fish, sole, and cod; lean white meat chicken breasts *(preferably organic)*; fresh or frozen non-citrus fruits, ideally berries only *(preferably organic)*; fresh vegetables *(preferably organic)*; fresh vegetable broth *(three to four cups per day)*; legumes *(lentils, navy beans, adzuki beans, mung beans, tofu and others)*; brown rice; nuts and seeds *(almonds, walnuts, pecans, macadamia nuts and pumpkin seeds)*; flaxseeds *(ground, preferably organic)*; lemons. - Eliminated foods: caffeine; processed and refined carbohydrates and sugar; high-fructose corn syrup, hydrogenated *(trans)* fats; processed, packaged, junk or fast foods; alcohol.	- *Can I get the food for this Ultra Simple Diet at my local grocery store?*
Volumetrics	- Promotes eating large quantities of food while still losing weight. - Utilizes low calories and high fiber foods that can be consumed in high volume.	
Warrior Diet	- Caters to the theory that humans are designed to be active hunters during the day and big eaters at night. - Eat one main meal at night. - Avoid chemicals. - Combine foods adequately. - Challenge your body physically.	- *I will hunt down a hot Krispy Kreme Doughnut, does that count?*

According to *Fat—Exploding the Myths* by Lisa Colles, Americans are reported to spend between $30-50 billion each year on diet and weight loss programs, products and pills; $6 billion of this is said to be spent on weight loss products and pills that don't work. Again, there is NO MAGIC BULLET, PILL, SHOT or PROCEDURE. However, prescription medications can be used as tools to help you in your weight loss efforts but lifestyle changes must be implemented or when you stop popping the pill or taking the shot—the weight will jump back on you. Additionally, you should never JUST take a pill or start a diet without working in exercise and increased activity.

What 10 Diet Plans Cost?

Found at www.moneycentral.msn.com/content/invest/forbes/P114424.asp
You can spend a little or you can spend a lot, but shedding those excess pounds doesn't depend on it.
By *Forbes*

It's no secret that Americans are fat—and getting fatter by the burger. Nearly one-third of U.S. adults are overweight, and another third are technically obese, as defined by a body-mass index of more than 30. And Americans aren't happy about it. Last year, we spent an estimated $46 billion on diet products and self-help books.

Much of that money is wasted. Indeed, a government review found that two-thirds of American dieters regained all the weight they had lost within a year, and 97% had gained it all back within five years. And following these regimes is significantly more expensive than the tried and true technique of eating less and exercising more.

How much more? To find out, we examined weekly menus—culled from official publications or company representatives—from 10 of the most popular diets on the market: Atkins, Jenny Craig, Ornish, NutriSystem, Slim Fast, South Beach, Subway, Sugar Busters!, Weight Watchers and The Zone. The median diet worked out to a costly $85.79 a week—that's 50% more than the $54.44 the average single American spends on food. Our price calculations for the foods on each menu were done on a per-serving basis. Prices came from New York City-based online grocer Fresh Direct and were adjusted to the national average to control for any price differential.

The cost of dieting for a week

Diet	Weekly menu cost ($)*	Percent over national average
Jenny Craig	137.65	152.8
NutriSystem	113.52	108.5
Atkins Diet	100.52	84.6
Weight Watchers	96.64	77.5
Zone Diet	92.84	70.5
Ornish Diet	78.74	44.6
South Beach Diet	78.61	44.4
Slim-Fast	77.73	42.8
Sugar Busters	69.62	27.9
Subway sandwich	68.60	26.0
No diet	54.44	-

Sources *(2005 article)*: *Forbes*, Fresh Direct, Amazon, Bureau of Labor Statistics * Adjusted for NYC prices. Includes the cost of associated book, if applicable, and any membership fees associated with the diet, averaged over a six-month period.

Dollars do not equal results

Jenny Craig dieters were the hardest hit. A week's worth of food, which included both Jenny Craig-supplied meals and supplemental snacks, cost $137.65. Jared Fogle's informal—but, for him, effective—Subway Sandwich Diet was the least expensive of the bunch at $68.60 a week. The Sugar Busters! Diet came in a close second, with its weekly menu costing $69.62.

Does it really cost more to eat healthfully?

It doesn't have to, says Dr. Pamela Peeke, a Pew Foundation scholar in nutrition and metabolism, "as long as you keep it simple." A typical, unfussy Sugar Busters! dinner of baked turkey breast with vegetables and a sweet potato on the side worked out to a mere $3.24. By contrast, one Ornish dinner had a shopping list 28 items long—and that's not counting herbs, spices or condiments. And an Atkins lobster salad lunch recipe called for one-quarter pound of lobster tail meat at $25.99 a pound.

"How many people know what orange roughy is? Give me a break," Dr. Peeke grumbles. "Give me a skinless, boneless chicken breast and call it a day."

And despite the extra cost, most diets currently on the market are not effective. "Let's face it," says Dr. Stephen Gullo, a New York City doctor and author of The Thin Commandments Diet, "this is the only growth industry in the United States where most of the customers fail."

"The very existence of the diet industry is proof of its ineffectiveness. If there were one safe, effective way to lose weight, then the others would be out of business," says Marilyn Wann, author of Fat! So?

According to Ernst Schaefer, a professor at Tufts University, "The fundamental misconception about diets is that most people are looking for a magic bullet." He—and many other nutritionists—claim that the most effective way of losing weight is to restrict caloric intake, and the most effective way to maintain the loss is through regular exercise.

Marian Nestle, professor of nutrition at New York University, agrees. "Eat less, move more," she suggests.

"One should eat to live, not live to eat." Cicero, Rhetoricorum LV

I told you from the beginning of this book that diets really don't work; but lifestyle changes do. However, you can choose your method and there are a lot of good programs, interventions out there that can help you in the struggle to life a healthier and lighter life. One thing that I HATE with a passion is hunger. Unfortunately, mentally when we say that we want to lose weight; we often think—"OMG, I'm gonna starve." Or we walk around like we're dying, with no energy and get up and go because we are STARVING. Then with these crazy diets which are unhealthy we begin to damage ourselves on the inside and out. Let's really make a decision that enough is ENOUGH!

Eat More, Weigh Less?

From the CDC, found at www.cdc.gov

How to manage your weight without being hungry.

Have you tried to lose weight by cutting down the amount of food you eat? Do you still feel hungry and not satisfied after eating? Or have you avoided trying to lose weight because you're afraid of feeling hungry all the time? If so, you are not alone. Many people throw in the towel on weight loss because they feel deprived and hungry when they eat less. But there is another way. Aim for a slow, steady weight loss by decreasing calorie intake while maintaining an adequate nutrient intake and increasing physical activity. You can cut calories without eating less nutritious food. The key is to eat foods that will fill you up without eating a large amount of calories.

If I cut calories, won't I be hungry?

Research shows that people get full by the *amount of food* they eat, not the *number of calories* they take in. You can cut calories in your favorite foods by lowering the amount of fat and or increasing the amount of fiber-rich ingredients, such as vegetables or fruit.

Let's take macaroni and cheese as an example. The original recipe uses whole milk, butter and full-fat cheese. This recipe has about 540 calories in one serving *(1 cup)*.

Here's how to remake this recipe with fewer calories and less fat:

- Use 2 cups non-fat milk instead of 2 cups whole milk.

- Use 8 oz. light cream cheese instead of 2 1/4 cups full-fat cheddar cheese.

- Use 1 tablespoon butter instead of 2 or use 2 tablespoons of soft trans-fat free margarine.

- Add about 2 cups of fresh spinach and 1 cup diced tomatoes *(or any other veggie you like)*.

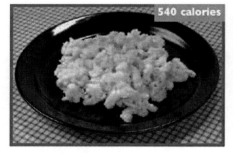

Your redesigned mac and cheese now has 315 calories in one serving *(1 cup)*. You can eat the same amount of mac and cheese with 225 fewer calories.

What foods will fill me up?

To be able to cut calories without eating less and feeling hungry, you need to replace some higher calorie foods with foods that are lower in calories and fat and will fill you up. In general, this means foods with lots of water and fiber in them. The chart below will help you make smart food choices that are part of a healthy eating plan.

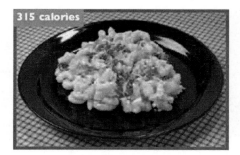

These foods will fill you up with fewer calories. Choose them more often...	These foods can pack more calories into each bite. Choose them less often...
Fruits and Vegetables *(prepared without added fat)*	Fried foods
Spinach, broccoli, tomato, carrots, watermelon, berries, apples	Eggs fried in butter, fried vegetables, French fries
Low-fat and fat-free milk products	Full-fat milk products
Low- or fat-free milk, low- or fat-free yogurt, low- or fat-free cottage cheese	Full-fat cheese, full-fat ice cream, whole and 2% milk
Broth-based soup	Dry snack foods
Vegetable-based soups, soups with chicken or beef broth, tomato soups *(without cream)*	Crackers or pretzels, cookies, chips, dried fruits
Whole grains	Higher-fat and higher-sugar foods
Brown rice, whole wheat bread, whole wheat pastas, popcorn	Croissants, margarine, shortening and butter, doughnuts, candy bars, cakes and pastries
Lean meat, poultry and fish	Fatty cuts of meat
Grilled salmon, chicken breast without skin, ground beef *(lean or extra lean)*	Bacon, brisket, ground beef (regular)
Legumes *(beans and peas)*	
Black, red kidney and pinto beans *(without added fat)*, green peas, black-eyed peas	

A healthy eating plan is one that:

- Emphasizes fruits, vegetables, whole grains and fat free or low fat milk and milk products.

- Includes lean meats, poultry, fish, beans, eggs and nuts.

- Is low in saturated fats, trans fats, cholesterol, salt *(sodium)* and added sugars.

- Stays within your calorie needs.

Technically speaking...

The number of calories in a particular amount or weight of food is called calorie density or energy density. Low-calorie-dense foods are ones that don't pack a lot of calories into each bite.

Foods that have a lot of water or fiber and little fat are usually low in calorie density. They will help you feel full without an unnecessary amount of calories.

Here are some more ideas for cutting back on calories without eating less and being hungry:

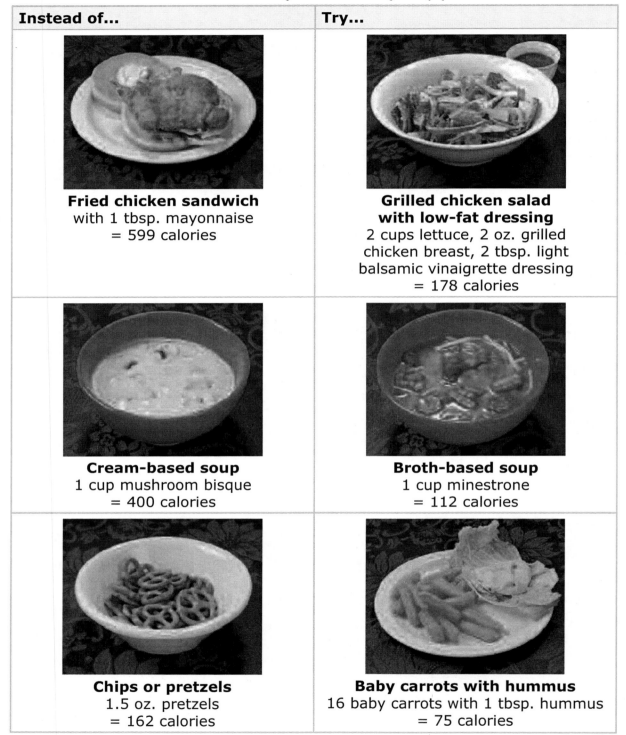

Instead of...	Try...
Fried chicken sandwich with 1 tbsp. mayonnaise = 599 calories	**Grilled chicken salad with low-fat dressing** 2 cups lettuce, 2 oz. grilled chicken breast, 2 tbsp. light balsamic vinaigrette dressing = 178 calories
Cream-based soup 1 cup mushroom bisque = 400 calories	**Broth-based soup** 1 cup minestrone = 112 calories
Chips or pretzels 1.5 oz. pretzels = 162 calories	**Baby carrots with hummus** 16 baby carrots with 1 tbsp. hummus = 75 calories

Good things can come in big packages!

People eat more than they realize when faced with large portion sizes. This usually means eating too many calories. But, not all large portions are created equal. Larger portions of water- and fiber-rich foods, like fruits, vegetables and broth-based soups, can fill you up with fewer calories. Start with an appetizer. Research shows that if you eat a low-calorie appetizer before a meal, you will eat fewer total calories during the meal. Start your meals with a broth-based soup or a green salad without a large amount of cheese, or croutons.

Fruits and Veggies: Keep It Simple!

Most fruits and veggies are low calorie and will fill you up, but the way you prepare them can change that. Breading and frying, and using high-fat creams or butter with vegetables and fruit will add extra calories. Try steaming vegetables and using spices and low-fat sauces for flavor. And enjoy the natural sweetness of raw fruit.

Dr. Sharon's Fruit and Vegetable Week For Your Health & Wellness

(and cuteness)

Found at www.drsharononline.com

Once a week or every two weeks I try to do an all fruit/veggie day to just feel better and as a way of keeping on track. It also does help drop the pounds. Well, one week I decided that I wanted to try to do a week *(Monday- Friday)* of all fruits and veggies and shared it on Facebook with my friends, many of whom had joined me on the fruit/veggie days.

What this is NOT:

1. A QUICK fix diet or fad. You should be eating, eating, eating and not starving. We're just making it healthier and yes—lighter.

2. A substitution for your physician's recommendations. DO NOT UNDER ANY CIRCUMSTANCES undertake any new eating plan if you have a chronic condition *(diabetes, etc.)* without consulting your physician *(see my disclaimer on the website)*.

What this IS:

1. A healthy kick in the bootie to get you or keep you on track. What's wrong with eating all fruits and vegetables? NOTHING; and yes if done correctly you will drop some pounds because fruits and veggies are generally lower in calories than other foods. What's wrong with bumping up exercise? NOTHING—you'll look and feel better.

2. A commitment and a test for you in discipline.

3. YOUR program, I put out guidelines but YOU make the tweaks and do what you need in order to reach your goals.

What I Expect:

1. This is FOR ME…you should write down what you expect this week according to your goals.

    a. I expect more energy and to feel lighter.

    b. I expect to crave chocolate and to have to pray my way through it!

    c. I expect to lose about 5-7 pounds.

    d. I expect to be down about ½-1 dress size.

    e. I expect that my exercise boost is going to be fun as I will try at least 2 new exercise classes—or ones that I haven't tried in a while.

    f. I expect to slip up in at least one area on at least one day, but I accept that I will forgive myself and move on.

    g. I expect to hear success stories from YOU and my FB friends.

    h. I expect that my assistant is going to kill me as she has to find another ½-1 hour out of my day that she can't touch because I'm adding more exercise time.

    i. I expect that I'll be feeling fabulous on Friday evening after I get into bed and await Saturday morning's weigh in.

What do you expect? Go for it. So here are the guidelines:

Step 1: The Mind and Your Focus

1. Get your mind right and wrapped around the fact that you will feel healthier and lighter.

2. It's not about what you can't have versus what you ARE eating/doing to benefit your body.

3. Be realistic, if you're going to have a rough week ahead, physically, emotionally, professionally, etc…that is out of the ordinary—you should probably hold off. But don't let being busy make you forgive being unhealthy. Be realistic but don't look for an excuse.

Step 2: The Fruit/Vegetable Portion

1. This is basically a total vegetarian eating plan.

    a. What does that mean???? From the American Heart Association's website: Some people follow a vegetarian diet, but there's no single vegetarian eating pattern. The vegan or total vegetarian diet includes only foods from plants: fruits, vegetables, legumes *(dried beans and peas)*, grains, seeds and nuts. The lacto vegetarian diet includes plant foods plus cheese and other dairy products. The ovo-lactovegetarian *(or lacto-ovovegetarian)* diet also includes eggs. Semi-vegetarians don't eat red meat but include chicken and fish with plant foods, dairy products and eggs.

2. Eat as much and as many fresh fruit as you wish.

    a. Fruits: Apples, grapes, cantaloupe, strawberries, blueberries and the list goes on. Have them with you as frequent snacks, make fresh berry mix *(my favorite)* and what about a nice green salad as a meal. You can have all the fruit that you like BUT this does not mean that you can have apple pie—or chocolate covered strawberries.

    b. Avoid canned fruits in syrup; the goal is to eat fresh fruits. Fruit cups in water are ok.

    c. Avoid fruits dripping in syrups, sugars, etc. Candied apples do not count and are a no!

    d. Vegetables: Eat as much and as many fresh vegetables as you want. Lightly steamed if necessary but AVOID the bacon grease, heavy butter, sauces, etc. Use *I Can't Believe it's Not Butter (light)*, sprays or Olive oil, etc. NO hollandaise sauces or pouring junk over fresh vegetables and don't fall for the salad dressing soup *(i.e., a little salad with tons of high fat dressing poured over it—let the salad breathe and not drown—SAVE THE SALAD!)*. Fresh mixed greens, carrots, broccoli and a host of great fiber veggies are a go alone or in a hearty salad. The dressings should be vinaigrette or the sprays are great and add no *(to very little)* calories. You can put beans on the salad to add protein and I LUV to put apples, nuts and fruit on salads.

    e. Beverages: WATER, WATER, WATER throughout the day and as the main choice for hydration. NO carbonated beverages—even diet beverages; NONE. I have a rule about drinking my calories; I don't drink calories…but that's just my rule and suggest that if you need to drop some pounds to follow it. If you want to add in limited fruit or vegetable juices, that's up to you. This would be if you are really only going for cleansing but either way; why not agree to avoid drinking more than 200 calories a day? Green Tea *(increases metabolism and is an antioxidant)* is my staple drink with Splenda. I am committing to increasing my water this week.

    f. Other: This is YOUR plan and you should customize it so you don't feel like you're sucking on lemons. I will have at least one-two days where I will allow some low fat cheese on this plan. Beans are a great source of protein and you may also want to allow 1-2 protein shakes during the week.

Step 3: The Fitness/Exercise Portion

1. **Exercise is a MUST:** I'll say it again— Exercise is a MUST for at LEAST 3 of the 5 days through Friday. It is preferred that you exercise EVERY day. If you're already exercising bump it up by 20-60 minutes. I am committing to 2.25-2.5 hours daily with at least one day of 3 hours, however, realize that 2 hours is not unusual for me—do what YOU do. If you don't exercise take it slowly— don't hurt yourself. If you KNOW that you can only walk for 10 minutes then start there; walk in place; do squats during commercials, do something—dancing, walking and cleaning *(vigorously)* all count! It is a process—check out my old pictures in the photo gallery and on the site—it is a PROCESS; originally I could only walk for about 15 minutes. *(New pics are coming)*

2. **Make sure that you're eating enough to fuel workouts.** Don't starve yourself and don't think that by working out for 45 minutes that you can eat the refrigerator.

3. **Try something new:** Walking outside if the weather permits, yoga, elliptical machines, spin class, pole dancing, dancing in your living room, etc., whatever is going to be fun and work for you. Remember that you need strength as well as cardio. LISTEN to your body and your doctor's advice. If you are a couch potato—don't try to run a marathon this week!

Final Thoughts:

1. We all want to feel, and let's tell the truth, LOOK better.

2. If you desire to lose weight then I suggest that you do weigh yourself at the start and pick out a pair of pants or dress, shirt that is a little snug and use that as a barometer and motivation. But don't use a picture of your husband/man or wife/girlfriend or the person that you are fatally attracted to (*i.e., Denzel*) as the motivation. This is about YOU! This is about YOU! And your health/wellness *as well as cuteness which comes in all shapes and sizes.*

3. If you don't want to lose weight but want to be healthier, make sure that you're really piling on the calories to maintain your weight.

4. Take time every day to do some meditation, deep breathing, prayer and searching into the inner you. This is a kick start but every day I have to exam my relationship with food and fitness. I don't care what anyone says; you have to be a little fanatical to fight all of the wars that rage against our health. YOU are the most important person to you and make time for YOU.

5. Exercise is an important aspect—I say it all over the country. "If you don't have time to exercise, then you don't have time to eat!" This means don't lie to yourself if you can shovel food in, you can run, walk, jog, dance or whatever it off.

   a. Sleep and rest are important!

   b. Expect that you're not perfect, and it's okay to slip up but jump back into it.

   c. Don't forget to take a multivitamin daily and any other supplements as directed by your doctor. I will try to take a multivitamin, calcium supplement, baby aspirin, Omega 3 and complex B as part of my continued regimen.

"If there is no struggle, there is no progress." Frederick Douglass

Dr. Sharon's Adaptation of Douglass's quote for this week: *"Lord, help me in my struggle to not have Godiva chocolate during this Fruit/Veggie week. Help me to just say no to the cheeses that I love. Help me to progress to better health and to that cute Escada dress that's hanging in my closet. Help me progress to the no jiggle zone. A Luta Continua—my struggle continues."*

I'm not the only one that loves fruits and vegetables; here's what the CDC has to say about fruits and vegetables.

How to Use Fruits and Vegetables to Help Manage Your Weight

From the CDC, found at www.cdc.gov

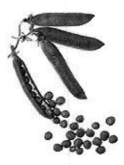

Fruits and vegetables are part of a well-balanced and healthy eating plan. There are many different ways to lose or maintain a healthy weight. Using more fruits and vegetables along with whole grains and lean meats, nuts and beans is a safe and healthy one. Helping control your weight is not the only benefit of eating more fruits and vegetables. Diets rich in fruits and vegetables may reduce the risk of some types of cancer and other chronic diseases. Fruits and vegetables also provide essential vitamins and minerals, fiber and other substances that are important for good health.

To lose weight, you must eat fewer calories than your body uses.

This doesn't necessarily mean that you have to eat less food. You can create lower-calorie versions of some of your favorite dishes by substituting low-calorie fruits and vegetables in place of higher-calorie ingredients. The water and fiber in fruits and vegetables will add volume to your dishes, so you can eat the same amount of food with fewer calories. Most fruits and vegetables are naturally low in fat and calories and are filling.

Here are some simple ways to cut calories and eat fruits and vegetables throughout your day:

Breakfast: Start the Day Right

- Substitute some spinach, onions, or mushrooms for one of the eggs or half of the cheese in your morning omelet. The vegetables will add volume and flavor to the dish with fewer calories than the egg or cheese.

- Cut back on the amount of cereal in your bowl to make room for some cut-up bananas, peaches or strawberries. You can still eat a full bowl, but with fewer calories.

Lighten Up Your Lunch

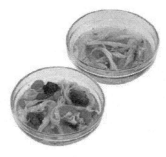

- Substitute vegetables such as lettuce, tomatoes, cucumbers, or onions for 2 oz. of the cheese and 2 oz. of the meat in your sandwich, wrap, or burrito. The new version will fill you up with fewer calories than the original.

- Add a cup of chopped vegetables, such as broccoli, carrots, beans, or red peppers, in place of 2 oz. of the meat or 1 cup of noodles in your favorite broth-based soup. The vegetables will help fill you up, so you won't miss those extra calories.

Dinner

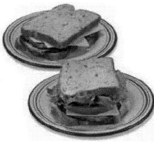

Add in 1 cup of chopped vegetables such as broccoli, tomatoes, squash, onions, or peppers, while removing 1 cup of the rice or pasta in your favorite dish. The dish with the vegetables will be just as satisfying but have fewer calories than the same amount of the original version.

Take a good look at your dinner plate. Vegetables, fruit and whole grains should take up the largest portion of your plate. If they do not, replace some of the meat, cheese, white pasta, or rice with legumes, steamed broccoli, asparagus, greens, or another favorite vegetable. This will reduce the total calories in your meal without reducing the amount of food you eat. BUT remember to use a normal- or small-size plate, not a platter. The total number of calories that you eat counts, even if a good proportion of them come from fruits and vegetables.

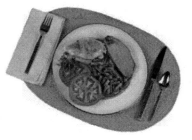

Smart Snacks

- Most healthy eating plans allow for one or two small snacks a day. Choosing most fruits and vegetables will allow you to eat a snack with only 100 calories.

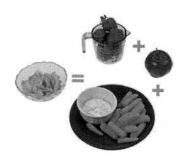

  About 100 Calories or Less
  - a medium-sized apple *(72 calories)*
  - a medium-sized banana *(105 calories)*
  - 1 cup steamed green beans *(44 calories)*
  - 1 cup blueberries *(83 calories)*
  - 1 cup grapes *(100 calories)*
  - 1 cup carrots *(45 calories)*, broccoli *(30 calories)* or bell peppers *(30 calories)* with 2 tbsp. hummus *(46 calories)*

Instead of a high-calorie snack from a vending machine, bring some cut-up vegetables or fruit from home. One snack-sized bag of corn chips *(1 oz.)* has the same number of calories as a small apple, 1 cup of whole strawberries AND 1 cup of carrots with ¼ cup of low calorie dip. Substitute one or two of these options for the chips and you will have a satisfying snack with fewer calories.

Remember: Substitution is the key. It's true that fruits and vegetables are lower in calories than many other foods, but they do contain some calories. If you start eating fruits and vegetables in addition to what you usually eat, you are adding calories and may gain weight. The key is substitution. Eat fruits and vegetables instead of some other higher calorie food.

More tips for making fruits and vegetables part of your weight management plan:

Eat fruits and vegetables the way nature provided—or with fat-free or low-fat cooking techniques.

Try steaming your vegetables, using low-calorie or low-fat dressings, and using herbs and spices to add flavor. Some cooking techniques, such as breading and frying, or using high-fat dressings or sauces will greatly increase the calories and fat in the dish. And eat your fruit raw to enjoy its natural sweetness.

Canned or frozen fruits and vegetables are good options when fresh produce is not available.

However, be careful to choose those without added sugar, syrup, cream sauces or other ingredients that will add calories.

Choose whole fruit over fruit drinks and juices. Fruit juices have lost fiber from the fruit.

It is better to eat the whole fruit because it contains the added fiber that helps you feel full. One 6-oz. serving of orange juice has 85 calories, compared to just 65 calories in a medium orange.

Whole fruit gives you a bigger size snack than the same fruit dried—for the same number of calories.

A small box of raisins *(¼ cup)* is about 100 calories. For the same number of calories, you can eat 1 cup of grapes.

Dr. Sharon's Favorite Fruit and Vegetable Tips/Recipes

1. Mixed Berries, I will NEVER give them up.

- Slice strawberries and mix with the berries that are in season—I love blueberries, blackberries and even will throw in grapes (*not a berry I know but I'm writing this so I can put it here*). Throw a little Splenda or other artificial sweetener on them if you choose (*don't write me about the harmful effects of sweeteners—I will only respond with the harmful effects of fat—just saying—YOU choose and you may not even need anything sprinkled on top*).

  - Now this can get costly and I tell you that often I'm about to cry at the grocery store when my blackberries, blueberries and strawberries are more than a Porterhouse steak with all the fixings. HOWEVER, it also costs to get clothes altered because you've been eating JUNK. YOU decide *Is It Worth It*!

2. Watermelon (when in season)

- Ice cold and sliced with just a tad of Splenda (*if needed*) on it makes a great breakfast, lunch or dinner. I mean REALLY eat it—I can eat an entire watermelon on the days that I'm committed to just fruits/vegetables.

3. Dr. Sharon's Ridiculously tasty green beans.

- **ONLY because I love you, will I give you my quick recipe**:

  - Ingredients: FRESH green beans, FRESH (*jar*) garlic and FRESH onions, sliced. Italian Seasonings, Kosher Salt and Paprika are the seasonings that I use. You will need Olive Oil (*2 tablespoons*) and have the spray can handy as well as one teaspoon of butter or butter spray as you desire.

  - Put the oil in a sauce pan, sauté the garlic, onions and add in Italian seasoning, paprika and a dash of Kosher salt just when you have finished the sauté.

  - Throw the green beans in the pan and mix it all up. I love lots of garlic (*great for cholesterol*) and lots of onions—I use red onions in this but it's your choice. Cook to desired consistency but do NOT overcook—don't kill the little green beans; they need firmness. Taste as you go and add seasoning (*go easy on the salt*) per your preference.

  - You can also be creative and add pine nuts, various mushrooms and have at it. (*Do NOT put MEAT in them.*)

  - I tell you that when I cook this, I can literally eat the whole pan over the course of the day. Great low calorie, low fat food that's full of great taste served alone or as a side dish. *Sidebar: get some peppermint and mouthwash; the garlic may get you.*

4. Dr. Sharon's Awesome spinach

- I won't give you this recipe now, I can't tell you EVERYTHING. However, sautéed spinach is low calorie and fabulous. If you DON'T like spinach; you'll like this—ask my brother Rod (*a.k.a. Attorney Roderick Allison and Comedian Rod of God—shameless family plug: www.rodofgodcomedy.com*).

5. One Word: SALAD

- There is a fine art to making salad, particularly if you're focused on fresh fruits and veggies. I will give you hints to help you in this journey. Mixed greens, carrots, onions, broccoli, strawberries, apples, nuts, tomatoes, mushrooms and the list goes on. If you like a vegetable or fruit alone, try it in a salad.

- I will decide later if I open my treasure chest of salad recipes. I'm struggling because I want to help us all in the struggle but I can't tell it all!

Beware of Beverages

As I've stated before in this book, in lectures and articles, I try my very best NOT to drink any calories. I am very fond of EATING and CHEWING, therefore if I pile up the calories by drinking them I will not be able to EAT them. A personal example, I love Starbucks. I am a regular at three of them; when I walk in they know what to get me immediately.

My OLD Starbucks Favorite: Caramel Macchiato with extra foam, 4 pumps of extra caramel and at least 4 packets of brown sugar and 3 of white sugar *(Venti = 20 oz.)*

The calories in this were *(at least):* 510 calories and 18 g fat

To burn off the 510 calories in this Caramel Macchiato, you would have to:

Activity	130 lbs	150 lbs	170 lbs	190 lbs	220 lbs	250 lbs	270 lbs
Aerobics, General	80 mins.	69 mins.	61 mins.	55 mins.	47 mins.	42 mins.	39 mins.
Bicycle, Stationary	74 mins.	64 mins.	57 mins.	51 mins.	44 mins.	39 mins.	36 mins.
Calisthenics *(push-ups, sit-ups, pull-ups, jumping jacks)*	65 mins.	56 mins.	50 mins.	44 mins.	38 mins.	34 mins.	72 mins.
Food Shopping	225 mins.	196 mins.	173 mins.	155 mins.	133 mins.	118 mins.	109 mins.
Gardening, General	130 mins.	112 mins.	99 mins.	89 mins.	76 mins.	68 mins.	63 mins.
Raking Lawn	121 mins.	105 mins.	92 mins.	83 mins.	71 mins.	63 mins.	58 mins.
Sex, General, Moderate	399 mins.	346 mins.	306 mins.	274 mins.	235 mins.	208 mins.	193 mins.
Shoveling Snow	86 mins.	75 mins.	66 mins.	59 mins.	51 mins.	45 mins.	42 mins.
Sweep Floors	157 mins.	136 mins.	120 mins.	108 mins.	93 mins.	82 mins.	76 mins.
Treadmill	58 mins.	50 mins.	44 mins.	40 mins.	34 mins.	30 mins.	28 mins.
Vacuum	148 mins.	129 mins.	114 mins.	102 mins.	87 mins.	77 mins.	72 mins.
Volleyball	130 mins.	112 mins.	99 mins.	89 mins.	76 mins.	68 mins.	63 mins.
Washing Dishes	225 mins.	196 mins.	173 mins.	155 mins.	133 mins.	118 mins.	109 mins.
Weight Lifting	173 mins.	150 mins.	132 mins.	119 mins.	102 mins.	90 mins.	84 mins.

This was a DRINK, not a meal, a DRINK that I often would have twice in one day. I could have made it better by doing the following:

- Change from whole milk to 2% milk or nonfat: Savings approx. 40 calories or even better with nonfat milk save 100 calories.

- Savings 80 calories.

- Decrease the size from a Venti *(20 oz.)* to a Grande *(16 oz.)* and save over 100 calories and even more if I made the other changes to the milk.

- Other obvious changes get rid of the sugar and use a no calorie sweetener.

By making just those simple changes I could easily turn my 510 calorie *cling to the hips* caramel macchiato to a better drink that is less than 200 calories.

My NEW Starbucks Favorite: *(usually at least twice EVERY day)*: Venti Green Ice Tea with no lemonade and no sweetener, shaken with 10 Splenda. Calories: 0, NADA, NUNCA, NEIN, Fat: 0, NADA, NUNCA, NEIN.

Let's take another look at other beverages and evaluate if they are *Worth It.*

Frappuccino

To burn off one frappuccino with whipped cream *(approx. 600 calories)* you would have to:

Activity	130 lbs	150 lbs	170 lbs	190 lbs	220 lbs	250 lbs	270 lbs
Aerobics, General	94 min.	81 min.	72 min.	64 min.	55 min.	49 min.	45 min.
Bicycle, Stationary	87 min.	76 min.	67 min.	60 min.	51 min.	46 min.	42 min.
Calisthenics *(push-ups, sit-ups, pull-ups, jumping jacks)*	76 min.	66 min.	58 min.	52 min.	45 min.	40 min.	37 min.
Food Shopping	265 min.	230 min.	203 min.	182 min.	157 min.	139 min.	128 min.
Gardening, General	153 min.	132 min.	117 min.	105 min.	90 min.	80 min.	74 min.
Raking Lawn	142 min.	123 min.	109 min.	97 min.	84 min.	74 min.	69 min.
Sex, General, Moderate	469 min.	407 min.	360 min.	322 min.	277 min.	245 min.	227 min.
Shoveling Snow	102 min.	88 min.	78 min.	70 min.	60 min.	53 min.	49 min.
Sweeping Floors	185 min.	160 min.	142 min.	127 min.	109 min.	97 min.	89 min.
Treadmill	68 min.	59 min.	52 min.	47 min.	40 min.	35 min.	33 min.
Vacuum	174 min.	151 min.	134 min.	120 min.	103 min.	91 min.	84 min.
Volleyball	153 min.	132 min.	117 min.	105 min.	90 min.	80 min.	74 min.
Washing Dishes	244 min.	230 min.	203 min.	182 min.	157 min.	139 min.	128 min.
Weight Lifting	203 min.	176 min.	156 min.	140 min.	120 min.	106 min.	98 min.

Apple Cider

To burn off 16 oz. of apple cider *(approx. 200 calories)* you would have to:

Activity	130 lbs	150 lbs	170 lbs	190 lbs	220 lbs	250 lbs	270 lbs
Aerobics, General	31 mins.	27 mins.	24 mins.	21 mins.	18 mins.	16 mins.	15 mins.
Bicycle, Stationary	29 mins.	25 mins.	22 mins.	20 mins.	17 mins.	15 mins.	14 mins.
Calisthenics *(push-ups, sit-ups, pull-ups, jumping jacks)*	25 mins.	22 mins.	19 mins.	17 mins.	15 mins.	13 mins.	12 mins.
Food Shopping	88 mins.	77 mins.	68 mins.	61 mins.	52 mins.	46 mins.	43 mins.
Gardening, General	51 mins.	44 mins.	39 mins.	35 mins.	30 mins.	27 mins.	25 mins.
Raking Lawn	47 mins.	41 mins.	36 mins.	32 mins.	28 mins.	25 mins.	23 mins.
Sex, General, Moderate	156 mins.	136 mins.	120 mins.	107 mins.	92 mins.	82 mins.	76 mins.
Shoveling Snow	34 mins.	29 mins.	26 mins.	23 mins.	20 mins.	18 mins.	16 mins.
Sweep Floors	62 mins.	53 mins.	47 mins.	42 mins.	36 mins.	32 mins.	30 mins.
Treadmill	23 mins.	20 mins.	17 mins.	16 mins.	13 mins.	12 mins.	11 mins.
Vacuum	58 mins.	50 mins.	45 mins.	40 mins.	34 mins.	30 mins.	28 mins.
Volleyball	51 mins.	44 mins.	39 mins.	35 mins.	30 mins.	27 mins.	25 mins.
Washing Dishes	88 mins.	77 mins.	68 mins.	61 mins.	52 mins.	46 mins.	43 mins.
Weight Lifting	68 mins.	59 mins.	52 mins.	47 mins.	40 mins.	35 mins.	33 mins.

Frozen Pina Colada

To burn off one small frozen pina colada *(approx. 250 calories)* you would have to:

Activity	130 lbs	150 lbs	170 lbs	190 lbs	220 lbs	250 lbs	270 lbs
Aerobics, General	39 mins.	34 mins.	30 mins.	27 mins.	23 mins.	20 mins.	19 mins.
Bicycle, Stationary	36 mins.	32 mins.	28 mins.	25 mins.	21 mins.	19 mins.	18 mins.
Calisthenics *(push-ups, sit-ups, pull-ups, jumping jacks)*	32 mins.	28 mins.	24 mins.	22 mins.	19 mins.	17 mins.	15 mins.
Food Shopping	111 mins.	96 mins.	85 mins.	76 mins.	65 mins.	58 mins.	53 mins.
Gardening, General	64 mins.	55 mins.	49 mins.	44 mins.	38 mins.	33 mins.	31 mins.
Raking Lawn	59 mins.	51 mins.	45 mins.	41 mins.	35 mins.	31 mins.	29 mins.
Sex, General, Moderate	196 mins.	170 mins.	150 mins.	134 mins.	115 mins.	102 mins.	95 mins.
Shoveling Snow	42 mins.	37 mins.	32 mins.	29 mins.	25 mins.	22 mins.	20 mins.
Sweep Floors	77 mins.	67 mins.	59 mins.	53 mins.	45 mins.	40 mins.	37 mins.
Treadmill	28 mins.	25 mins.	22 mins.	19 mins.	17 mins.	15 mins.	14 mins.
Vacuum	73 mins.	63 mins.	56 mins.	50 mins.	43 mins.	38 mins.	35 mins.
Volleyball	64 mins.	55 mins.	49 mins.	44 mins.	38 mins.	33 mins.	31 mins.
Washing Dishes	111 mins.	96 mins.	85 mins.	76 mins.	65 mins.	58 mins.	53 mins.
Weight Lifting	85 mins.	74 mins.	65 mins.	58 mins.	50 mins.	44 mins.	41 mins.

Looking further at my beloved Starbucks, compare the following at www.starbucks.com. This is using WHOLE milk in a Grande *(16 oz.)* size beverage.

Product	Serving Size *(fl oz.)*	Calories	Fat Calories *(g)*	Total Fat *(g)*	Saturated Fat *(g)*	Trans Fat *(g)*	Cholesterol	Sodium *(mg)*	Total Carbohydrates *(g)*	Fiber *(g)*	Sugars *(g)*	Protein *(g)*
Caffè Americano	16	15	0	0	0	0	0	10	3	0	0	1
Caffè Latte	16	220	100	11	7	0	35	140	18	0	16	12
Caffè Mocha - no whip	16	290	110	12	6	0	30	120	40	2	31	13
Caffè Mocha - whip	16	360	170	19	10	0	55	125	42	2	32	13
Cappuccino	16	140	60	7	4	0	20	85	11	0	9	7
Caramel Brulee Latte - no whip	16	390	90	10	6	0	30	240	64	0	48	11
Caramel Brulee Latte - whip	16	470	150	17	10	0	55	240	70	0	53	11
Caramel Macchiato	16	270	90	10	6	0	30	130	34	0	31	10
Cinnamon Dolce Latte - no whip	16	290	90	10	6	0	30	130	39	0	37	11
Cinnamon Dolce Latte - whip	16	370	160	17	10	0.5	60	140	41	0	39	11
Cinnamon Dolce Latte with Sugar-Free Syrup	16	210	100	11	6	0	35	160	17	0	15	11
Eggnog Latte	16	480	200	22	13	0	145	220	53	0	48	16
Espresso Truffle - no whip	16	370	100	11	7	0	15	135	54	6	37	15
Espresso Truffle - whip	16	440	160	18	11	0	40	140	56	6	38	15
Gingerbread Latte - no whip	16	280	90	10	6	0	30	130	37	0	35	11
Gingerbread Latte - whip	16	350	160	17	10	0	60	140	39	0	36	11
Peppermint Mocha - no whip	16	350	100	11	6	0	25	110	59	2	51	12
Peppermint Mocha - whip	16	440	170	19	11	0	55	120	62	2	53	12
Peppermint White Chocolate Mocha - no whip	16	470	120	14	9	0	30	210	74	0	71	13
Peppermint White Chocolate Mocha - whip	16	550	190	21	14	0	55	220	77	0	74	13

JUST make a substitution to Nonfat Milk and see the difference:

Product	Serving Size (fl oz.)	Calories	Fat Calories (g)	Total Fat (g)	Saturated Fat (g)	Trans Fat (g)	Cholesterol	Sodium (mg)	Total Carbohy-drates (g)	Fiber (g)	Sugars (g)	Protein (g)
Caffè Americano	16	15	0	0	0	0	0	10	3	0	0	1
Caffè Latte	16	130	5	0	0	0	5	150	19	0	18	13
Caffè Mocha - no whip	16	220	20	2.5	0.5	0	5	125	42	2	32	13
Caffè Mocha - whip	16	290	90	10	5	0	30	135	44	2	34	13
Cappuccino	16	80	0	0	0	0	5	90	12	0	10	8
Caramel Brulee Latte - no whip	16	310	5	0	0	0	5	240	66	0	50	11
Caramel Brulee Latte - whip	16	400	70	7	4.5	0	30	250	71	0	54	12
Caramel Macchiato	16	190	10	1	0.5	0	10	135	35	0	32	11
Cinnamon Dolce Latte - no whip	16	210	0	0	0	0	5	135	41	0	39	11
Cinnamon Dolce Latte - whip	16	280	70	7	4.5	0	30	140	43	0	40	12
Cinnamon Dolce Latte with Sugar-Free Syrup	16	130	0	0	0	0	5	170	19	0	17	12
Eggnog Latte	16	450	170	18	11	0	135	230	53	0	49	16
Espresso Truffle - no whip	16	370	100	11	7	0	15	135	54	6	37	15
Espresso Truffle - whip	16	440	160	18	11	0	40	140	56	6	38	15
Gingerbread Latte - no whip	16	200	0	0	0	0	5	140	38	0	36	11
Gingerbread Latte - whip	16	270	70	7	4.5	0	30	150	40	0	37	12
Peppermint Mocha - no whip	16	290	25	2.5	1.5	0	5	115	61	2	52	12
Peppermint Mocha - whip	16	370	90	10	6	0	30	125	64	2	54	13
Peppermint White Chocolate Mocha - no whip	16	400	50	5	4.5	0	10	220	75	0	73	13
Peppermint White Chocolate Mocha - whip	16	480	120	13	9	0	35	230	78	0	75	14

My goal in writing this book is to somehow make us all THINK about what passes on our lips and how we can keep ourselves in balance with a healthy lifestyle that includes exercise. I must say again, EXERCISE is NOT PUNISHMENT for eating. Exercise should be a way of life for you and you should enjoy all the happy hormones that are produced when you do it. Don't think of the *Worth It* model as, if I want to eat this and enjoy it I have to torture myself with exercise and burn it off. No, make rationale, informed decisions and then do the work! If that means ordering your favorite drink and throwing half of it away, then do that. Let me share information from the CDC.

Rethink Your Drink

From the CDC, found at www.cdc.gov

When it comes to weight loss, there's no lack of diets promising fast results. There are low-carb diets, high-carb diets, low-fat diets, grapefruit diets, cabbage soup diets and blood type diets, to name a few. But no matter what diet you may try, to lose weight, you must take in fewer calories than your body uses. Most people try to reduce their calorie intake by focusing on food, but another way to cut calories may be to think about what you drink.

What Do You Drink? It Makes More Difference Than You Think!

Calories in drinks are not hidden *(they're listed right on the Nutrition Facts label)*, but many people don't realize just how many calories beverages can contribute to their daily intake. As you can see in the example below, calories from drinks can really add up. But there is good news: you have plenty of options for reducing the number of calories in what you drink.

Occasion	Instead of...	Calories	Try...	Calories
Morning coffee shop run	Medium café latte *(16 oz.)* made with whole milk	265	Small café latte *(12 oz.)* made with fat-free milk	125
Lunchtime combo meal	20-oz. bottle of non diet cola with your lunch	227	Bottle of water or diet soda	0
Afternoon break	Sweetened lemon iced tea from the vending machine *(16 oz.)*	180	Sparkling water with natural lemon flavor *(not sweetened)*	0
Dinnertime	A glass of non diet ginger ale with your meal *(12 oz.)*	124	Water with a slice of lemon or lime, or seltzer water with a splash of 100% fruit juice	0 calories for the water with fruit slice, or about 30 calories for seltzer water with 2 oz. of 100% orange juice.
Total beverage calories:		796		125-155

(USDA National Nutrient Database for Standard Reference)

Substituting no or low calorie drinks for sugar-sweetened beverages cuts about 650 calories in the example above.

Of course, not everyone drinks the amount of sugar-sweetened beverages shown above. Check the list below to estimate how many calories you typically take in from beverages.

Type of Beverage	Calories in 12 oz.	Calories in 20 oz.
Fruit punch	192	320
100% apple juice	192	300
100% orange juice	168	280
Lemonade	168	280
Regular lemon/lime soda	148	247
Regular cola	136	227
Sweetened lemon iced tea *(bottled, not homemade)*	135	225
Tonic water	124	207
Regular ginger ale	124	207
Sports drink	99	165
Fitness water	18	36
Unsweetened iced tea	2	3
Diet soda *(with aspartame)*	0*	0*
Carbonated water *(unsweetened)*	0	0
Water	0	0

*Some diet soft drinks can contain a small number of calories that are not listed on the nutrition facts label.
(USDA National Nutrient Database for Standard Reference)

Milk contains vitamins and other nutrients that contribute to good health, but it also contains calories.

Choosing low fat or fat free milk is a good way to reduce your calorie intake and still get the nutrients that milk contains.

Type of Milk	Calories per cup (8 oz.)
Chocolate milk (whole)	208
Chocolate milk (2% reduced-fat)	190
Chocolate milk (1% low-fat)	158
Whole Milk (unflavored)	150
2% reduced-fat milk (unflavored)	120
1% low-fat milk (unflavored)	105
Fat-free milk (unflavored)	90
* Some diet soft drinks can contain a small number of calories that are not listed on the nutrition facts label. (USDA National Nutrient Database for Standard Reference)	

Learn To Read Nutrition Facts Labels Carefully

Be aware that the Nutrition Facts label on beverage containers may give the calories for only part of the contents. The example below shows the label on a 20-oz. bottle. As you can see, it lists the number of calories in an 8-oz. serving (100) even though the bottle contains 20 oz. or 2.5 servings. To figure out how many calories are in the whole bottle, you need to multiply the number of calories in one serving by the number of servings in the bottle (100 x 2.5). You can see that the contents of the entire bottle actually contain 250 calories even though what the label calls a serving only contains 100. This shows that you need to look closely at the serving size when comparing the calorie content of different beverages.

NUTRITION FACTS LABEL	
Serving Size 8 fl. oz. Servings Per Container **2.5**	
Amount per serving	
Calories **100**	

Sugar by Any Other Name: How To Tell Whether Your Drink Is Sweetened

Sweeteners that add calories to a beverage go by many different names and are not always obvious to anyone looking at the ingredients list. Some common caloric sweeteners are listed below. If these appear in the ingredients list of your favorite beverage, you are drinking a sugar-sweetened beverage.

- High-fructose corn syrup
- Fructose
- Fruit juice concentrates
- Honey
- Sugar
- Syrup
- Corn syrup
- Sucrose
- Dextrose

High-Calorie Culprits in Unexpected Places

Coffee drinks and blended fruit smoothies sound innocent enough, but the calories in some of your favorite coffee-shop or smoothie-stand items may surprise you. Check the website or in-store nutrition information of your favorite coffee or smoothie shop to find out how many calories are in different menu items. And when a smoothie or coffee craving kicks in, here are some tips to help minimize the caloric damage:

At the coffee shop:

- Request that your drink be made with fat-free or low-fat milk instead of whole milk

- Order the smallest size available.

- Forgo the extra flavoring—the flavor syrups used in coffee shops, like vanilla or hazelnut, are sugar-sweetened and will add calories to your drink.

- Skip the Whip. The whipped cream on top of coffee drinks adds calories and fat.

- Get back to basics. Order a plain cup of coffee with fat-free milk and artificial sweetener or drink it black.

At the smoothie stands:

- Order a child's size if available.

- Ask to see the nutrition information for each type of smoothie and pick the smoothie with the fewest calories.

- Hold the sugar. Many smoothies contain added sugar in addition to the sugar naturally in fruit, juice, or yogurt. Ask that your smoothie be prepared without added sugar: the fruit is naturally sweet.

Better Beverage Choices Made Easy

Now that you know how much difference a drink can make, here are some ways to make smart beverage choices:

- Choose water, diet, or low-calorie beverages instead of sugar-sweetened beverages.

- For a quick, easy and inexpensive thirst-quencher, carry a water bottle and refill it throughout the day.

- Don't stock the fridge with sugar-sweetened beverages. Instead, keep a jug or bottles of cold water in the fridge.

- Serve water with meals.

- Make water more exciting by adding slices of lemon, lime, cucumber or watermelon, or drink sparkling water.

- Add a splash of 100% juice to plain sparkling water for a refreshing, low-calorie drink.

- When you do opt for a sugar-sweetened beverage, go for the small size. Some companies are now selling 8-oz. cans and bottles of soda, which contain about 100 calories.

- Be a role model for your friends and family by choosing healthy, low-calorie beverages.

It's not just beverages that we need to rethink. I love to cook and there are several ways for us to shave calories in the kitchen.

A Lighter and Healthier Kitchen

Dr. Sharon's FIVE Quick Tips for Reducing Calories in Your Kitchen

1.   Have cooking spray *(a variety)* on hand at all times.

   a.   I love the olive oil, butter and baking sprays, they definitely have less calories and fat than butter or margarine.

2.   Cook with egg whites and/or substitutes.

   a.   Do you really need to cook with and eat eggs every day? Can you enjoy the taste of egg whites or substitutes *(my favorite—Egg beaters)*? Have you ever tried?

   b.   You save calories and fat while still getting protein.

   c.   One quick tip, use 1 egg and mix in the egg substitute. Now, I must admit every once in a while, a girl has got to have a hardboiled egg and even I can't possibly throw away the entire egg yolk.

3.   Reduced calorie BREAD. Let me say that again—REDUCED calorie bread.

   a.   To some I have just committed a major sin by even suggesting that you TRY a low calorie version of bread. Okay, eat it—and just be prepared to buy larger clothes; I'm just saying.

   b.   If you don't buy reduced calorie bread, what about an open faced sandwich. Interpretation, a sandwich with just one slice of bread.

   c.   For the love of all that is HOLY! Do NOT do what I did years ago, buy a bread maker and make my own *healthy* bread. I gained 15 pounds in that month of foolishness. I wanted cinnamon and raisin bread but also threw in pecans, walnuts, syrup and anything else that I could. I felt like I was IT because I made my own bread which would literally call to me in the middle of the night and demand butter and jelly. *Somebody may say that they make only healthy bread in their bread maker…repent now because you're lying.*

4.   Avoid the use of regular *(heart attack in a jar)* mayonnaise.

   a.   If you're serious about losing and maintaining your proper weight *(and not even talking about your cholesterol)*, why bother putting these extra calories in your food? What about no fat, low calorie mayonnaise on your sandwiches and in your potato salad? I know someone just said, "I gotta have my mayo, she's crazy. Ok, look at the lumpy mayonnaise and then look at your right hip; any resemblance? I'm just saying.

5.   Buy bags of mixed greens/salad.

   a.   A salad is traditionally filled with mixed greens, veggies and healthy stuff or so it should be. Don't take a wonderful salad and drown it in high fat/high calorie salad dressing. For my sanity…please don't do it!

   b.   A quick check of your salad; if you have more meat, chicken, shrimp, boiled eggs, cheeses and other food on your mixed greens, you're not having a salad, you're having STUFF with parsley *(i.e., mixed greens)*.

   c.   Keep bags of mixed greens in the fridge and learn to really try to create great salads. My family will tell you that I am the queen of a salad. *Email me and I'll give you one of Dr. Sharon's best salads which are good to you and for you.*

There are lots of great websites and places to get information on making healthier choices in the kitchen. I applaud anyone that regularly cooks because it does take time and energy. Further, most studies show that people eat healthier if they cook their foods versus eating out. However, I don't know if that's true of southern cooking. How can you make a pig's foot healthy? **Here are three great articles that I wanted to share with you.**

Ingredient Substitutions: Make the Switch for Healthier Recipes

Cook up healthier recipes by swapping one ingredient for another. These substitution tips can help.
By Mayo Clinic staff, found at www.mayoclinic.com

You stock healthy foods in your pantry, but what do you do with them? And how do you modify favorite family recipes so that they're more in line with your healthy-eating plan? It's not as hard as you may think. The key is to incorporate healthier alternatives into your daily eating routine.

The following suggestions can help you lower fat, salt, sugar and calories and increase fiber in your recipes.

If your recipe calls for:	Try substituting:
All-purpose *(plain)* flour	Whole-wheat flour for half of the called-for all-purpose flour in baked goods Note: Whole-wheat pastry flour is less dense and works well in softer products like cakes and muffins.
Bacon	Canadian bacon, turkey bacon, smoked turkey or lean prosciutto *(Italian ham)*
Butter, shortening or oil in baked goods	Applesauce or prune puree for half of the called-for butter, shortening or oil Note: To avoid dense, soggy or flat baked goods, don't substitute oil for butter or shortening.
Butter, margarine, shortening or oil to prevent sticking	Cooking spray or nonstick pans
Creamed soups	Fat-free milk-based soups, mashed potato flakes, or pureed carrots, potatoes or tofu for thickening agents
Dry bread crumbs	Rolled oats or crushed bran cereal
Eggs	Two egg whites or ¼ cup egg substitute for each whole egg
Enriched pasta	Whole-wheat pasta
Evaporated milk	Evaporated skim milk
Fruit canned in heavy syrup	Fruit canned in its own juices or in water, or fresh fruit
Fruit-flavored yogurt	Plain yogurt with fresh fruit slices
Full-fat cream cheese	Fat-free or low-fat cream cheese, Neufchatel or low-fat cottage cheese pureed until smooth
Full-fat sour cream	Fat-free or low-fat sour cream, plain fat-free or low-fat yogurt
Ground beef	Extra-lean or lean ground beef, chicken or turkey breast *(make sure no poultry skin has been added to the product)*
Iceberg lettuce	Arugula, chicory, collard greens, dandelion greens, kale, mustard greens, spinach or watercress
Margarine in baked goods	Trans fat-free butter spreads or shortenings that are specially formulated for baking Note: If ingredient lists include the term "partially hydrogenated," it may have up to 0.5 grams of trans fat in one serving. To avoid dense, soggy or flat baked goods, don't substitute diet, whipped or tub-style margarine for regular margarine.
Mayonnaise	Reduced-calorie mayonnaise-type salad dressing or reduced-calorie, reduced-fat mayonnaise
Meat as the main ingredient	Three times as many vegetables as the meat on pizzas or in casseroles, soups and stews
Oil-based marinades	Wine, balsamic vinegar, fruit juice or fat-free broth
Salad dressing	Fat-free or reduced-calorie dressing or flavored vinegars
Seasoning salt, such as garlic salt, celery salt or onion salt	Herb-only seasonings, such as garlic powder, celery seed or onion flakes, or use finely chopped herbs or garlic, celery or onions
Soups, sauces, dressings, crackers, or canned meat, fish or vegetables	Low-sodium or reduced-sodium versions
Soy sauce	Sweet-and-sour sauce, hot mustard sauce or low-sodium soy sauce
Syrup	Pureed fruit, such as applesauce, or low-calorie, sugar-free syrup
Table salt	Herbs, spices, fruit juices or salt-free seasoning mixes or herb blends
White bread	Whole-wheat bread
White rice	Brown rice, wild rice, bulgur or pearl barley
Whole milk	Reduced-fat or fat-free milk

"The biggest seller is cookbooks and the second is diet books - how not to eat what you've just learned how to cook." *Andy Rooney*

Recipe makeovers: 5 ways to create healthy recipes

Use these techniques to reduce the fat, calories and sodium in your favorite recipes. *By Mayo Clinic staff, found at www.mayoclinic.com.*

You love your grandmother's bread pudding. But her recipe calls for 4 cups of whole milk, 1 stick of butter and 4 eggs—ingredients that raise the calorie count and fat content of this dessert. The solution? Redo the recipe by switching or reducing certain ingredients.

Many recipes can tolerate a healthy renovation without affecting the taste or texture of the food. So whether you're trying to stick to a healthy-eating plan or you're following a special diet, use these techniques to make your recipes—including your time-honored family favorites—healthier.

1. Reduce the amount of fat, sugar and sodium

With most recipes, you can reduce the amount of fat, sugar and sodium without losing the flavor. By cutting fat and sugar, you also cut calories. How much can you leave out without affecting the flavor and consistency of the food? Apply the following general guidelines:

- **Fat.** For baked goods, use half the butter, shortening or oil and replace the other half with unsweetened applesauce, mashed banana or prune puree. You can also use commercially prepared fruit-based fat replacers found in the baking aisle of your local grocery store.

- **Sugar.** Reduce the amount of sugar by one-third to one-half. When you use less sugar, add spices such as cinnamon, cloves, allspice and nutmeg or flavorings such as vanilla extract or almond flavoring to enhance the sweetness of the food.

- **Sodium.** Reduce salt by one-half in baked goods that don't require yeast. For foods that require yeast, don't reduce the amount of salt, which is necessary for leavening. Without salt, the foods may become dense and flat. For most main dishes, salads, soups and other foods, however, you can reduce the salt by one-half or eliminate it completely.

Other ingredients may contain sugar, fat and sodium, and you can decrease them as well. For example, if the recipe calls for 1 cup shredded cheddar cheese, use ½ cup instead. Or use less soy sauce than is indicated to decrease the amount of sodium in the food.

2. Make a healthy substitution

Healthy substitutions not only reduce the amount of fat, calories and sodium in your recipes, but also can boost the nutritional content. For example, use whole-wheat pasta in place of enriched pasta. You'll triple the fiber and reduce the number of calories. Prepare a dessert with fat-free milk instead of whole milk to save 63 calories and almost 8 g fat per cup.

3. Delete an ingredient

In some recipes, you can delete an ingredient altogether; likely candidates include items you add out of habit or for appearance, such as frosting, coconut or nuts, which are high in fat and calories. Other possibilities include optional condiments, such as pickles, olives, butter, mayonnaise, syrup, jelly and mustard, which can have large amounts of sodium, sugar, fat and calories.

4. Change the method of preparation

Healthy cooking techniques—such as braising, broiling, grilling and steaming—can capture the flavor and nutrients of your food without adding excessive amounts of fat, oil or sodium. If your recipe calls for frying the ingredients in oil or butter, try baking, broiling or poaching the food instead. If the directions say to baste the meat or vegetables in oil or drippings, use wine, fruit juice, vegetable juice or fat-free vegetable broth instead. Using nonstick pans or spraying pans with nonstick cooking spray will further reduce the amount of fat and calories added to your meals.

5. Change the portion size

No matter how much you reduce, switch or omit ingredients, some recipes may still be high in sugar, fat or salt. In these cases, reduce the amount of that food you eat. Smaller portions have less fat, calories and sodium and allow you to eat a wider variety of foods during a meal. Eating a variety of foods will ensure that you get all the energy, protein, vitamins, minerals and fiber you need.

Putting it all together

As you look over your recipe, decide what to change and how to change it. Make notes of any alterations, so you can refer to them the next time you prepare the food. You may have to make the recipe a few times, adjusting your alterations, before you get the results you want. But finding the right combination of ingredients—for the desired taste, consistency and nutrients—is well worth the trouble.

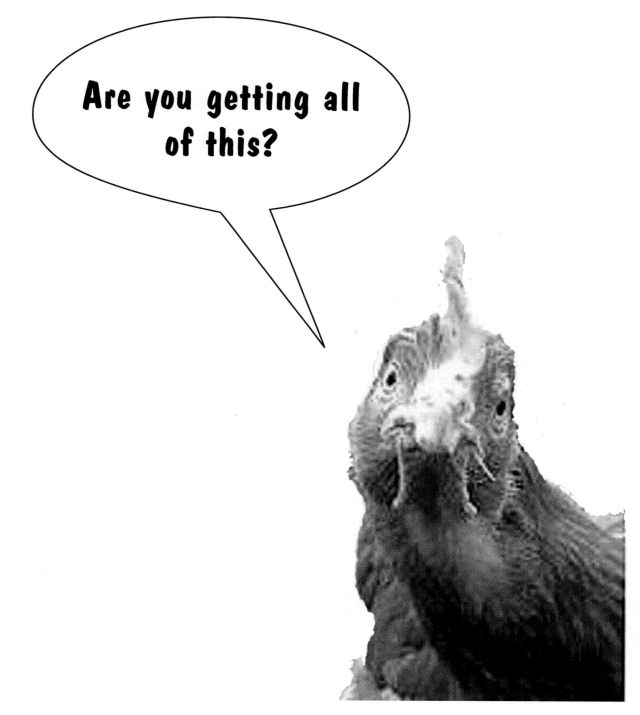

From Cooking Light:
Lighten Up Secrets Revealed!

20 of our most innovative techniques for making any dish more healthful.

Found at www.cookinglight.com

By: Brandi Rushing

When it comes to making food delicious and light, our *(Cooking Light)* Test Kitchens professionals have learned all the tricks. Here, they share some of their tried-and-true techniques for making dishes more nutritious without sacrificing an oz. flavor.

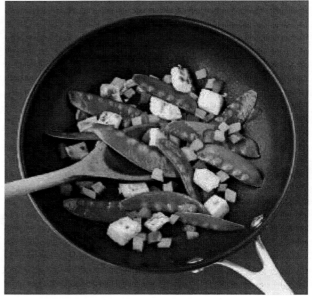

FOR ALL RECIPES

1. **Study the recipe.** Closely examine the original to see where changes can be made. "You can't just wing it, no matter how familiar you are with the recipe," says Test Kitchens Professional Kathryn Conrad. "Look at each ingredient to see where you can take away, add or substitute."

2. **Reference lightened versions** of similar recipes before starting. Check out past issues of *Cooking Light* cookbooks or visit *CookingLight*.com.

3. **Limit sodium.** Try the recipe with half the recommended sodium.

4. **Reduce portion sizes.** When plating, start with a smaller amount and see if that satisfies you.

5. **Give yourself some slack.** "We try different versions of the same recipe three or four times," says Test Kitchens Professional Jan Moon. "Recipes are a science; you may need a few attempts to get it just right."

Read on for tips on toppings and baking.

FOR TOPPINGS

6. **Choose a flavorful cheese.** "Use a variety with more flavor, such as Parmigiano-Reggiano," says Assistant Food Editor Kathy Kitchens Downie, RD. "The stronger the flavor, the less you have to use."

7. **Sprinkle cheese, chocolate or nuts on top** rather than mixing into batters. As toppings, they deliver concentrated flavor.

8. **Reduce sugar-crumb toppings.** Half the amount is often enough.

9. **Substitute panko,** extra crisp Japanese breadcrumbs, for ordinary bread or cracker crumbs. Doing so can reduce the crust's fat, calories and sodium by half.

FOR BAKED GOODS

10. **Think beyond fat-free.** Sometimes no-fat foods don't satisfy. "To account for this, we often use a blend of reduced-fat and fat-free varieties," says Vanessa Johnson, Test Kitchens director.

11. **Use egg substitute** in recipes that call for more than one egg. A quarter cup equals one egg, cutting 5 g fat and 213 milligrams of cholesterol from your recipe.

12. **Increase low-calorie ingredients.** For example, add extra vegetables to casseroles and fruits to breads, muffins or snack cakes. This will increase the yield of your recipe without adding fat.

13. **Finely chop** nuts, bacon, olives and other high-fat or high-sodium ingredients. They will distribute more evenly, allowing you to use less without sacrificing taste.

Read on for tips on meats, veggies and soups...

FOR MEATS AND VEGETABLES

14. **Opt for leaner meats;** such as center-cut or loin meats and skinless, white-meat poultry. "For example, a slice of center-cut bacon has slightly less sodium and fat than regular cured bacon," Downie says. In some cases, pork can be a leaner option than chicken.

15. **Add zing with citrus.** A squeeze of fresh lemon juice can help brighten the flavors of veggies and meats without added sodium.

FOR SAUTÉING

16. **Use nonstick pans** and cooking spray in place of oil or butter.

17. **When you need oil, use canola,** which has nearly half the saturated fat and more healthful, unsaturated fat than other oils.

FOR SOUPS AND STEWS

18. **Opt for low-sodium broths** and no-salt-added tomatoes; always rinse canned beans in a strainer under cold water, which cuts sodium by up to 40 percent.

19. **Puree vegetables to add body.** For example, mash some of the beans in a chili or the potatoes in a chowder.

20. **Trade 1 percent milk for whole** or half-and-half for heavy cream, in creamy soups.

We've focused a lot on the FORK portion of our lives, we have to focus on the SNEAKERS as well and bring them all together. In the diet table, you saw some absolutely stupid things that people do with a goal of weight loss. However, it just doesn't stop with the meals/eating plan; there are CRAZY exercise fads/ gimmicks. You know the ones—we usually see them on late night TV and get hooked as we gulp down yet another bowl of ice cream.

- The silver sweat suit that you wear while working out around the house. You feel so good because you see sweat pouring off of you. It also has a cousin which is the rubber thing that you wrap around your waist to get a slim waistline.

  - *Sidebar: When you drink water, guess what—it comes back. The worst thing is to see people, usually men, walking or running on the street decked out in the suit and about to pass out. A Dr. Sharon plea—leave it ALONE, especially in the summer time please do this for me. I have hurt myself laughing on more than one occasion.*

  - The abdominal roller that you can use for 5 minutes a day and get rock hard abs.

  - *Let me ask a simple question, even if you get rock hard abs—can you see them under layers of fat? Just asking.*

- The cords that you put on the door handle put our feet and arms in and pull. *I have personally pulled a many a door handle almost completely off trying to work this thing.*

- The over the counter, all natural, fat blocker pill that has the money back guarantee. The claim is eat whatever you want and these magic bullets fight the fat. *Ahhhhh, okay I have some stock in the Suez Canal that I would love to sell you—CALL ME.*

The list goes on and on and if we are honest; most of us have been desperate enough to try a lot of them. The end result is the same, we initially lose some pounds, if we're lucky, but soon the starvation or drastic measures become too much to continue and we eat the whole refrigerator. This leads to even more weight gain and the yo-yo continues. DIETS DON'T WORK! Even if you take on more drastic measures like surgical intervention such as gastric bypass, stapling or even having your mouth wired shut; unless you really commit to changing your lifestyle, the pounds will hunt you down and find you. I don't care if you've been overweight for a day or for 70 years—there is always hope and a way for you to make changes. Let's talk about some things that CAN work! You might want to memorize these, they are from Prevention magazine and they are Winners!

100 Smartest Diet Tips Ever

By the American Dietetic Association, as printed online by *Prevention Magazine*

Courtesy of the American Dietetic Association *(ADA)*, *Prevention Magazine* took their readers' 11 toughest diet problems and ran them by some of the top dietitians in the U.S.: RDs who, in addition to their private careers, serve as media spokespersons or heads of specialty practice groups for the ADA.

Here's what they told us, in their own words. These tips are solid gold, learned from successful experience with thousands of clients. Some tips are new. Some you've heard before, but they're repeated because they work. This treasure trove of RD wisdom could change your life, starting today.

I Can Only Handle One Diet Change Right Now—What Should I Do?

1. Add just one fruit or veggie serving daily. Get comfortable with that, then add an extra serving until you reach 8 to 10 a day.
2. Eat at least two servings of a fruit or veggie at every meal.
3. Resolve never to supersize your food portions—unless you want to supersize your clothes.
4. Make eating purposeful, not mindless. Whenever you put food in your mouth, peel it, unwrap it, plate it and sit. Engage all of the senses in the pleasure of nourishing your body.
5. Start eating a big breakfast. It helps you eat fewer total calories throughout the day.
6. Make sure your plate is half veggies and/or fruit at both lunch and dinner.

Are There Any Easy Tricks to Help Me Cut Calories?

7. Eating out? Halve it, and bag the rest. A typical restaurant entree has 1,000 to 2,000 calories, not even counting the bread, appetizer, beverage and dessert.
8. When dining out, make it automatic: Order one dessert to share.
9. Use a salad plate instead of a dinner plate.
10. See what you eat. Plate your food instead of eating out of the jar or bag.
11. Eat the low-cal items on your plate first, then graduate. Start with salads, veggies and broth soups, and eat meats and starches last. By the time you get to them, you'll be full enough to be content with smaller portions of the high-calorie choices.
12. Instead of whole milk, switch to 1 percent. If you drink one 8-oz glass a day, you'll lose 5 lbs in a year.
13. Juice has as many calories, oz. for oz., as soda. Set a limit of one 8-oz glass of fruit juice a day.
14. Get calories from foods you chew, not beverages. Have fresh fruit instead of fruit juice.
15. Keep a food journal. It really works wonders.
16. Follow the Chinese saying: "Eat until you are eight-tenths full."
17. Use mustard instead of mayo.
18. Eat more soup. The noncreamy ones are filling but low-cal.
19. Cut back on or cut out caloric drinks such as soda, sweet tea, lemonade, etc. People have lost weight by making just this one change. If you have a 20-oz bottle of Coca-Cola every day, switch to Diet Coke. You should lose 25 lbs in a year.
20. Take your lunch to work.
21. Sit when you eat.
22. Dilute juice with water.
23. Have mostly veggies for lunch.
24. Eat at home.
25. Limit alcohol to weekends.

More Smartest Diet Tips

How Can I Eat More Veggies?

26. Have a V8 or tomato juice instead of a Diet Coke at 3 p.m.

27. Doctor your veggies to make them delicious: Dribble maple syrup over carrots, and sprinkle chopped nuts on green beans.

28. Mix three different cans of beans and some diet Italian dressing. Eat this three-bean salad all week.

29. Don't forget that vegetable soup counts as a vegetable.

30. Rediscover the sweet potato.

31. Use prebagged baby spinach everywhere: as lettuce in sandwiches, heated in soups, wilted in hot pasta and added to salads.

32. Spend the extra few dollars to buy vegetables that are already washed and cut up.

33. Really hate veggies? Relax. If you love fruits, eat plenty of them; they are just as healthy *(especially colorful ones such as oranges, mangoes and melons)*.

34. Keep seven bags of your favorite frozen vegetables on hand. Mix any combination, microwave, and top with your favorite low-fat dressing. Enjoy 3 to 4 cups a day. Makes a great quick dinner.

Can You Give Me a Mantra That Will Help Me Stick to My Diet?

35. "The best portion of high-calorie foods is the smallest one. The best portion of vegetables is the largest one. Period."

36. "I'll ride the wave. My cravings will disappear after 10 minutes if I turn my attention elsewhere."

37. "I want to be around to see my grandchildren, so I can forgo a cookie now."

38. "I am a work in progress."

39. "It's more stressful to continue being fat than to stop overeating."

I Eat Healthy, but I'm Overweight - What Mistakes Could I Be Making Without Realizing It?

40. Skipping meals: Many healthy eaters diet by day and binge by night.

41. Don't graze yourself fat. You can easily munch 600 calories of pretzels or cereal without realizing it.

42. Eating pasta like crazy: A serving of pasta is 1 cup, but some people routinely eat 4 cups.

43. Eating supersize bagels of 400 to 500 calories for snacks.

44. Ignoring Serving Size on the Nutrition Facts panel.

45. Snacking on bowls of nuts. Nuts are healthy but dense with calories. Put those bowls away, and use nuts as a garnish instead of a snack.

46. Thinking all energy bars and fruit smoothies are low-cal.

What Can I Eat for a Healthy Low-Cal Dinner if I Don't Want to Cook?

47. A smoothie made with fat-free milk, frozen fruit and wheat germ.

48. Have the smallest fast-food burger *(with mustard and ketchup, not mayo)* and a no-cal beverage. Then at home, have an apple or baby carrots.

49. A peanut butter sandwich on whole wheat bread with a glass of 1 percent milk and an apple.

50. Precooked chicken strips and microwaved frozen broccoli topped with Parmesan cheese.

51. A healthy frozen entree with a salad and a glass of 1 percent milk.

52. Scramble eggs in a nonstick skillet. Pop some asparagus in the microwave, and add whole wheat toast. If your cholesterol levels are normal, you can have seven eggs a week!

53. A bag of frozen vegetables heated in the microwave, topped with 2 tablespoons of Parmesan cheese

and 2 tablespoons of chopped nuts.

54. Prebagged salad topped with canned tuna, grape tomatoes, shredded reduced-fat cheese, and low-cal Italian dressing.

55. Keep lean sandwich fixings on hand: whole wheat bread, sliced turkey, reduced-fat cheese, tomatoes and mustard with horseradish.

56. Heat up a can of good soup.

57. Cereal, fruit and fat-free milk make a good meal anytime.

58. Try a veggie sandwich from Subway.

59. Precut fruit for a salad and add yogurt.

What's Your Best Advice for Avoiding Those Extra Holiday Pounds?

60. Don't tell yourself, "It's OK, it's the holidays." That opens the door to six weeks of splurging.

61. Remember, eat before you meet. Have this small meal before you go to any parties: a hardboiled egg, apple and a thirst quencher *(water, seltzer, diet soda, tea)*.

62. As obvious as it sounds, don't stand near the food at parties. Make the effort, and you'll find you eat less.

63. At a buffet? Eating a little of everything guarantees high calories. Decide on three or four things, only one of which is high in calories. Save that for last so there's less chance of overeating.

64. For the duration of the holidays, wear your snuggest clothes that don't allow much room for expansion. Wearing sweats is out until January.

65. Give it away! After company leaves, give away leftover food to neighbors, doormen, or delivery people, or take it to work the next day.

66. Walk around the mall three times before you start shopping.

67. Make exercise a nonnegotiable priority.

68. Dance to music with your family in your home. One dietitian reported that when she asks her patients to do this, initially they just smile, but once they've done it, they say it is one of the easiest ways to involve the whole family in exercise.

How Can I Control a Raging Sweet Tooth?

69. Once in a while, have a lean, mean salad for lunch or dinner, and save the meal's calories for a full dessert.

70. Are you the kind of person who does better if you make up your mind to do without sweets and just not have them around? Or are you going to do better if you have a limited amount of sweets every day? One RD reported that most of her clients pick the latter and find they can avoid bingeing after a few days.

71. If your family thinks they need a very sweet treat every night, try to strike a balance between offering healthy choices but allowing them some free will. Compromise with low-fat ice cream and fruit or sometimes just fruit with a dollop of whipped cream.

72. Try two weeks without sweets. It's amazing how your cravings vanish.

73. Eat more fruit. A person who gets enough fruit in his diet doesn't have a raging sweet tooth.

74. Eat your sweets, just eat them smart! Carve out about 150 calories per day for your favorite sweet. That amounts to about an oz. of chocolate, half a modest slice of cake, or ½ cup of regular ice cream.

75. Try these smart little sweets: sugar-free hot cocoa, frozen red grapes, fudgsicles, sugar-free gum, Nutri-Grain chocolate fudge twists, Tootsie Rolls and hard candy.

How Can I Conquer My Downfall: Bingeing at Night?

76. Eat breakfast, lunch and dinner. The large majority of people who struggle with night eating are those who skip meals or don't eat balanced meals during the day. This is a major setup for overeating at night.

77. Eat your evening meal in the kitchen or dining room, sitting down at the table.

78. Drink cold unsweetened raspberry tea. It tastes great and keeps your mouth busy.

79. Change your nighttime schedule. It will take effort, but it will pay off. You need something that will occupy your mind and hands.

80. If you're eating at night due to emotions, you need to focus on getting in touch with what's going on and taking care of yourself in a way that really works. Find a nonfood method of coping with your stress.

81. Put a sign on the kitchen and refrigerator doors: Closed After Dinner.

82. Brush your teeth right after dinner to remind you: No more food.

83. Eat without engaging in any other simultaneous activity. No reading, watching TV, or sitting at the computer.

84. Eating late at night won't itself cause weight gain. It's how many calories—not when you eat them—that counts.

How Can I Reap Added Health Benefits From My Dieting?

85. Fat-free isn't always your best bet. Research has found that none of the lycopene or alpha- or beta-carotene that fight cancer and heart disease is absorbed from salads with fat-free dressing. Only slightly more is absorbed with reduced-fat dressing; the most is absorbed with full-fat dressing. But remember, use your dressing in moderate amounts.

86. Skipping breakfast will leave you tired and craving naughty foods by midmorning. To fill up healthfully and tastefully, try this sweet, fruity breakfast full of antioxidants. In a blender, process 1 c nonfat plain or vanilla yogurt, 1 ⅓ c frozen strawberries *(no added sugar)*, 1 peeled kiwi and 1 peeled banana. Pulse until mixture is milkshake consistency. Makes one 2-cup serving; 348 calories and 1.5 g fat.

87. If you're famished by 4 p.m. and have no alternative but an office vending machine, reach for the nuts. The same goes if your only choices are what's available in the hotel minibar.

88. Next time you're feeling wiped out in late afternoon, forgo that cup of coffee and reach for a cup of yogurt instead. The combination of protein, carbohydrate, and fat in an 8-oz. serving of low-fat yogurt will give you a sense of fullness and well-being that coffee can't match, as well as some vital nutrients. If you haven't eaten in 3 to 4 hours, your blood glucose levels are probably dropping, so eating a small amount of nutrient-rich food will give your brain and your body a boost.

89. Making just a few changes to your pantry shelves can get you a lot closer to your weight loss goals. Here's what to do: If you use corn and peanut oil, replace it with olive oil. Same goes for breads—go for whole wheat. Trade in those fatty cold cuts like salami and bologna and replace them canned tuna, sliced turkey breast, and lean roast beef. Change from drinking whole milk to fat-free milk or low-fat soy milk. This is hard for a lot of people so try transitioning down to 2 percent and then 1 percent before you go fat-free.

90. Nothing's less appetizing than a crisper drawer full of mushy vegetables. Frozen vegetables store much better, plus they may have greater nutritional value than fresh. Food suppliers typically freeze veggies just a few hours after harvest, locking in the nutrients. Fresh veggies, on the other hand, often spend days in the back of a truck before they reach your supermarket.

91. Worried about the trans-fat content in your peanut butter? Good news: In a test done on Skippy, JIF, Peter Pan and a supermarket brand, the levels of trans fats per 2-tablespoon serving were far lower than 0.5 g—low enough that under proposed laws, the brands can legally claim zero trans fats on the label. They also contained only 1 g more sugar than natural brands—not a significant difference.

Eating Less Isn't Enough—Which Exercising Tips Will Help Me Shed Pounds?

92. Overeating is not the result of exercise. Vigorous exercise won't stimulate you to overeat. It's just the opposite. Exercise at any level helps curb your appetite immediately following the workout.

93. When you're exercising, you shouldn't wait for thirst to strike before you take a drink. By the time you feel thirsty, you're already dehydrated. Try this: Drink at least 16 oz. of water, sports drinks or juices two hours before you exercise. Then drink 8 oz. an hour before and another 4 to 8 oz. every 15 to 20 minutes during your workout. Finish with at least 16 oz. after you're done exercising.

94. Tune in to an audio book while you walk. It'll keep you going longer and looking forward to the next walk—and the next chapter! Check your local library for a great selection. Look for a whodunit; you might walk so far you'll need to take a cab home!

95. Think yoga's too serene to burn calories? Think again. You can burn 250 to 350 calories during an hour-long class *(that's as much as you'd burn from an hour of walking)*! Plus, you'll improve muscle strength, flexibility, and endurance.

96. Drinking too little can hamper your weight loss efforts. That's because dehydration can slow your metabolism by 3 percent, or about 45 fewer calories burned a day, which in a year could mean weighing 5 pounds more. The key to water isn't how much you drink, it's how frequently you drink it. Small amounts sipped often work better than 8 oz. gulped down at once.

How Can I Manage My Emotional Eating and Get the Support I Need?

97. A registered dietitian *(RD)* can help you find healthy ways to manage your weight with food. To find one in your area who consults with private clients call 800.366.1655.

98. The best place to drop pounds may be your own house of worship. Researchers set up healthy eating and exercise programs in 16 Baltimore churches. More than 500 women participated and after a year the most successful lost an average of 20 lbs. Weight-loss programs based on faith are so successful because there's a built-in community component that people can feel comfortable with.

99. Here's another reason to keep level-headed all the time: Pennsylvania State University research has found that women less able to cope with stress—shown by blood pressure and heart rate elevations—ate twice as many fatty snacks as stress-resistant women did, even after the stress stopped *(in this case, 25 minutes of periodic jackhammer-level noise and an unsolvable maze)*.

100. Sitting at a computer may help you slim down. When researchers at Brown University School of Medicine put 92 people on online weight-loss programs for a year, those who received weekly email counseling shed 5 ½ more pounds than those who got none. Counselors provided weekly feedback on diet and exercise logs, answered questions and cheered them on. Most major online diet programs offer many of these features.

Other Nutrition/Food Tips

There are some shockers here and great tips!
(Found from a variety of sources like Shape, Fitness, Women's Day, Good Housekeeping *and* Health *magazine as well as online sites.)*

- **Counting calories is essential as reported in *Women's Day* magazine:**

  - Why you resist: Because you've been told time and again that cutting carbs matters, not calories.

  - Why experts insist: Many diets cut out whole food groups, so you lose weight just by eating fewer calories—which is what really counts.

    - "Total calories are far and away the most important aspect of weight gain or loss," says Brad Schoenfield, S.C.S., author of *28-Day Body Shapeover*. "If you take in more calories than you expend you'll gain weight, and if you take in fewer, you'll lose weight—period," he says. "You can lose weight on an ice cream diet if you eat only 1,200 calories of ice cream while you're burning 1,500 calories a day—not that I'd advocate it."

- **Severely restricting your food intake can backfire**, says Brad Crump, health services manager at Red Mountain Spa in St. George, Utah. When you don't consume enough calories, your metabolism slows and so does the rate at which you burn calories. Aim for at least 1,500 calories per day *(up to 200 more if you exercise regularly)*; concentrate on getting a mix of good carbs like produce and whole grains, lean protein, such as chicken and fish and healthy fats, like olive oil or avocado, with each meal.

- **Dirty dishes:** People who saw proof of how much food they were eating *(e.g., a pile of chicken-wing bones)* ate 27 percent less than those whose tables were bused while they noshed, reveals research from Cornell University in Ithaca, New York. Take a mental snapshot of your meal before you bite.

- **Is grapefruit really the main squeeze?** Grapefruit has always been a diet classic; now a study in the Journal of Medicinal Food proves how the sweet-and-sour citrus may aid weight loss. Simply eating grapefruit or drinking a glass of fresh juice daily could help you drop 3½ pounds in 12 weeks according to researchers, who say the fruit keeps insulin levels low, which might help your body burn more fat.

- **Salad does the body good:** Pump up your intake with a salad at your next meal. A study in the journal of the American Dietetic Association shows that eating just one salad doubles your chances of getting your daily dose of folic acid and vitamins A and C.

- ***Shape* magazine published 5 easy ways to slim down any holiday recipe:**

  - *Skip the heavy cream* - Try fat-free chicken stock or nonfat milk in place of cream or whole milk in gratins and creamed dishes. To thicken, whisk ½ teaspoon of cornstarch into 1 cup of liquid at room temperature just before adding to your recipe.

  - *Swap out the butter* - Substitute equal amounts of low fat plain yogurt or fat free pureed cottage cheese for the cream or butter in mashed potatoes.

  - *Roast a leaner bird* - Instead of slathering the turkey with better; rub it with mixture of olive oil and crushed herbs *(try rosemary, sage, a little garlic, and black pepper)*. Or slip herbs or seasonings under the skin of the turkey. Use a roasting rack to allow the fat to drain from the roast. Baste with fat-free chicken stock mixed with orange or cranberry juice instead of turkey drippings, which contain a lot of fat.

- *Defat your gravy*- for easy, low fat gravy, stir 1 teaspoon of cornstarch into ¼ cup of fat-free chicken broth at room temperature. Bring another 1-½ cups of broth to a simmer, and whisk in the cornstarch mixture. Allow gravy to simmer, stirring until clear and thickened.

  - *Lose the yolks*- Substitute 2 egg whites for 1 whole egg or 3 whites for 2 whole eggs.
  - *Stir in fruit*- Replace half the oil or butter in your baked good with applesauce or other pureed fruit. Your guests will never know their treats are low fat!

- **Last Call:** Experts say the evening is a prime time for bingeing, which can tack hundreds of calories onto your daily tally. What's more, a study in the journal Obesity reveals that people who ate 25 percent or more of their daily calories—about 400 calories for most women—after their evening meal were twice as likely to be obese than those who consumed less in the evening. Researchers say eating before bedtime can cause you to toss and turn at night and lose sleep, which increases the levels of an appetite-stimulating hormone called ghrelin. **So next time you want to snack after dinner, try sipping a cup of herbal tea first.** If you're still hungry, have a 100- to 200-calories treat that contains protein and carbs, like nonfat milk and graham crackers, to help fill you up without keeping you up.

- **The kitchen is full of landmines:** According to new research from Brain Wanskin, PhD, author of *Mindless Eating: Why We Eat More Than We Think.*

  - *Food lighting.* Bright lights put you in the mood to race through meals.

  - *TV trouble.* Distractions like the television, music, even dinner companions can lead you to take in 100 additional calories each meal.

  - *Clear and present danger.* Treats in see-through containers tempt you to indulge.

  - *Platter-size plates.* Huge, 12-inch dinner plates beg to be filled with oversize portions.

  - *Grabbable goodies.* Snacks within easy reach are hard to resist.

- **Mindless Munching adds pounds:** A study shows that *people eat significantly more when watching any TV show.* Researchers gave 45 subjects a bowl of potato chips for 5 minutes with no TV, and then in front of both Leno and letterman monologues. Participants ate 41.9 percent more chips and 44.2 percent more while Letterman was on. "Watching TV while eating causes a distraction, so you're less aware of smells, tastes. And how full you feel," says lead study author Alan Hirsch, MD "The more engaging the show, the more you'll eat."

- **The Movie Theater's concession stand in NOT your friend:**

  - 66% of moviegoers buy something from the concession stand

  - 1,220 calories in a large movie-theater popcorn with butter

  - 162 minutes you'd have to swim to burn off that popcorn

  - 483 calories in a soft pretzel

75 Cents is the price difference between a large and a jumbo popcorn
420 Calorie difference between a large and a jumbo popcorn

Movie Theater Snacks

To burn off 1 large popcorn with butter 170 oz. 1 large soda and 1 box of candy
(approx. 1940 calories) you would have to:

Activity	130 lbs	150 lbs	170 lbs	190 lbs	220 lbs	250 lbs	270 lbs
Aerobics, General	304 min.	263 min.	233 min.	208 min.	179 min.	158 min.	147 min.
Bicycle, Stationary	282 min.	245 min.	216 min.	193 min.	166 min.	147 min.	136 min.
Calisthenics *(push-ups, sit-ups, pull-ups, jumping jacks*	247 min.	214 min.	189 min.	169 min.	146 min.	129 min.	119 min.
Food Shopping	858 min.	744 min.	657 min.	588 min.	506 min.	448 min.	415 min.
Gardening, General	493 min.	428 min.	378 min.	338 min.	291 min.	258 min.	239 min.
Raking Lawn	459 min.	398 min.	352 min.	315 min.	271 min.	240 min.	222 min.
Sex, General, Moderate	1518 min.	1317 min.	1163 min.	1041 min.	895 min.	792 min.	734 min.
Shoveling Snow	329 min.	285 min.	252 min.	226 min.	194 min.	172 min.	159 min.
Sweep Floors	598 min.	519 min.	458 min.	410 min.	353 min.	312 min.	289 min.
Treadmill	219 min.	190 min.	168 min.	150 min.	129 min.	114 min.	106 min.
Vacuum	564 min.	489 min.	432 min.	387 min.	333 min.	294 min.	273 min.
Volleyball	493 min.	428 min.	378 min.	338 min.	291 min.	258 min.	239 min.
Washing Dishes	858 min.	744 min.	657 min.	588 min.	506 min.	448 min.	415 min.
Weight Lifting	658 min.	571 min.	504min.	451 min.	388 min.	343 min.	318 min.

- ## Grilling and Americans from *Fitness* magazine

  76% of women like to grill

  150 Millions of hot dogs Americans eat over Memorial Day weekend

  100 Calories in a turkey dog

  148 Calories in a regular hot dog

  49% of grillers who think it's acceptable to bring their own sauce to a barbecue

  121 Calories you save by grilling a chicken breast instead of frying it

- ## Fish is the single most important food for good health, a review of studies from the Harvard School of Public Health in Boston reveals. Approximately 2 grams of omega-3 fatty acids from oily fish weekly cut the risk of dying from heart disease by 36 percent. And fish oil reduced death from other diseases by 17 percent. Shoot for at least two servings of low-mercury fish a week.

- ## Salt smarts Scaling back on salt consumption may help you lose weight, a study in Progress in Cardiovascular Diseases suggests. Eating salty processed food makes you thirsty—which might prompt you to reach for sugary drinks. The average person's salt intake jumped 55 percent in the past 20 years; carbonated drinks increased by 135 %. Opt for fresh foods, and sip water.

- ## Healthy Salad How-To's from *Fitness* magazine.

  - Punch up the color. Toss your lettuce *(spinach, romaine and field greens are the most nutritious)* with a rainbow of veggies, such as tomatoes, yellow bell peppers, carrots and cucumbers.

  - Pick a protein. Tofu, beans chicken, turkey, fish—all of these are good sources to keep you satisfied. Stick with one and you won't go overboard.

  - Watch the add-ons. A sprinkle of cheese or nuts is okay, but skip the calorie bombs, like bacon bits and croutons.

  - Dress for success. Instead of mayo-based toppings, like ranch, opt for vinaigrette made with olive or canola oil.

- ## Swap it Out: Three Smart Swaps as printed in *Fitness* magazine

  SWITCH FROM...

  Regular bacon to turkey or Canadian bacon. "Pork bacon is loaded with saturated fat," says Emily Rubin, RD Canadian and turkey bacon are much leaner choices.

  *Stick margarine to tub-*or even better, to butter. Stick margarine can have three times the trans fats the tub version does. Butter has no trans fats.

  Premium ice cream to low fat. "Two scoops of the premium kind can have 11 grams of saturated fat-about half the amount you should eat for the entire day," warns Rubin. Low-fat ice cream can have less than one gram.

- ## The Shocking Fat Trap: Surprise: It's wedge-shaped food. "Most people have no idea how big a serving one slice is," says Sandria Godwin, PhD, RD, a professor at Tennessee State University in Nashville. Add to this the facts that foods served in slices tend to be high in fat and sugar *(think pizza and cake)*, and you may have the reason for your tighter pants. Even with the aid of a measuring tool, people's size estimates were off by more than 25 percent, Godwin found. Here, her guidelines for three common wedge-shaped foods.

  - **Pizza:** Generally, if you cut a regular-crust medium-size pizza *(12 inches)* into eight equal pieces, one slice will be one serving. A large pizza *(14 inches)* should be divided into 10 slices; an extra *(16 inches)*, into 12. **Sample serving: one slice of little Caesars Original Round Pepperoni regular-crust pizza, 230 calories and 8 g fat.**
  - **Cake:** Since you can't easily eye a slice that's one-thirty-sixth of the cake *(which is one serving of a three-inch-tall, nine-inch-wide cake)*, Godwin recommends slicing yourself the thinnest sliver possible that doesn't break apart. "It'll be close to one serving, no matter how many layers the cake has," she says. **Sample serving: one slice of yellow cake with chocolate frosting, 243 calories and 11 g fat.**
  - **Cheese:** In general, if you slice the cheese a quarter of an inch thick and in a two-inch square, and you cut two slices; you'll have one serving. **Sample serving: two slices of cheddar, 226 calories and 19 g fat.**

- ## What is a Vegan? I typically have a day a week in which I only eat fruits or vegetables. Additionally, as I shared I've incorporated a Dr. Sharon's Fruit and Veggie Week into my life. **So what is a vegetarian?** There are several types, here are a few:

  - **Vegans -**They eliminate all animal food: red meat, poultry, fish, dairy and eggs;

  - **Lacto-Vegetarians -** These basic vegetarians exclude meat, poultry, fish and eggs but do eat dairy;

  - **Lacto-ovo Vegetarians -** They follow the lacto guidelines but are slightly less restrictive, allowing eggs;

  - **Pesca-Vegetarians -** Lacto-ovo vegetarians who include fish in their diet;

  - **Flexitarians -** Lots of wiggle room here—a mostly lacto-ovo vegetarian diet with meat, poultry or fish now and then;

  - **Fruitarians -** Eat mostly fruit but include some seeds and nuts. Most nutritionists consider this an extreme diet;

  - **Raw Foodists Vegans -** Eat all food raw on the theory that cooking destroys a food's living nature.

  - **Airitarians -** Rumored but never seen *(like Bigfoot!)*, they purportedly have learned to live off the nutrients in oxygen.

- ### 26 Ways to cut calories from "Good Housekeeping" magazine

Instead of	Try	Instead of	Try	Instead of	Try
A strawberry daiquiri	A glass of white wine	Porterhouse steak	Flank steak	20 peanut M&M's	20 regular M&M's
Instead of	Try	Instead of	Try	Instead of	Try
1 oz. Cheddar on 5 Triscuits	2 tablespoons goat cheese on 1 Wasa Crisp'n Cracker bread	A sandwich made with 2 slices of regular bread	A sandwich made with 2 slices of light bread	A 20-oz. bottle of Vitamin water	Water with a daily multivitamin pill

- ### Holiday weight gain, beat it with info from *Self* magazine. Afraid you're doomed to elastic waistbands come January 1?

  - 90 Number of extra calories you'd have to eat per day in order gain a pound between Thanksgiving and New Year's

  - 148 calories burned in one hour of vigorous mall shopping

  - 11% drop in visits to Gold's Gym locations from November to December

  - 340 calories in a Starbucks Grande Eggnog Latte with skim milk

  - 4 pound gained if you drank an eggnog latte every day from Thanksgiving until New Year's

  - 56% of women who blame special occasions for cheating on their diets

  - 309 calories burned in an hour of breaking it down on the dance floor rather than loitering around the buffet table

- ### SLASH Calories with these GREAT tips from *Women's Health* magazine.

Cut 100 calories—**At Breakfast**

- Ditch the Pop-Tart for a slice of high-fiber toast with strawberry jam.

- Gotta have crabs? Split a bagel with a coworker.

- Drink you two cups of Joe black. Or order a single espresso instead of your usual latte.

- Swap OJ for the real deal—one fresh orange.

- Trade a side of regular sausage for turkey.

- Top your waffles with Redi-wip instead of syrup *(or use sugar-free)*.

- Skip the whip on any Caribou Coffee 16-oz. drink.

- Eat your granola from a 4-oz. mug, not an 8-oz. bowl.

- Lose the Yoplait Thick & Creamy and have a Yoplait Fiber 1.

- Order pancakes, but hold the butter.

- Scramble together 4 egg whites instead of 2 whole eggs.

Sub nonfat cream cheese for regular on your bagel.

Cut 100 calories—**At Lunch**

- Leave the Swiss cheese out of your sandwich.

- Slather your bread with mustard rather than mayo and save 80 calories per tablespoon.

- Pass up croutons at the salad bar.

- Use up to 10 pumps of ranch dressing spray instead of pouring 2 tablespoons from a bottle.

- Devour a slice of Pizza Hut cheese pan pizza instead of the meat lover's variety.

- Take your iced tea unsweetened.

- Reach for a Snapple raspberry white tea instead of a Snapple raspberry iced tea,

- Stuff chicken salad into a whole-wheat pita instead of between slices of multigrain bread.
- Make your burger turkey, not beef.
- Slurp minestrone soup instead of cream of anything.
- Go bunless—shed your hamburger roll.
- Use south-of-the-border savvy: Have a quesadilla made with two 6-inch corn, not flour, tortillas.

Two or more slices? Blot off the grease with a napkin.

Cut 100 calories—**At happy Hour**

- Nurse a single glass of wine instead of downing 2 beers.
- Ask for your rum and cokes in a highball glass. Bartenders pour an average of 20 percent less liquid into taller tumblers, so you'll swig less per round.
- Drizzle extra hot sauce, not blue cheese or ranch dressing, on your wings.
- Ordering a cocktail? Make it on the rocks instead of frozen. Slushy fruit drinks tend to be made with bottled mixers that contain added sugar and syrups.
- Blending your own? Have a daiquiri, not a pina colada.
- Pop the cap off of an MGD 64 instead of a bottle of Killian's Irish Red.
- Sip a glass of water between drinks—pacing yourself can help you cut back by a glass or more.
- Dip your nachos in salsa rather than guacamole.
- For automatic portion control, sip wine from a Champagne flute, not an oversize goblet.

Mix your vodka with Red Bull Sugar free, not cranberry juice.

Cut 100 calories—**On Your Snack Break**

- Drink sparkling water instead of soda.
- Move your stash of Hershey's Kisses at least 6 feet away from your desk—you'll dip in half as often.
- Drain the heavy syrup from your can of fruit cocktail and then rinse the fruit with water before digging in.
- Have ½ cup of fresh grapes instead of that little snack box of raisins.
- Lay off the Lay's Classis potato chips and have a handful of Rold Gold pretzels.
- Munch on a bag of Orville Redenbacher's Smart Pop Kettle Korn, not Movie Theater Butter.
- Chase down the ice-cream truck for a Good Humor vanilla sandwich, not a King Cone.

Satisfy a crunch craving with baby carrots, not potato chips.

Cut 100 calories—**During Dessert**

- Stop eating when you hit the crust. The edges and bottoms of baked goods are especially caloric because they absorb the butter used to grease the pan.
- Fill your bowl with sorbet instead of ice cream—you can have an extra ½ cup of the former and still slash calories.
- Next time a cocoa craving hits, ditch the dish of chocolate ice cream *(about ¾ cup)* for a Fudgsicle.
- Have sugar-free Jell-O instead of pudding. Better your nighttime treat jiggle than your thighs.
- Go ahead and have that piece of birthday cake—just scrape off the chocolate frosting first.
- Eat 5 meringue cookies instead of 2 chocolate chips ones.
- Pass on the a la mode and savor that brownie au naturel.
- Can the cone. Have your ice cream in a bowl.

Top your dessert with ½ cup of fresh berries instead of 2 teaspoons of chocolate syrup.

Cut 100 calories—In The Kitchen

- Substitute nonfat Greek yogurt for a serving of sour cream.
- Use chicken broth *(low-sodium is best)* instead of oil to sauté meat and veggies.
- Making homemade mac'n cheese? Cut 2 tablespoons of butter from the recipe.
- Replace the oil or butter in cakes with Sunweet Lighter Bake prune-and-apple mixture or any brand of unsweetened applesauce.
- Next time you make meatballs, meatloaf, or burgers, go half-and-half with ground beef and turkey.
- When preparing packaged foods that call for butter or oil, like rice and stuffing, use a broth instead.
- Swap low-fat cottage cheese for whole-milk ricotta when you make lasagna or stuffed shells.

Use tuna packed in water, not oil.

Cut 100 calories—At The Drive-Thru

- Pass up Wendy's baked potato with sour cream and chives and chow down on value fries instead. Amazing but true.
- Have a McDonald's cheeseburger instead of a Quarter Pounder with cheese.
- Downsize your drink: Trade a larger fountain soda *(with ice)* for a medium.
- Go for grill marks. Order a flame-broiled chicken sandwich rather than one that's breaded *(and usually fried in oil).*
- Treat yourself to an ice-cream cone at McDonald's instead of Dairy Queen.
- Crunch on one Taco bell regular taco instead of a Ranchero Chicken Soft Taco. And all the hot sauce you want.
- Slurp a cup of Panera Bread's low-fat chicken noodle soup instead of the cream of chicken with wild rice.
- Make your daily pick-me-up at Starbucks a skinny vanilla latte, not a regular.

Skip the two packets of BBQ sauce—eat your burger and fries plain.

Cut 100 calories—When You're Not Cooking

- Request the lemon chicken with white rice, not fried.
- Skip the crunchy noodles with your bowl of wonton soup.
- Ask for an order of Szechuan Shrimp instead of your usual General Tso's.
- Choose the pasta with ½ cup of marinara instead of ½ cup Alfredo sauce.
- Indulge your inner carnivore with beef stroganoff, not meat lasagna.
- Go with the baked potato *(butter only)*, not the mashed, as your side of choice.
- Dip your dinner roll in marinara sauce instead of olive oil.
- Avoid anything breaded. Flour and bread crumbs not only add calories but also absorb more cooking oil.

Pop 12 pieces of sashimi and ⅓ cup of edamame, not 12 pieces of spicy tuna roll.

Making Sure that Take Out Doesn't Take You Out!

"The journey of a thousand pounds begins with a single burger." Chris O'Brien

"Believe it or not, Americans eat 75 acres of pizza a day."
Boyd Matson, TV journalist

"We live in an age when pizza gets to your home before the police." Jeff Arder

The reality is that many of us live very busy lives and neither time nor energy permits us the luxury of preparing all of our meals at home. We depend upon the fast food and restaurant industry to meet our nutritional needs.

Is That Fast Food Really Worth It? *(nutritional info from various sources including the restaurant chain, if available)*

French Fries

Fast Food Restaurant	Size/Special Info.	Calories	Total Fat (g)	Carbs (g)	Sodium (mg)
A&W	Regular	430	18	61	640
A&W	Chili	370	16	49	780
A&W	Cheese	380	19	50	870
A&W	Chili Cheese	400	19	51	990
Arby's	Homestyle	566	37	82	1029
Arby's	Curly	631	37	73	1476
Burger King	Regular	500	28	57	820
Burger King	Salt Not Added	500	28	57	530
Carl's Jr.	Regular	620	29	80	380
Dairy Queen	Regular	730	33	100	1530
Hardee's	Regular	610	28	78	370
Hardee's	Crispy Curls	480	23	60	1190
Jack In The Box	Natural Cut	640	33	77	1180
Jack In The Box	Seasoned Curly	550	31	60	1200
McDonald's	Regular	570	30	70	330
Sonic	Regular	280	11	42	135
Sonic	Cheese	380	19	44	600
Sonic	Chili/Cheese	450	25	48	610
Wendy's	Regular	540	26	69	550
White Castle	Regular	700	34	89	560

Sandwiches/Hamburgers

Fast Food Restaurant	Type	Serving Size (g)	Calories	Total Fat (g)	Carbs (g)	Sodium (mg)
A&W	Papa Burger	288	720	42	46	1390
A&W	Bacon Double Cheeseburger	303	800	48	47	1610
A&W	Double Cheeseburger	288	720	42	46	1370
A&W	Bacon Cheeseburger	223	570	33	41	1200
Burger King	Regular	121	290	12	30	560
Burger King	Whopper	290	670	39	51	1020
Burger King	Whopper *(cheese)*	315	760	47	52	1450

Fast Food Restaurant	Type	Serving Size (g)	Calories	Total Fat (g)	Carbs (g)	Sodium (mg)
Burger King	Double Whopper	373	900	57	51	1090
Burger King	Double Whopper (cheese)	398	990	64	52	1520
Burger King	Triple Whopper	456	1130	74	51	1160
Burger King	Triple Whopper (cheese)	480	1230	82	52	1590
Burger King	Whopper Jr.	158	370	21	31	570
Burger King	Whopper Jr. (cheese)	170	410	24	32	780
Burger King	Double Hamburger	164	410	21	30	600
Burger King	Double Stacker	190	610	39	32	1100
Burger King	Triple Stacker	250	800	54	33	1450
Burger King	Quad Stacker	311	1000	68	34	1800
Burger King	Double Cheeseburger	189	500	29	31	1030
Carl's Jr	Big Hamburger	209	470	17	54	1060
Carl's Jr.	Six Dollar Burger	430	1010	68	60	1980
Carl's Jr.	Western Bacon Six Dollar Burger	382	1130	66	83	2540
Carl's Jr.	Bacon Cheese Six Dollar Burger	409	1070	76	50	1910
Carl's Jr.	Double Six Dollar Burger	602	1520	111	60	2760
Carl's Jr.	Low Carb Six Dollar Burger	267	490	37	6	1290
Carl's Jr.	Famous Star (cheese)	278	660	39	53	1260
Carl's Jr.	Super Star (cheese)	385	930	59	54	1600
Carl's Jr.	Philly Cheesesteak Burger	297	830	55	52	1510
Carl's Jr.	Western Bacon Cheeseburger	241	710	33	70	1480
Carl's Jr.	Double Western Bacon Cheeseburger	323	970	52	71	1820
Carl's Jr.	Jalapeno Burger	286	720	45	50	1320
Dairy Queen	Homestyle Burger	140	350	14	33	400
Dairy Queen	Homestyle Double Cheeseburger	226	640	34	34	950
Dairy Queen	Homestyle Bacon Double Cheeseburger	245	730	41	35	1270
Dairy Queen	Ultimate Burger	259	780	48	33	1110
Dairy Queen	¼ lb FlameThrower GrillBurger	245	780	54	41	1490
Dairy Queen	½ lb FlameThrower GrillBurger	344	1030	73	41	2020
Dairy Queen	Classic GrillBurger	212	470	23	42	1020
Dairy Queen	Classic GrillBurger (cheese)	231	560	30	42	1160
Dairy Queen	½ lb GrillBurger	297	670	37	42	1310
Dairy Queen	½ lb GrillBurger (cheese)	330	820	49	47	1510
Dairy Queen	Bacon Cheddar GrillBurger	229	650	37	41	1480
Dairy Queen	Mushroom Swiss GrillBurger	210	630	40	39	950
Del Taco	Double Del Cheeseburger	202	560	35	35	960
Del Taco	Bacon Double Del Cheeseburger	212	610	39	35	1130
Hardee's	Regular	118	310	12	36	560
Hardee's	Thickburger	349	910	64	53	1560
Hardee's	Cheeseburger	254	680	39	52	1450
Hardee's	Mushroom N' Swiss Thickburger	276	720	42	48	1570
Hardee's	Bacon Cheese Thickburger	334	910	64	50	1550
Hardee's	Low Carb Thickburger	245	420	32	5	1010
Hardee's	Six Dollar Burger	412	1060	73	58	1950
Hardee's	Grilled Sourdough Thickburger	381	1030	77	42	1910
Hardee's	Double Thickburger	471	1250	90	54	2160
Hardee's	Double Bacon Cheese Thickburger	463	1300	97	50	2200

Fast Food Restaurant	Type	Serving Size (g)	Calories	Total Fat (g)	Carbs (g)	Sodium (mg)
Hardee's	Monster Thickburger	413	1420	108	46	2770
Hardee's	Double Cheeseburger	186	510	26	38	1120
Hardee's	Double Hamburger	161	420	19	37	670
In-N-Out Burger	Regular	243	390	19	39	650
In-N-Out Burger	Double-Double	330	670	41	39	1440
Jack in the Box	Regular	118	310	14	30	600
Jack in the Box	Bacon Ultimate Cheeseburger	338	1090	77	53	2040
Jack in the Box	Bacon n' Cheese Ciabatta Burger	395	1120	76	66	1670
Jack in the Box	Jumbo Jack	261	600	35	51	940
Jack in the Box	Jumbo Jack (cheese)	286	690	42	54	1310
Jack in the Box	Junior Bacon Cheeseburger	131	430	25	30	820
Jack in the Box	Single Bacon n' Cheese Ciabatta Burger	308	870	54	66	1550
Jack in the Box	Sirloin Cheeseburger	421	1070	71	61	1850
Jack in the Box	Sirloin Bacon n' Cheese Burger	422	1120	73	63	2620
Jack in the Box	Sourdough Jack	245	710	51	36	1230
Jack in the Box	Sourdough Ultimate Cheeseburger	291	950	73	36	1360
Jack in the Box	Ultimate Cheeseburger	323	1010	71	53	1580
McDonald's	Regular	100	250	9	31	520
McDonald's	Quarter Pounder	169	410	19	37	730
McDonald's	Quarter Pounder (cheese)	198	510	26	40	1190
McDonald's	Double Quarter Pounder (cheese)	279	740	42	40	1380
McDonald's	Big Mac	214	540	29	43	1040
McDonald's	Double Cheeseburger	165	440	23	34	1150
McDonald's	Big N' Tasty	206	460	24	37	720
McDonald's	Big N' Tasty (cheese)	220	510	28	38	960
Sonic	Jr. Burger	117	310	15	30	610
Sonic	Bacon Cheeseburger	279	780	48	57	1300
Sonic	SuperSonic Cheeseburger (mayo)	343	980	64	58	1430
Sonic	Sonic Burger (mayo)	248	650	37	55	720
Sonic	Sonic Cheeseburger (mayo)	266	720	42	56	1040
Sonic	Dixie Burger	255	660	37	55	810
Sonic	Dixie Cheeseburger	273	720	42	56	1120
Sonic	California Cheeseburger	266	690	39	57	1060
Sonic	SuperSonic Jalapeno Cheeseburger	313	890	53	56	1600
Sonic	Thousand Island Cheeseburger	266	680	38	58	1130
Sonic	Jalapeno Cheeseburger	215	610	31	53	930
Sonic	Jalapeno Burger	197	550	26	52	610
Sonic	Green Chili Cheeseburger	287	630	31	56	1070
Sonic	Chili Cheeseburger	226	660	35	56	990
Sonic	Hickory Cheeseburger	236	640	31	61	1170
Sonic	Jr. Double Cheeseburger	190	570	35	33	1290
Wendy's	Jr. Hamburger	Unknown	230	8	26	500
Wendy's	Single	Unknown	430	20	37	900
Wendy's	Double (cheese)	Unknown	700	40	38	1500
Wendy's	Triple (cheese)	Unknown	980	59	38	2090
Wendy's	Baconator	Unknown	830	51	35	1920

Fast Food Restaurant	Type	Serving Size (g)	Calories	Total Fat (g)	Carbs (g)	Sodium (mg)
White Castle	Regular	58	140	7	14	210
White Castle	Bacon Cheeseburger	71	200	11	15	480
White Castle	Double White Castle	104	250	13	22	340
White Castle	Double Cheeseburger	118	300	17	23	590
White Castle	Double Jalapeno Cheeseburger	122	320	19	23	680
White Castle	Double Bacon Cheeseburger	130	370	22	23	880

Chicken (*nuggets, strips, etc.*)

Fast Food Restaurant	Type	Serving Size (g)	Calories	Total Fat (g)	Carbs (g)	Sodium (mg)
Arby's	Chicken Tenders *(5pc)*	218	630	31	47	1977
Arby's	Popcorn Chicken *(large)*	184	531	26	39	1666
Burger King	Chicken Tenders *(6pc)*	92	250	15	16	720
Burger King	Chicken Fries *(6pc)*	85	260	15	18	650
Carl's Jr.	Chicken Breast Strips *(5pc)*	215	710	41	46	2020
Dairy Queen	Chicken Strip Basket *(6pc)*	531	1270	67	121	2910
Hardee's	Chicken Strips *(5pc)*	241	630	34	45	2260
KFC	Popcorn Chicken *(large)*	160	550	35	30	1600
McDonald's	Chicken McNuggets *(6pc)*	96	250	15	15	670
McDonald's	Chicken Selects Premium Strips *(5pc)*	221	630	33	46	1550
Wendy's	Chicken Nuggets *(5pc)*	Unknown	230	15	12	520
White Castle	Chicken Rings *(6pc)*	110	340	23	15	670

Chicken Sandwiches

Fast Food Restaurant	Type	Serving Size (g)	Calories	Total Fat (g)	Carbs (g)	Sodium (mg)
A&W	Grilled	213	440	19	34	860
A&W	Crispy	219	590	29	54	1170
Arby's	Crispy Fillet	238	526	30	50	901
Arby's	Grilled Fillet	233	414	17	36	913
Burger King	TENDERGRILL *(with mayo)*	258	510	19	49	1180
Burger King	TENDERCRISP	284	790	44	68	1640
Burger King	Original	219	660	40	52	1440
Burger King	Chick'n Crisp *(with mayo)*	144	480	31	36	870
Boston Market	Boston Carver	321	700	29	68	1560
Boston Market	Half Boston Carver	199	340	15	29	710
Carl's Jr.	Charbroiled BBQ	239	360	4.5	48	1150
Carl's Jr.	Charbroiled Club	264	550	25	43	1410
Carl's Jr.	Charbroiled Santa Fe	264	610	32	43	1540
Carl's Jr.	Spicy	213	560	30	59	1480
Chick-fil-A	Chicken Sandwich	170	410	16	38	1300
Chick-fil-A	Chargrilled Chicken Sandwich	193	270	3.5	33	940
Chick-fil-A	Chargrilled Chicken Club Sandwich	221	380	11	33	1240
Chick-fil-A	Chicken Salad Sandwich	153	350	15	32	880

Fast Food Restaurant	Type	Serving Size (g)	Calories	Total Fat (g)	Carbs (g)	Sodium (mg)
Dairy Queen	Crispy	198	540	29	47	700
Dairy Queen	Grilled	177	350	16	49	780
Hardee's	Charbroiled Club	277	560	30	32	1430
Hardee's	Charbroiled BBQ	242	340	4	40	1070
Hardee's	Low Carb Charbroiled Club	250	370	21	10	1170
Hardee's	Big Fillet	351	800	37	76	1890
Hardee's	Spicy	159	470	25	46	1220
Jack In The Box	Regular	145	400	21	38	730
Jack In The Box	Jack's Spicy	270	620	31	61	1100
Jack In The Box	Sourdough Grilled	266	530	28	34	1430
KFC	Snacker	119	290	13	29	680
KFC	Honey BBQ Snacker	101	210	3	32	530
KFC	Double Crunch	213	470	23	38	1190
KFC	Crispy Twister	252	550	28	49	1500
KFC	Oven Roasted Twister	269	420	17	40	1250
KFC	Tender Roast	236	380	13	29	1180
KFC	Honey BBQ	147	280	3.5	40	780
McDonald's	McChicken	147	360	16	40	790
McDonald's	Premium Grilled Chicken Classic	226	420	10	51	1190
McDonald's	Premium Crispy Chicken Classic	229	500	17	61	1330
McDonald's	Premium Grilled Chicken Club	260	570	21	52	1720
McDonald's	Premium Crispy Chicken Club	263	660	28	63	1860
Popeyes	Deluxe	265	630	31	53	1480
Sonic	Club Toaster	257	740	46	55	1740
Subway	Oven Roasted	238	310	5	48	830
Wendy's	Ultimate Chicken Grill	Unknown	320	7	36	950
Wendy's	Spicy Chicken Fillet	Unknown	440	16	46	1320
Wendy's	Homestyle Chicken Fillet	Unknown	430	16	48	1140
Wendy's	Chicken Club	Unknown	540	25	49	1410
Wendy's	Crispy	Unknown	320	14	34	660
White Castle	Breast (with cheese)	82	200	8	21	720
White Castle	Supreme	88	230	10	21	860

Onion Rings

Fast Food Restaurant	Serving Size (g)	Calories	Total Fat (g)	Carbs (g)	Sodium (mg)
A&W	113	350	16	45	710
Burger King (King Size)	150	500	25	62	720
Carl's Jr.	128	430	21	53	550
Dairy Queen (Large)	142	590	37	56	930
Jack In The Box	119	500	30	51	420
Sonic (Large)	227	640	31	80	300
White Castle (Sack)	178	410	20	53	400
White Castle (Homestyle, Sack)	178	790	44	91	860

Breakfast Sandwiches/Biscuits/Croissants/Wraps Compared

Fast Food Restaurant	Type	Serving Size (g)	Calories	Total Fat (g)	Carbs (g)	Sodium (mg)
Arby's	Bacon & Egg Croissant	120	337	22	23	651
Arby's	Bacon Biscuit	95	340	21	29	1028
Arby's	Bacon, Egg & Cheese Biscuit	158	461	28	30	1446
Arby's	Bacon, Egg & Cheese Croissant	133	378	22	23	850
Arby's	Bacon, Egg & Cheese Sourdough	173	437	16	40	1220
Arby's	Bacon, Egg & Cheese Wrap	193	515	29	50	1367
Arby's	Egg & Cheese Sourdough	164	392	12	40	1058
Arby's	Sausage, Egg & Cheese Biscuit	185	557	38	30	1579
Arby's	Sausage, Egg & Cheese Sourdough	191	514	27	40	1232
Arby's	Ham & Cheese Croissant	113	274	12	22	842
Arby's	Ham Biscuit	125	316	17	29	1240
Arby's	Ham, Egg & Cheese Biscuit	188	437	23	31	1658
Arby's	Ham, Egg & Cheese Croissant	213	434	24	25	1282
Arby's	Ham, Egg & Cheese Sourdough	296	679	35	42	2104
Arby's	Ham, Egg & Cheese Wrap	242	568	31	51	1929
Arby's	Sausage & Egg Croissant	147	433	32	23	784
Arby's	Sausage Biscuit	122	436	31	28	1160
Arby's	Sausage Gravy Biscuit	238	961	68	107	3755
Arby's	Sausage, Egg & Cheese Croissant	160	475	32	23	982
Arby's	Sausage, Egg & Cheese Wrap	239	689	45	50	1849
Burger King	Croissan'wich Egg & Cheese	115	300	17	26	740
Burger King	Croissan'wich Sausage & Cheese	106	370	25	23	810
Burger King	Croissan'wich Sausage, Egg & Cheese	159	470	32	26	1060
Burger King	Croissan'wich Ham, Egg & Cheese	149	340	18	26	1230
Burger King	Croissan'wich Bacon, Egg & Cheese	122	340	20	26	890
Burger King	Double Croissan'wich Sausage, Egg & Cheese	215	680	51	26	1590
Burger King	Double Croissan'wich Bacon, Egg & Cheese	142	430	27	27	1250
Burger King	Double Croissan'wich Ham, Egg & Cheese	196	420	23	27	2210
Burger King	Double Croissan'wich Sausage, Bacon, Egg & Cheese	179	550	39	27	1420
Burger King	Double Croissan'wich Ham, Bacon, Egg & Cheese	169	420	24	27	1600
Burger King	Double Croissan'wich Ham, Sausage, Egg & Cheese	206	550	37	27	2040
Burger King	Enormous Omelet Sandwich	266	730	45	44	1940
Burger King	Ham Omelet Sandwich	139	330	14	35	1130
Burger King	Sausage Biscuit	118	390	26	28	1020
Burger King	Ham, Egg & Cheese Biscuit	156	390	22	31	1410
Burger King	Sausage, Egg & Cheese Biscuit	183	530	37	31	1490
Burger King	Bacon, Egg & Cheese Biscuit	146	410	25	31	1320
Carl's Jr.	Breakfast Burger	309	830	47	65	1580
Carl's Jr.	Sourdough Breakfast Sandwich	193	460	21	39	1050
Carl's Jr.	Sunrise Croissant	172	560	41	27	970

Fast Food Restaurant	Type	Serving Size (g)	Calories	Total Fat (g)	Carbs (g)	Sodium (mg)
Carl's Jr.	Bacon & Egg Burrito	208	570	33	37	990
Carl's Jr.	Loaded Breakfast Burrito	328	820	51	52	1530
Carl's Jr.	Steak & Egg Burrito	322	660	36	44	1690
Chick-fil-A	Chicken Burrito	191	410	16	42	940
Chick-fil-A	Sausage Burrito	191	450	23	39	860
Chick-fil-A	Chicken, Egg & Cheese (sunflower multi-grain bagel)	215	500	20	49	1260
Chick-fil-A	Hot Buttered Biscuit	79	270	12	38	660
Chick-fil-A	Chicken Biscuit	145	420	19	44	1270
Chick-fil-A	Bacon, Egg & Cheese Biscuit	163	470	26	39	1190
Chick-fil-A	Sausage & Egg Biscuit	198	570	37	39	1130
Chick-fil-A	Biscuit (with gravy)	192	330	15	43	950
Hardee's	Egg Biscuit	152	450	51	35	940
Hardee's	Bacon Biscuit	120	430	28	35	1110
Hardee's	Sausage Biscuit	142	530	38	36	1240
Hardee's	Country Ham Biscuit	144	440	26	36	1710
Hardee's	Breaded Chicken Fillet Biscuit	226	600	34	50	1680
Hardee's	Breaded Country Steak Biscuit	180	620	41	44	1360
Hardee's	Breaded Pork Chop Biscuit	222	690	42	48	1330
Hardee's	Sausage & Egg Biscuit	185	610	44	36	1290
Hardee's	Country Steak & Egg Biscuit	223	690	47	44	1800
Hardee's	Bacon, Egg & Cheese Biscuit	174	560	38	37	1360
Hardee's	Ham, Egg & Cheese Biscuit	220	560	35	37	1800
Hardee's	Loaded Omelet Biscuit	198	640	44	37	1510
Hardee's	Monster Biscuit	212	710	51	37	2250
Hardee's	Sunrise Croissant (Ham)	164	430	26	28	1050
Hardee's	Sunrise Croissant (Bacon)	138	450	29	28	900
Hardee's	Sunrise Croissant (Sausage)	161	550	38	29	1030
Hardee's	Frisco Breakfast Sandwich	185	420	20	37	1340
Hardee's	Loaded Breakfast Burrito	258	780	51	38	1620
Jack In The Box	Bacon, Egg & Cheese Biscuit	149	430	25	34	1100
Jack In The Box	Bacon Breakfast Jack	113	300	14	29	730
Jack In The Box	Breakfast Jack	125	290	12	29	760
Jack In The Box	Chicken Biscuit	154	450	24	42	980
Jack In The Box	Ciabatta Breakfast Sandwich	278	710	36	63	1730
Jack In The Box	Extreme Sausage Sandwich	213	670	48	31	1300
Jack In The Box	Meaty Breakfast Burrito	183	480	29	29	1210
Jack In The Box	Sausage Biscuit	131	440	29	32	870
Jack In The Box	Sausage Breakfast Jack	154	450	28	29	840
Jack In The Box	Sausage Croissant	174	580	39	37	770
Jack In The Box	Sausage, Egg & Cheese Biscuit	234	740	55	35	1430
Jack In The Box	Sirloin Steak & Egg Burrito	289	790	48	52	1320
Jack In The Box	Spicy Chicken Biscuit	169	460	22	44	1020
Jack In The Box	Supreme Croissant	151	450	25	36	860
Jack In The Box	Ultimate Breakfast Sandwich	249	570	27	49	1700
McDonald's	Egg McMuffin	139	300	12	30	820

Fast Food Restaurant	Type	Serving Size (g)	Calories	Total Fat (g)	Carbs (g)	Sodium (mg)
McDonald's	Sausage McMuffin	114	370	22	29	850
McDonald's	Sausage McMuffin (egg)	164	450	27	30	920
McDonald's	Bacon, Egg & Cheese Biscuit (regular)	144	450	25	36	1360
McDonald's	Sausage Biscuit (egg, regular)	159	500	32	35	1130
McDonald's	Sausage Biscuit (regular)	113	410	27	33	1040
McDonald's	Biscuit (regular)	72	250	11	32	700
McDonald's	Bacon, Egg & Cheese McGriddles	173	460	21	48	1360
McDonald's	Sausage, Egg & Cheese McGriddles	202	560	32	48	1360
McDonald's	Sausage McGriddles	141	420	22	44	1030
Sonic	Bacon, Egg & Cheese Bistro	162	510	30	37	1060
Sonic	Ham, Egg & Cheese Bistro	181	460	24	36	1320
Sonic	Sausage, Egg & Cheese Bistro	189	590	40	37	1000
Sonic	Sausage, Egg & Cheese Toaster	194	620	42	40	1380
Sonic	Bacon, Egg & Cheese Toaster	167	530	32	40	1440
Sonic	Ham, Egg & Cheese Toaster	186	490	26	40	1700
Sonic	Sausage, Egg & Cheese Burrito	167	470	30	38	1140
Sonic	Bacon, Egg & Cheese Burrito	157	450	26	38	1240
Sonic	Ham, Egg & Cheese Burrito	183	440	23	37	1630
Sonic	SuperSonic Breakfast Burrito	216	550	34	47	1340
Subway	Cheese Sandwich	167	400	17	43	940
Subway	Chipotle Steak & Cheese Sandwich	259	580	31	48	1400
Subway	Double Bacon & Cheese Sandwich	185	500	25	44	1310
Subway	Honey Mustard Ham & Cheese Sandwich	216	460	19	51	1430
Subway	Western Sandwich (cheese)	207	440	18	45	1320
Subway	Cheese Wrap	159	390	19	37	1050
Subway	Chipotle Steak & Cheese Wrap	251	570	33	41	1510
Subway	Double Bacon & Cheese Wrap	177	480	27	38	1420
Subway	Honey Mustard Ham & Cheese Wrap	208	450	21	45	1540
Subway	Western Wrap (cheese)	199	420	20	39	1430

Mozzarella Sticks

Fast Food Restaurant	Type	Serving Size (g)	Calories	Total Fat (g)	Carbs (g)	Sodium (mg)
Arby's	4 pc (Regular)	137	426	28	38	1370
Arby's	8 pc (Large)	273	849	56	75	2730
Jack In The Box	3 pc	71	240	12	21	420
Jack In The Box	6 pc	138	483	27	39	1018
Sonic	Unknown	140	440	22	40	1050
White Castle	3 pc	79.2	250	14	22	750
White Castle	5 pc	132	420	23	37	1240
White Castle	10 pc	264	820	46	73	2490

Breadsticks, Cheesy Bread, Cheese Breadsticks Compared

Fast Food Restaurant	Type	Serving Size	Calories	Total Fat (g)	Carbs (g)	Sodium (mg)
Domino's Pizza	Breadsticks	1 pc	130	7	14	90
Domino's Pizza	Cheesy Bread	1 pc	140	7	14	140
Little Caesars	Crazy Bread	1 pc	100	3	15	150
Little Caesars	Italian Cheese Bread	1 pc	130	7	13	230
Little Caesars	Pepperoni Cheese Bread	1 pc	150	8	13	280
Papa John's	Breadsticks	1 pc	140	2	26	260
Papa John's	Cheesesticks	2 pc	370	16	42	830
Pizza Hut	Breadsticks	1 pc	150	6	20	230
Pizza Hut	Cheese Breadsticks	1 pc	200	10	21	370

"14 Inch Large Cheese Pizza" *(1 slice, no toppings)*

Fast Food Restaurant	Type	Serving Size (g)	Calories	Total Fat (g)	Carbs (g)	Sodium (mg)
Domino's Pizza	14" Classic Hand-Tossed	121	290	9	42	470
Little Caesers	14" Round Hot-N-Ready Pizza	94	200	7	25	340
Papa John's	14" Original Crust Pizza	132	300	11	39	750
Pizza Hut	14" Large Pan Pizza	146	390	19	38	800

All is not lost; there are choices that can be made when choosing a fast food restaurant. Here is a surprising article from *Fitness* magazine.

24 Surprisingly Healthy Fast Foods

Burgers, tacos, pizza—find out which of your fast-food favorites aren't so bad after all. Our list includes picks from KFC, McDonald's, Taco Bell and more, plus healthy fast-food desserts.

By H.K. Jones, RD published in *Fitness* magazine

Kentucky Fried Chicken Picks

Is the drive-thru the fast lane to a heart attack? On the one hand, it's true: One slipup *("okay, sure, I'll take the large fries and apple pie with that")* and you can add more than 800 high-in-saturated-fat calories to your takeout. But there is good news. Some of the burgers, sides, sandwiches, and even desserts aren't as bad for you as you might think. In fact, some are downright light! Here are 24 fast-food picks that are all figure-friendly, unless of course you order them all at once.

KFC Mashed Potatoes with Gravy

120 calories
4.5 g fat, 1 g saturated fat

Even when made with milk and butter *(some KFCs use these ingredients; others don't)*, mashed is always better than fried. Don't worry about the gravy; it adds only a few calories and just half a gram of fat.

KFC Original Recipe Drumstick

140 calories
8 g fat, 2g saturated fat

Order one regular drumstick *(avoid the Extra Crispy, which is just fast-food speak for "extra high in saturated and trans fats")* and fill up on the chain's better-for-you sides, such as corn on the cob, baked beans, or a small helping of the next two choices on our list.

KFC Potato Salad

180 calories
9 g fat, 1.5 g saturated fat

Made with red bell peppers, onions, celery and about a tablespoon of mayo, this is a tasty, trans-fat-free alternative to the deep-fried Potato Wedges.

KFC Cole Slaw

190 calories

11 g fat, 2 g saturated fat

Cole slaw's two main ingredients have a lot going for them: Cabbage is an excellent source of vitamin C and fiber; carrots are chock-full of vitamins A, K, C and potassium.

KFC Honey BBQ Sandwich

300 calories

6 g fat, 1.5 g saturated fat

Don't let the thick, sweet sauce fool you: This Southern specialty is actually the lowest-calorie full-size sandwich on the menu.

McDonald's Picks

McDonald's Chicken McNuggets with Sweet 'N Sour Sauce

4 pieces, 220 calories

10 g fat, 2 g saturated fat

The sauce is low in calories and sodium. But since you get only four measly nuggets, go ahead and add a Fruit & Walnut Salad *(310 calories, with yogurt dressing)* for additional sustenance.

McDonald's Hamburger

260 calories

9 g fat, 3.5 g saturated fat

This less-than-two-oz. burger is pretty small, so it's one of the diet-friendliest sandwiches in the biz. Pair it with a Side Salad drizzled with a packet of Newman's Own Low Fat Balsamic Vinaigrette *(60 calories total)* and a bottle of water.

McDonald's Egg McMuffin

300 calories

12 g fat, 4.5 g saturated fat

With its lean Canadian-style bacon and English muffin, this breakfast sandwich is a better choice than the 500-calorie Sausage Biscuit with Egg.

McDonald's McChicken

370 calories

16 g fat, 3.5 g saturated fat

Its size and small portion of mayo mean this crispy, fried sandwich is lower in calories than the grilled-chicken options.

Taco Bell Picks

Taco Bell Fresco Style Crunchy Taco

150 calories

7 g fat, 2.5 g saturated fat

When you ask for your meal Fresco Style, you get fresh salsa *(packed with cancer-fighting lycopene)* instead of fatty cheese and sauce. Pair your taco with a safe but filling side *(like beans or rice)*, so you won't be hungry again before you leave the parking lot.

Taco Bell Fresco Style Grilled Steak Soft Taco

170 calories

5 g fat, 1.5 g saturated fat

Although red meat does deliver a little fat, it also adds protein, zinc, iron, and vitamin B12.

Taco Bell Fresco Style Tostada

200 calories

6 g fat, 1 g saturated fat

A flat corn shell topped with fiber-rich beans, Fiesta salsa, tangy red sauce, and lettuce makes a healthy taco alternative.

Taco Bell Gordita Nacho Cheese—Chicken

270 calories

10 g fat, 2.5 g saturated fat

Not all our picks come from the healthier Fresco Style menu. This one is smothered in cheese but still manages to squeeze in under 300 calories.

Pizza Hut and Wendy's Picks

Pizza Hut 12" Fit 'N Delicious Pizza with Diced Chicken, Red Onion, and Green Pepper

2 slices, 340 calories

9 g fat, 4 g saturated fat

A dietitian's dream: thin crust, lean chicken, and vegetable toppings, plus half the cheese of the regular Thin 'N Crispy Pizza.

Pizza Hut 12" Veggie Lover's Hand-Tossed Pizza

1 slice, 220 calories

6 g fat, 3 g saturated fat

One slice is sometimes just as satisfying as more, as long as it has a thick crust and a full allotment of cheese. Though not quite as light as the Fit 'N Delicious, the Hut's Hand-Tossed pies are still lower in calories than its deep-dish pan pizzas.

Wendy's Jr. Hamburger

280 calories

9 g fat, 3.5 g saturated fat

This junior-size sandwich is almost as low-cal as the McDonald's burger. Skip the side of fries and have a Low-Fat Strawberry Flavored Yogurt with Granola Topping *(250 calories)* for dessert.

Wendy's Large Chili

330 calories

9 g fat, 3.5 g saturated fat

Packed with folate-, iron- and fiber-rich beans, the 12-oz. serving will fill you up. Round out your meal with a Mandarin Orange Cup *(80 calories)*.

Wendy's Ultimate Chicken Grill

360 calories

7 g fat, 1.5 g saturated fat

It has half the fat of Wendy's other non-burger sandwiches, thanks to Honey Mustard Sauce instead of mayo and grilling instead of deep-frying.

6 Diet-Friendly Desserts

McDonald's Vanilla Reduced Fat Ice Cream Cone

150 calories

3.5 g fat, 2 g saturated fat

With their velvety vanilla flavor, McDonald's perfectly sized cones don't taste like they're made with reduced-fat ice cream, but thank goodness they are!

Taco Bell Cinnamon Twists

160 calories

5 g fat, 1 g saturated fat

The airy puffed corn underneath all the cinnamon and sugar makes this treat guilt-free.

Wendy's Jr. Frosty

160 calories

4 g fat, 2.5 g saturated fat

Thicker than a milk shake but thinner than a sundae, the four-oz. Jr. Frosty packs plenty of satisfaction into a quarter-pint cup.

KFC Lil' Bucket Strawberry Shortcake

200 calories

6 g fat, 4 g saturated fat

With significantly fewer calories than most other KFC desserts, this is one sweet find.

Pizza Hut Cherry Dessert Pizza

1 slice, 240 calories

3.5 g fat, 0.5 g saturated fat

It's not as virtuous as a bowl of cherries, but Pizza Hut's dessert pie has half the calories and less than a quarter of the fat of homemade cherry pie.

KFC Lemon Meringue Pie Slice

240 calories

9 g fat, 2.5 g saturated fat

Traditional shortening- or butter-packed crusts make home-baked lemon meringue pie a dieter's nightmare. But KFC's lemon meringue has fewer than three grams of artery-clogging saturated fat, putting it a slice above the rest.

5 Drive-Thru Disasters

You'll need to order a side of cholesterol-lowering statin drugs with any of these artery-clogging menu items.

Wendy's Big Bacon Classic: 580 calories, 29 g fat, 12 g saturated fat

McDonald's Double Quarter Pounder with Cheese: 730 calories, 40 g fat, 19 g saturated fat

KFC Chicken Pot Pie: 770 calories, 40 g fat, 15 g saturated fat

Burger King Triple Whopper with Cheese: 1,230 calories, 82 g fat, 32 g saturated fat

Taco Bell Fiesta Taco Salad: 860 calories, 46 g fat, 14 g saturated fat

Dr. Sharon's Let's Get REAL Moment: It is nearly impossible for us to totally avoid fast food restaurants. I want to make sure that we are practical in our approach to health/wellness. This also means that you really may want to get that Taco Bell Fiesta Taco Salad with 860 calories at some point. If you do, what do you do? Do you jump out a window with your cellulite flying? Or do you get back on track and make the decision to do better while you allow yourself occasional splurges. It was important to me to show you that there are good choices to be made in fast food. However, now we must see utter foolishness again as it relates to our meals.

The 30 Worst Fast Food Restaurant Choices

(from fitnessmagazine.com)

Reader beware: the 30 unhealthiest choices at fast food restaurant chains—and the healthier substitutions you can make to avoid the calorie bomb.

By Melissa Roth

The 30 Worst Restaurant Menu Items

In recent years, American restaurants have been piling on layers of fat, salt and sugar to their creations—all of which tricks our brain into craving more food, says former FDA commissioner David Kessler, MD, in his book *The End of Overeating*. "Even lettuce has become a vehicle for fat," he says, citing the cream-based dressings, cheese chunks, bacon bits and oil-soaked croutons that turn many restaurants salads into health hazards.

That said, prepare yourself—and your gag reflex for some surprising calorie bombs *(presented in no particular order)*.

1. Quizno's Tuna Melt with Cheese and Dressing *(large)*

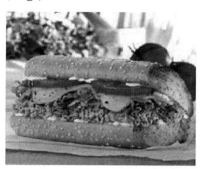

1760 calories
133 g fat
25 g saturated fat
200 mg cholesterol
2120 mg sodium

It looks so harmless: tuna salad, cheddar, lettuce, tomato.

But the combination of mayo, cheese and fatty tuna—not to mention the sheer size of this monster—adds up to more fat grams than four Big Macs, says Debi Silber, MS, RD, WHC, a Long Island, NY-based nutritionist and author of *The Lifestyle Fitness Program*.

Even the small sub contains more fat *(55 grams!)* than most of us should be consuming in an entire day.

2. Quizno's Classic Italian Sandwich

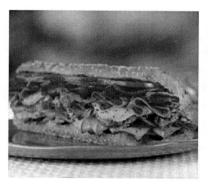

Large size, with cheese and dressing:
1330 calories
68 g fat
24.5 g saturated fat
135 mg cholesterol
3760 mg sodium

This salami-pepperoni-capicola-ham combo comes with a light vinaigrette and still eats up nearly a day's calories and two days worth of sodium.

If that's not enough to scare you, "We have clear and convincing evidence that sodium is associated with high blood pressure, and high blood pressure is a major risk factor for stroke—and it is pretty consistent across populations and ethnic groups," Dr. David Katz, a preventive medicine specialist at Yale University Medical School, told the *Los Angeles Times* in June. "It is unconscionable that a single meal would have 2,000 milligrams or more of sodium."

"Meats like salami, pepperoni, capicola and ham are loaded in fat, saturated fat, cholesterol, sodium and calories," adds Silber. "These foods are caloric time bombs—offering little nutrient value for the amount of calories and fat they have."

3. Quizno's Chicken with Honey Mustard Flatbread Chopped Salad

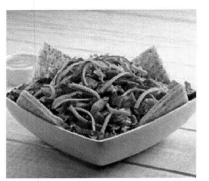

1070 calories
71 g fat
13.5 g saturated fat
135 mg cholesterol
1770 mg sodium

This salad looks healthy enough, with chicken breast, tomatoes and red onion. However, the biggest calorie culprit isn't even the bacon in the salad—it's the honey mustard dressing, which clocks in at 500 calories all on its own. And the skinny-sounding "flatbread"? That adds an additional 330 calories.

4. TGI Friday's Jack Daniels Ribs & Shrimp

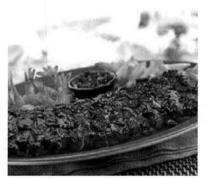

1910 calories

A "full rack" of baby back pork ribs—flinch-inducing on its own—is basted in the chain's Jack Daniel's glaze, accompanied by "battered and fried shrimp" and fries. There are so many kinds of wrong here, someone oughta write a country-Western song about it.

5. TGI Friday's Pecan Crusted Chicken Salad

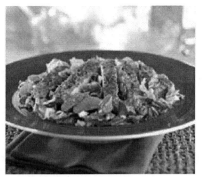

1360 calories

Sure, there are good ingredients in here: pecans, chicken breast, dried cranberries. And the choice in dressing *(balsamic vinaigrette)* is wise.

But watch out for the word "glazed," which just means the nuts are covered in sugar. And adding blue cheese to an already-dressed salad is yet another example of the "conditioned hyper-eating" referred to by Dr. Kessler.

6. TGI Friday's Loaded Potato Skins appetizer

1430 calories

Potato skins are nothing but "fat on fat on fat on fat, much of it loaded with salt," as Dr. Kessler puts it, and nowhere is this more evident than at Friday's.

The hollowed-out skins are fried, giving the surface area extra "fat pickup"—which is then loaded up with bacon, cheese and sour cream.

7. California Pizza Kitchen Thai Crunch Salad

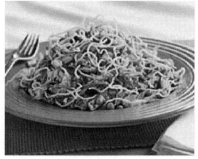

2115 calories

If only they'd stopped at the shredded cabbage, grilled chicken, cucumbers, edamame, carrots, green onions and lime-cilantro dressing—this would be a healthy, crunchy salad. But the peanuts, crispy wontons, crispy rice sticks and peanut dressing *(yes, again with the* double *dressings)* turn this salad into three meals worth of calories.

Note: California Pizza Kitchen plans to reduce the calories of this salad down to 1253 by November 2009.

8. California Pizza Kitchen Avocado Club Egg Rolls appetizer

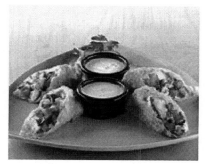

1180 calories

The avocado, chicken, tomato, and Monterey Jack cheese sounds good. But then you see the rest: bacon, deep fried wontons, and a double whammy that is the ranchito sauce *and* herb ranch dressing. You don't even want one ranch, much less two.

9. California Pizza Kitchen Blue Crab Cakes

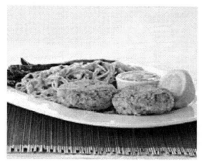

1567 calories

Crab cakes are usually small enough to make for a reasonable lunch entrée. But not when they come extra-large, are served with remoulade sauce *and* an accompaniment of "spaghettini in a creamy lemon-caper sauce."

Don't let the word lemon fool you into thinking it's light—this is what the Center for Science in the Public Interest would call "discomfort food.

10. Denny's Cheesy Three Pack appetizer

1940 calories
125 g fat
23 g saturated fat
100 g cholesterol
3840 mg sodium

"But they're so *cute!*"

Not everything that comes in "mini" size is adorable. You'd be better off ordering the Fit Fare Boca burger *(410 calories)*, or even their Classic Burger *(770 calories)* than this three-pack of mini cheeseburgers served with onion rings—a frightening overdose of calories, saturated fat and sodium.

11. Denny's Granola *(4oz)* with milk *(8oz)*

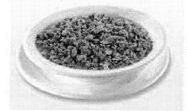

690 calories
12 g fat
2 g saturated fat
20 mg cholesterol
430 mg sodium

A bowl of cereal that adds up to nearly half a day's calories? And this is supposed to be a breakfast "side"?

Take heed: "People don't realize there's a ton of fat and sugar in granola, and restaurants serve oversized portions," says New York-based nutritionist Richter, who tells her clients to avoid granola altogether, not just at Denny's. "Opt for oatmeal instead—or Cheerios."

12. Denny's Heartland Scramble

1150 calorie
66 g fat
20 g saturated fat
530 mg cholesterol
2800 sodium

There's only *two* eggs in this breakfast entrée—yet the bacon, fried potatoes and cheddar cheese send this one into the danger zone, especially when you factor in the sodium content.

13. Applebee's Quesadilla Burger

1820 calories
46 g saturated fat
4410 mg sodium

This new menu item stuffs a burger into an already stuffed bacon-cheddar-pepper Jack quesadilla, then adds a Mexi-ranch sauce.

With fries *(440 calories)*, this full day's worth of calories adds up to 46 grams of saturated fat—the equivalent of two jumbo steak burritos at Chipotle. And with 4,410 milligrams of sodium, the Center for Science in the Public Interest *(CSPI)* calls this one "a prime candidate for Applebee's Don't-Have-a-Stroke *(on our property)* Special."

14. Applebee's Grilled Shrimp Pesto Alfredo Fettuccine

1790 calories

The Center for Science in the Public Interest *(CSPI)* once referred to fettuccine Alfredo as "heart attack on a plate." This entrée takes the heart attack and finishes it off with a bullet of highly-caloric pesto and high-cholesterol shrimp.

15. Applebee's Spinach and Artichoke Dip appetizer

1590 calories

Even though it's an appetizer, it still packs more punch than an entrée should. "'Spinach dip' is a misnomer," says Dr. Kessler, author of *The End of Overeating.*

"The spinach provides little more than color and a bit of appeal; a high-fat, high-salt dairy product is the main ingredient. It's a tasty dish of salt on fat."

16. On the Border Dos XX® Fish Tacos w/ Creamy Red Chile Sauce

2350 calories
152 g fat
31 g saturated fat
4060 mg sodium

No, those numbers aren't typos. Yes, this is all meant for one person.

Though fish is generally considered a healthy option, these three fish tacos stuffed with Dos XX beer-battered, golden fried fish, creamy red chili sauce, and cheese are far from that. What it all means, in plain English: fat on salt on fat on deep-fried-fat on alcohol and fat, in a fat-soaked shell… with a little bit of fish hidden inside it all.

In one single meal, you are getting 2 to 3 times the maximum daily dose of fat, saturated fat and sodium. "When our levels of sodium are too high, our blood volume increases which puts more pressure on the arteries and blood vessels," says Silber. "This makes the heart work harder than it needs to." The effects can be cumulative, and it's worth noting that heart disease is the number one killer of women over 65.

17. On the Border Grande Taco Salad with Taco Beef and Smoked Chipotle Vinaigrette Dressing

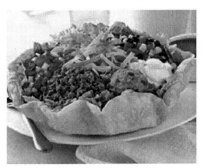

1,680 calories
121 g fat
40 g saturated fat
2,660 mg sodium

This salad was chosen by *Men's Health* as the Worst Salad in America in 2008—perhaps because it contains "as much saturated fat as 40 strips of bacon and more calories than 11 Taco Bell Fresco Tacos."

How's that even *possible*? Watch out for the bowl —it's made of deep-fried tortilla. That's fat-onto-fat-onto-fat, holding up a whole pile of fat.

18. On the Border Big Beef Bordurrito

1,600 calories
110 g fat
27 g saturated fat
3840 mg sodium

The word "stuffed" is a big red flag, because not only is the Bordurrito filled to bursting, but *you* probably will be too after ingesting it.

In this case, it's stuffed with fajita steak or chicken, Mexican rice, cheese, black beans, caramelized onions and red peppers, and sour cream sauce. Oh, wait, what's that noise? Probably your digestive tract staging a pre-emptive rebellion.

19. Outback Steakhouse Bloomin' Onion appetizer

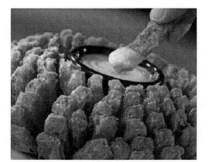

1560 calories

This could be called "The Bloomin' Butt."

Outback representatives say this is meant to be shared with a group, but the onion—healthy and flavorful on its own—provides a whole lot of surface area to absorb fat, Dr. Kessler explains. Here it's fried in batter and topped with "spicy signature bloom sauce"—layering salt on sugar on fat.

20. Outback Steakhouse Aussie Cheese Fries appetizer

2140 calories

Make sure there are at least 5 of you digging into this plate!

Cheese fries come under particular condemnation from Kessler. "The potato base is a simple carbohydrate, which quickly breaks down to sugar in the body. Once it's fried and layered with cheese, we're eating salt on fat on fat on sugar." And that's not even to mention the bacon and the ranch dressing.

21. Outback Steakhouse Baby Back Ribs *(full rack)*

2580 calories

Can you count the sins in here? A full rack of ribs smoked, grilled, coated in BBQ sauce, and served with Aussie fries. That's what's known as fat on fat on sugar on fat on fat.

22. Baja Fresh Breaded Fish Quesadilla

1400 calories
770 g fat
38 g saturated fat
170 mg cholesterol
2350 mg sodium

More than half the calories in this entrée are from fat *(770)*, and 38 grams of saturated fat is more than twice the maximum amount you want to be digesting in an entire day—much less in one meal.

The red flag here is the word "breaded"—and the irony is you'll hardly taste it since the fish is buried in a cheesy quesadilla. Avoid this and your heart will pump with pride *(and relief)*.

23. Baja Fresh Shrimp Bean & Cheese Burrito

950 calories
34 g fat
17 g saturated fat
310 mg cholesterol
2320 g sodium
Enchilada Style: 1580 calories, 74 g fat, 36 g saturated fat, 385 mg cholesterol, 3770 mg sodium

Shrimp and black beans = good. This burrito = bad.

It's the size of a linebacker, for one, and if you order the enticing "Enchilado Style"—melted jack and cheddar *on top* of the cheese that's already in the burrito, plus nachos and sour cream on the side—you could find yourself consuming a day's worth of calories *(1580 calories)*, roughly two days

worth of fat *(74 grams)* and enough sodium *(3770 mg)* to bloat you into the next dress size.

24. Baja Fresh Charbroiled Steak Tostada Salad

1230 calories
63 g fat
17 g saturated fat
140 mg cholesterol
2380 mg sodium

Be afraid of the word "tostada"—it involves a whole lot of surface area that's deep fried into an edible shell, designed to be eaten after you consume the steak, cheese, sour cream and guacamole it will contain. The only *actual* salad ingredients you'll find in here are some *(buried)* lettuce and tomato.

25. PF Chang's Chicken Chopped Salad with Ginger Dressing

940 calories
68 g fat
10 g saturated fat
2225 mg sodium

According to the menu, this salad is simply grilled chicken with house greens tossed with the restaurant's "signature ginger dressing." But they add, "for a lighter touch, try it with our sesame vinaigrette dressing" and that should be your cue that their signature tosser is anything but light.

Eater beware: not all salads are made equal.

26. PF Chang's Crispy Honey Shrimp

2110 calories
70 g fat
10 g saturated fat
1815 mg sodium

Though shrimp is relatively low in calories *(three oz. contains around 90 calories)*, the two words "crispy" and "honey" spell bad news. This is the fat on sugar concept, and it works like crack. Remember, kids: just say no!

27. PF Chang's Lo Mein Combo

1968 calories
24 g fat
3 g saturated fat
1465 mg sodium

We're used to seeing our lo mein noodles in a small, harmless-looking white cardboard box. This is something else entirely.

Intended to be shared by three people, a big pile of lo mein noodles are stir-fried in oil with large portions of beef, pork, chicken and shrimp. To avoid keeling over from cardiac arrest, ask for a "vegetable stock velveted" preparation to replace the oil, and remember to split this one!

28. Olive Garden Create Your Own Pizza appetizer *(cheese and sauce only)*

930 calories
910 calories
28 g fat
12 g saturated fat
2970 mg sodium

Before you even add a tomato, you're looking at nearly 1,000 calories and *gasp* 2970 mg of sodium! The 12 grams of saturated fat also clogged our arteries just thinking about it.

29. Olive Garden Pork Milanese

1510 calories
87 g fat
37 g saturated fat
3100 g sodium

Milan may be the fashion capital of Italy, but you can be sure those runway models aren't eating anything "Milanese": pan-seared pork scaloppini covered in Italian herb breadcrumbs, accompanied by "asiago cheese-filled tortelloni pasta tossed in a garlic-butter sauce with fresh spinach."

Step away from this entrée, and no one gets hurt.

30. Olive Garden Tour of Italy pasta

1450 calories
74 g fat
33 g saturated fat
3830 mg sodium

For the indecisive hedonist, this entrée includes lasagna, "lightly breaded" chicken parmigiana and fettuccine Alfredo—all with a meat sauce made of beef and Italian sausage. In other words, your tour of Italy begins and ends with "The Last Supper."

How to Navigate the Menu

If you're watching your calories—or your life expectancy—there are a few fast rules to follow if you eat out at a popular restaurant chain:

- Avoid anything with the word sampler or platter, unless you plan to share it with three or more people and make it your main course.

- Skip anything that comes in an edible bowl or includes the words stacked, stuffed, double, triple, slammed or dunked.

- Nachos are something best shared with a group, and subs are something best measured in calories, fat and sodium—not inches.

- When you see the words crispy or glazed, realize that's what will happen to your arteries and your eyes, respectively, if you consume too many of these items.

- Dressing and sauces are among the major calorie culprits of many restaurant choices, sometimes doubling the fat and sodium content of an entrée. Ask for all sauces on the side, and try replacing cream-based dressings with mustard (straight mustard, not sugar-loaded honey mustard), suggests New York City-based nutritionist Sharon Richter, MS, RD. Other good alternatives: lemon and grated cheese *(25 calories per tbsp)*.

- Just because an item falls under the word appetizers does not mean it should be followed by more food. Not even in the same day. Some of the country's most ubiquitous food establishments serve appetizers that would stuff a Sumo wrestler.

And remember, the average woman needs 1500 to 1800 calories a day to maintain weight *(depending upon activity level and frequency)*, and the American Heart Association recommends limiting dietary fat to 30 percent of total calories.

All nutritional information is from the restaurants' online menus, their respective publicists, and/or Men's Health magazine (NYS ordinance/their NYC menu, and the Center for Science in Public Interest).

Dr. Sharon's Six Quick Tips to Fast Food Restaurants

1. **The more time that you devote in the morning to planning your meals, the better.** Take a few minutes to THINK about what you need to eat and don't allow yourself to become so hungry that you throw all of the rules out the window as you roll it down in the drive thru.

2. **TRY your very best to avoid breakfast food at a fast food restaurant, unless you're traveling and there is no option.**

    a. The goal should be for there to be nutritious food at your home that is quick and easy for you to prepare. What about grits with some butter spray, egg beaters and a slice of whole wheat toast and jam? That's less than 10 minutes and you have sustenance that will carry you through the morning. Always have fresh fruit in the house, you can grab an apple on your way out the door and now you've added fiber.

3. **Fried is NEVER a good option.**

    a. Choose fast food chains that at least ATTEMPT to look like they want to have a healthy option.

    b. When in doubt, Chick-fil-A.

        i. Salads, grilled foods and my personal favorite the 4 piece kid's nugget meal.

4. **If you want a burger, make sure that you order it without mayo and other condiments that add on the calories.** AVOID the combinations unless you can add something lower in calories like a fruit cup.

    I can't eat a burger without cheese so I can't in good conscious tell you to do so. However, if you can…go for it! What I can do is take the burger and cut it in half—saving ½ of the calories. One big tip is to only order a regular burger/cheeseburger. Do not order a triple decker 50 pound beef monster and have the audacity to tell them to hold the mayo. Your heart, hips and wallet will thank you.

    Who says that you HAVE to have burger and fries—what about ordering one or the other. My personal favorite is a Medium McDonald's fry with water.

    SHARE with your coworker, spouse or the trash can. You don't have to finish all of the fries, you also don't have to upsize because it's cheaper. In the long run it is more expensive and detrimental to your health (*how much is a heart attack worth to you?*).

    Drink water NOT soda, sweetened tea, lemonade, etc. You're already having fast food, why continue the downward spiral.

To back up my #2 Tip on breakfast here is an excerpt from an article at www.webmd.com. I even have issues with what they identify as their best choices as they seem to have a significant portion of the daily caloric goal.

The Best and Worst Fast Food Breakfasts

Found at www.webmd.com

No matter which fast food chain you visit high fat and high-calorie breakfast choices abound. But there are some better choices out there. Here are some of the best and worst-case scenarios at several major chains:

McDonald's BEST Breakfast Choices:

*   **Egg McMuffin**: 300 calories, 12 grams fat, 5 g saturated fat, 260 mg cholesterol, 820 mg sodium, 2 g fiber.

*   **Hotcakes** (*without syrup and margarine*): 350 calories, 9 grams fat, 2 g saturated fat, 20 mg cholesterol, 590 mg sodium, 3 g fiber.

McDonald's WORST Choices:

*   **Deluxe Breakfast with regular size biscuit,** without syrup & margarine: 1070 calories, 55 g fat, 18 g saturated fat, 575 milligrams cholesterol, 2090 mg sodium, 6 g fiber.

*   **Deluxe Breakfast with large size biscuit,** without syrup & margarine: 1140 calories, 59 g fat, 20 g saturated fat, 575 mg cholesterol,

2250 mg sodium, 7 g fiber.

- **Big Breakfast** *(large size biscuit)*: 790 calories, 51 g fat, 18 g saturated fat, 555 mg cholesterol, 1,660 mg sodium, 4 g fiber.

Burger King's BEST Breakfast Choices:

- **Ham Omelet Sandwich**: 290 calories, 13 g fat 4.5 g saturated fat, 85 mg cholesterol, 870 mg sodium, 1 g fiber.
- **French Toast Sticks**, 3 piece: 240 calories, 13 g fat, 2.5 g saturated fat, 4 g protein, 0 mg cholesterol, 260 mg sodium, 1 g fiber.

Burger King's WORST Choices:

- **Double Croissan'Wich with sausage, egg, & cheese**: 680 calories, 51 g of fat, 18 g saturated fat, and 220 mg cholesterol, 1,590 mg sodium.
- **Enormous Omelet Sandwich**: 730 calories, 45 g of fat, 16 g of saturated fat, 330 mg of cholesterol, 1,940 mg sodium.

Jack in the Box BEST Breakfast Choices:

- **Breakfast Jack**: 290 calories, 12 g fat, 4.5 g saturated fat, 220 mg cholesterol, 760 mg sodium, 1 g fiber.
- **Bacon Breakfast Jack**: 300 calories, 14 g fat, 5 g saturated fat, 215 mg cholesterol, 730 mg sodium, 1 g fiber.

Jack in the Box WORST Choices:

- **Extreme Sausage Sandwich**: 670 calories, 48 g fat, 17 g saturated fat, 290 mg cholesterol, 1,300 mg sodium, 2 g fiber.
- **Sausage, Egg & Cheese Biscuit**: 740 calories, 55 g fat, 17 g saturated fat, 280 mg cholesterol, 1,430 mg sodium, 2 g fiber.
- **Sirloin Steak & Egg Burrito with Fire Roasted Tomato Salsa**: 790 calories, 48 g fat, 15 g saturated fat, 450 mg cholesterol, 1,440 mg sodium, 6 g fiber.

Carl's Jr. BEST Breakfast Choices:

- **French Toast Dips** *(5 pieces, no syrup)*: 430 calories, 18 g fat, 2.5 g saturated fat, 0 mg cholesterol, 530 mg sodium, 1 g fiber.

Carl's Jr. WORST Choices:

- **Loaded Breakfast Burrito**: 820 calories, 51 g fat, 16 g saturated fat, 595 mg cholesterol, 1,530 mg sodium, 2 g fiber.
- **Breakfast Burger**: 830 calories, 47 g fat, 15

g saturated fat, 275 mg cholesterol, 1,580 mg sodium, 3 g fiber.

Dunkin' Donuts BEST Breakfast Choices:

- **Blueberry Bagel**: 330 calories, 2.5 g fat, .5 g saturated fat, 10 g protein, 0 mg cholesterol, 600 mg sodium, 2 g fiber.
- **Wheat Bagel**:, 330 calories, 4 g fat, 1 g saturated fat, 12 g protein, 0 mg cholesterol, 610 mg sodium, 4 g fiber.
- **Reduced Fat Blueberry Muffin**: 400 calories, 5 g fat, 2 g saturated fat, 8 g protein, 60 mg cholesterol, 490 mg sodium, 3 g fiber.
- **Honey Bran Raisin Muffin**: 480 calories, 15 g fat, 2.5 g saturated fat, 8 g protein, 60 mg cholesterol, 480 mg sodium, 5 g fiber.

Dunkin' Donuts WORST Choices

- **Triple Chocolate Muffin**: 660 calories, 33 g fat, 7 g saturated fat, 10 mg cholesterol, 460 mg sodium, 4 g fiber.
- **Peanut Butter Cup Cookie**: 590 calories, 29 g fat, 13 g saturated fat, 50 mg cholesterol, 530 mg sodium, 3 g fiber.

Subway BEST Breakfast Choices:

- **Cheese Breakfast Sandwich** on 6" bread: 410 calories, 18 g fat, 8 g saturated fat, 190 mg cholesterol, 1,010 mg sodium, 5 g fiber.

Subway WORST Choices:

- **Chipotle Steak & Cheese Breakfast Sandwich** on 6" bread: 600 calories, 32 g fat, 11 g saturated fat, 220 mg cholesterol, 1,470 mg sodium, 6 g fiber.

A Starbucks on Every Corner

And what about the Starbucks Coffee cafes you'll find on nearly every corner in cities across America? Here are some of the healthier items you might find at your local Starbucks *(keeping in mind that bakery items vary regionally)*:

- **Low Fat Bran Muffins**: 360 calories, 4.5 g fat, 0 g saturated fat, 40 g cholesterol, 290 mg sodium, 7 g fiber
- **Reduced Fat Cranberry Apple Muffin:** 310 calories, 9 g fat, 1 g saturated fat, 60 mg cholesterol, 460 mg sodium, 5 g fiber.
- **Low-Fat Oat Fruit Scone**: 310 calories, 2.5 g fat, 1 g saturated fat, 9 g protein, 30 mg cholesterol, 280 mg sodium, 3 g fiber
- **Spinach Roasted Tomato, Feta & Egg**

Wrap: 240 calories, 10g fat, 3.5 g saturated fat, 140 mg cholesterol, 730 mg sodium, 7 g fiber.

- **Reduced Fat Blueberry Coffee Cake**: 320 calories, 6 g fat, 4.5 g saturated fat, 4 g protein, 10 mg cholesterol, 390 mg sodium, 1 g fiber.

- **Reduced-Fat Cherry Lemon Coffee Cake with Oatmeal-Pecan Streusel**: 370 calories, 9 g fat, 2.5 g saturated fat, 7 g protein, 50 mg cholesterol, 540 mg sodium, 3 g fiber.

- **Reduced Fat Cinnamon Swirl Coffee Cake**: 290 calories, 4 g fat, 3 g saturated fat, 4 g protein, <5 mg cholesterol, 330 mg sodium, <1 g fiber.

When all is said and done, it really continues to boil down to *Is it Worth It?* It's not only about the weight—what about your cholesterol, heart health, risk of diabetes and other health related issues. Further, if you have children and you're feeding them fast food several times a week—chances are little junior is getting bigger by the day. So, I ask again— *Is It Worth It?* Let's look at some of the food and what you would have to do to burn calories off.

McDonald's Deluxe Breakfast

To burn off scrambled eggs, hash browns, sausages, pancakes and syrup *(approx. 1120 calories)* you would have to:

Activity	130 lbs	150 lbs	170 lbs	190 lbs	220 lbs	250 lbs	270 lbs
Aerobics, General	175 mins.	152 mins.	134 mins.	120 mins.	103 mins.	91 mins.	85 mins.
Bicycle, Stationary	163 mins.	141 mins.	125 mins.	112 mins.	96 mins.	85 mins.	79 mins.
Calisthenics *(push-ups, sit-ups, pull-ups, jumping jacks)*	142 mins.	124 mins.	109 mins.	98 mins.	84 mins.	74 mins.	69 mins.
Food Shopping	495 mins.	430 mins.	379 mins.	340 mins.	292 mins.	259 mins.	239 mins.
Gardening, General	285 mins.	247 mins.	218 mins.	195 mins.	168 mins.	149 mins.	138 mins.
Raking Lawn	265 mins.	230 mins.	203 mins.	182 mins.	156 mins.	138 mins.	128 mins.
Sex, General, Moderate	876 mins.	760 mins.	671 mins.	601 mins.	517 mins.	457 mins.	424 mins.
Shoveling Snow	190 mins.	165 mins.	145 mins.	130 mins.	112 mins.	99 mins.	92 mins.
Sweep Floors	345 mins.	299 mins.	264 mins.	237 mins.	204 mins.	180 mins.	167 mins.
Treadmill	127 mins.	110 mins.	97 mins.	87 mins.	75 mins.	66 mins.	61 mins.
Vacuum	325 mins.	262 mins.	249 mins.	223 mins.	192 mins.	170 mins.	157 mins.
Volleyball	285 mins.	247 mins.	218 mins.	195 mins.	168 mins.	149 mins.	138 mins.
Washing Dishes	495 mins.	430 mins.	379 mins.	340 mins.	292 mins.	259 mins.	239 mins.
Weight Lifting	380 mins.	329 mins.	291 mins.	260 mins.	224 mins.	198 mins.	184 mins.

McDonald's Lunch

To burn off 1 McChicken sandwich, large fries and 1 large coke *(approx. 1240 calories)* you would have to:

Activity	130 lbs	150 lbs	170 lbs	190 lbs	220 lbs	250 lbs	270 lbs
Aerobics, General	194 mins.	168 mins.	149 mins.	133 mins.	114 mins.	101 mins.	94 mins.
Bicycle, Stationary	180 mins.	156 mins.	138 mins.	124 mins.	106 mins.	94 mins.	87 mins.
Calisthenics *(push-ups, sit-ups, pull-ups, jumping jacks)*	158 mins.	137 mins.	121 mins.	108 mins.	93 mins.	82 mins.	76 mins.
Food Shopping	548 mins.	476 mins.	420 mins.	376 mins.	323 mins.	286 mins.	265 mins.
Gardening, General	315 mins.	274 mins.	242 mins.	216 mins.	186 mins.	165 mins.	152 mins.
Raking Lawn	293 mins.	254 mins.	225 mins.	201 mins.	173 mins.	153 mins.	142 mins.
Sex, General, Moderate	970 mins.	842 mins.	743 mins.	665 mins.	572 mins.	506 mins.	469 mins.
Shoveling Snow	210 mins.	182 mins.	161 mins.	144 mins.	124 mins.	110 mins.	102 mins.
Sweep Floors	382 mins.	332 mins.	293 mins.	262 mins.	225 mins.	200 mins.	185 mins.
Treadmill	140 mins.	122 mins.	107 mins.	96 mins.	83 mins.	73 mins.	68 mins.

Vacuum	360 mins.	313 mins.	276mins.	247 mins.	213 mins.	188 mins.	174 mins.
Volleyball	315 mins.	274 mins.	242mins.	216 mins.	186 mins.	165 mins.	152 mins.
Washing Dishes	548 mins.	476 mins.	420 mins.	376 mins.	323 mins.	286 mins.	265 mins.
Weight Lifting	420 mins.	365 mins.	322 mins.	288 mins.	248 mins.	219 mins.	203 mins.

Taco Bell Lunch

To burn off 1 taco, 1 burrito and 1 large Pepsi *(approx. 860 calories)* you would have to:

Activity	130 lbs	150 lbs	170 lbs	190 lbs	220 lbs	250 lbs	270 lbs
Aerobics, General	135 mins.	117 mins.	103 mins.	92 mins.	79 mins.	70 mins.	65 mins.
Bicycle, Stationary	125 mins.	108 mins.	96 mins.	86 mins.	74 mins.	65 mins.	60 mins.
Calisthenics *(push-ups, sit-ups, pull-ups, jumping jacks)*	109 mins.	95 mins.	84 mins.	75 mins.	64 mins.	57 mins.	53 mins.
Food Shopping	380 mins.	330 mins.	291 mins.	261 mins.	224 mins.	199 mins.	184 mins.
Gardening, General	219 mins.	190 mins.	168 mins.	150 mins.	129 mins.	114 mins.	106 mins.
Raking Lawn	203 mins.	176 mins.	156 mins.	140 mins.	120 mins.	106 mins.	98 mins.
Sex, General, Moderate	673 mins.	584 mins.	515 mins.	462 mins.	397 mins.	351 mins.	325 mins.
Shoveling Snow	146 mins.	126 mins.	112 mins.	100 mins.	86 mins.	76 mins.	70 mins.
Sweep Floors	265 mins.	230 mins.	203 mins.	182 mins.	156 mins.	138 mins.	128 mins.
Treadmill	97 mins.	84 mins.	74 mins.	67 mins.	57 mins.	51 mins.	47 mins.
Vacuum	250 mins.	217 mins.	191 mins.	171 mins.	147 mins.	130 mins.	121 mins.
Volleyball	219 mins.	190 mins.	168 mins.	150 mins.	129 mins.	114 mins.	106 mins.
Washing Dishes	380 mins.	330 mins.	291 mins.	261 mins.	224 mins.	199 mins.	184 mins.
Weight Lifting	292 mins.	253 mins.	223 mins.	200 mins.	172 mins.	152 mins.	141 mins.

Taco Bell Dinner

To burn off 1 double decker taco supreme, 1 beef gordita supreme, 1 cheese quesadilla and 1 large Pepsi *(approx. 1350 calories)* you would have to:

Activity	130 lbs	150 lbs	170 lbs	190 lbs	220 lbs	250 lbs	270 lbs
Aerobics, General	211 mins.	183 mins.	162 mins.	145 mins.	125 mins.	110 mins.	102 mins.
Bicycle, Stationary	196 mins.	170 mins.	150 mins.	135 mins.	116 mins.	102 mins.	95 mins.
Calisthenics *(push-ups, sit-ups, pull-ups, jumping jacks)*	172 mins.	149 mins.	131 mins.	118 mins.	101 mins.	90 mins.	83 mins.
Food Shopping	597 mins.	518 mins.	457 mins.	410 mins.	352 mins.	312 mins.	289 mins.
Gardening, General	343 mins.	298 mins.	263 mins.	235 mins.	202 mins.	179 mins.	166 mins.
Raking Lawn	319 mins.	277 mins.	245 mins.	219 mins.	188 mins.	167 mins.	154 mins.
Sex, General, Moderate	1056 mins.	916 mins.	809 mins.	725 mins.	623 mins.	551 mins.	511 mins.
Shoveling Snow	229 mins.	199 mins.	175 mins.	157 mins.	135 mins.	119 mins.	111 mins.
Sweep Floors	416 mins.	361 mins.	319mins.	285 mins.	245 mins.	217 mins.	201 mins.
Treadmill	153 mins.	132 mins.	117 mins.	105 mins.	90 mins.	80 mins.	74 mins.
Vacuum	392 mins.	340 mins.	301 mins.	269 mins.	231 mins.	205 mins.	190 mins.
Volleyball	343 mins.	298 mins.	263 mins.	235 mins.	202 mins.	179 mins.	166 mins.
Washing Dishes	597 mins.	518 mins.	457mins.	410 mins.	352 mins.	312 mins.	289 mins.
Weight Lifting	458 mins.	397 mins.	351 mins.	314 mins.	270 mins.	239 mins.	221 mins.

Burger King Breakfast

To burn off 1 Croissan'wich w/ Sausage, Egg & Cheese, 1 large hash brown, and 1 large coffee *(approx. 900 calories)* you would have to:

Activity	130 lbs	150 lbs	170 lbs	190 lbs	220 lbs	250 lbs	270 lbs
Aerobics, General	141 mins.	122 mins.	108 mins.	97 mins.	83 mins.	74 mins.	68 mins.
Bicycle, Stationary	131 mins.	113 mins.	100 mins.	90 mins.	77 mins.	68 mins.	63 mins.
Calisthenics *(push-ups, sit-ups, pull-ups, jumping jacks)*	114 mins.	99 mins.	88 mins.	78 mins.	68 mins.	60 mins.	55 mins.
Food Shopping	398 mins.	345 mins.	305 mins.	273 mins.	235 mins.	208 mins.	192 mins.
Gardening, General	229 mins.	199 mins.	175 mins.	157 mins.	135 mins.	119 mins.	111 mins.
Raking Lawn	213 mins.	185 mins.	163 mins.	146 mins.	126 mins.	111 mins.	103 mins.
Sex, General, Moderate	704 mins.	611 mins.	539 mins.	483 mins.	415 mins.	368 mins.	340 mins.
Shoveling Snow	153 mins.	132 mins.	117 mins.	105 mins.	90 mins.	80 mins.	74 mins.
Sweep Floors	277 mins.	241 mins.	213 mins.	190 mins.	164 mins.	145 mins.	134 mins.
Treadmill	102 mins.	88 mins.	78 mins.	70 mins.	60 mins.	53 mins.	49 mins.
Vacuum	262 mins.	227 mins.	200 mins.	179 mins.	154 mins.	137 mins.	126 mins.
Volleyball	229 mins.	199 mins.	175 mins.	157 mins.	135 mins.	119 mins.	111 mins.
Washing Dishes	398 mins.	345 mins.	305 mins.	273 mins.	235 mins.	208 mins.	192 mins.
Weight Lifting	305 mins.	265 mins.	234 mins.	209 mins.	180 mins.	159 mins.	148 mins.

Burger King Lunch

To burn off 1 Double Whopper w/ Cheese, large onion rings and 1 large Coke *(approx. 1510 calories)* you would have to:

Activity	130 lbs	150 lbs	170 lbs	190 lbs	220 lbs	250 lbs	270 lbs
Aerobics, General	236 mins.	205 mins.	181 mins.	162 mins.	139 mins.	123 mins.	114 mins.
Bicycle, Stationary	219 mins.	190 mins.	168 mins.	150 mins.	129 mins.	115 mins.	106 mins.
Calisthenics *(push-ups, sit-ups, pull-ups, jumping jacks)*	192 mins.	167 mins.	336 mins.	132 mins.	113 mins.	100 mins.	93 mins.
Food Shopping	668 mins.	579 mins.	512 mins.	458 mins.	394 mins.	349 mins.	323 mins.
Gardening, General	384 mins.	333 mins.	294 mins.	263 mins.	226 mins.	200 mins.	186 mins.
Raking Lawn	357 mins.	310 mins.	274 mins.	245 mins.	211 mins.	186 mins.	173 mins.
Sex, General, Moderate	1181 mins.	1025 mins.	905 mins.	810 mins.	697 mins.	617 mins.	571 mins.
Shoveling Snow	256 mins.	222 mins.	196 mins.	176 mins.	151 mins.	134 mins.	124 mins.
Sweep Floors	465 mins.	404 mins.	357 mins.	319 mins.	275 mins.	243 mins.	225 mins.
Treadmill	171 mins.	148 mins.	131 mins.	117 mins.	101 mins.	89 mins.	83 mins.
Vacuum	439 mins.	381 mins.	336 mins.	301 mins.	259 mins.	229 mins.	212 mins.
Volleyball	384 mins.	333 mins.	294 mins.	263 mins.	226 mins.	200 mins.	186 mins.
Washing Dishes	668 mins.	579 mins.	512 mins.	458 mins.	394 mins.	349 mins.	323 mins.
Weight Lifting	512 mins.	444 mins.	392 mins.	351 mins.	302 mins.	267 mins.	248 mins.

Hardees Breakfast

To burn off 1 Big Country Breakfast Platter-Country Steak *(approx. 1150 calories)* you would have to:

Activity	130 lbs	150 lbs	170 lbs	190 lbs	220 lbs	250 lbs	270 lbs
Aerobics, General	180 mins.	156 mins.	138 mins.	123 mins.	106 mins.	94 mins.	87 mins.
Bicycle, Stationary	167 mins.	145 mins.	128 mins.	115 mins.	99 mins.	87 mins.	81 mins.
Calisthenics *(push-ups, sit-ups, pull-ups, jumping jacks)*	146 mins.	127 mins.	112 mins.	100 mins.	86 mins.	76 mins.	71 mins.
Food Shopping	508 mins.	441 mins.	390 mins.	349 mins.	300 mins.	265 mins.	246 mins.
Gardening, General	292 mins.	254 mins.	224 mins.	201 mins.	172 mins.	153 mins.	141 mins.
Raking Lawn	272 mins.	236 mins.	208 mins.	187 mins.	160 mins.	142 mins.	132 mins.
Sex, General, Moderate	900 mins.	781 mins.	689 mins.	617 mins.	531 mins.	470 mins.	435 mins.
Shoveling Snow	195 mins.	169 mins.	149 mins.	134 mins.	115 mins.	102 mins.	94 mins.
Sweep Floors	354 mins.	307 mins.	272 mins.	243 mins.	209 mins.	185 mins.	171 mins.
Treadmill	130 mins.	113 mins.	100 mins.	89 mins.	77 mins.	68 mins.	63 mins.
Vacuum	334 mins.	290mins.	256 mins.	229 mins.	197 mins.	174 mins.	162 mins.
Volleyball	292 mins.	254 mins.	224 mins.	201 mins.	172 mins.	153 mins.	141 mins.
Washing Dishes	508 mins.	441 mins.	390 mins.	349 mins.	300 mins.	265 mins.	246 mins.
Weight Lifting	390 mins.	338 mins.	299 mins.	267 mins.	230 mins.	204 mins.	189 mins.

Hardees Lunch

To burn off 1 Charbroiled Chicken Club Sandwich, Crispy Curls-Large and 1 large Coke *(approx. 1050 calories)* you would have to:

Activity	130 lbs	150 lbs	170 lbs	190 lbs	220 lbs	250 lbs	270 lbs
Aerobics, General	164 mins.	143 mins.	126 mins.	113 mins.	97 mins.	86 mins.	79 mins.
Bicycle, Stationary	153 mins.	132 mins.	117 mins.	105 mins.	90 mins.	80 mins.	74 mins.
Calisthenics *(push-ups, sit-ups, pull-ups, jumping jacks)*	133 mins.	116 mins.	102 mins.	92 mins.	79 mins.	70 mins.	65 mins.
Food Shopping	464 mins.	403 mins.	356 mins.	319 mins.	274 mins.	242 mins.	225 mins.
Gardening, General	267 mins.	232 mins.	205 mins.	183 mins.	158 mins.	139 mins.	129 mins.
Raking Lawn	248 mins.	215 mins.	190 mins.	170 mins.	147 mins.	130 mins.	120 mins.
Sex, General, Moderate	821 mins.	713 mins.	629 mins.	564 mins.	485 mins.	429 mins.	397 mins.
Shoveling Snow	178 mins.	154 mins.	136 mins.	122 mins.	105 mins.	93 mins.	86 mins.
Sweep Floors	324 mins.	281 mins.	248 mins.	222 mins.	191 mins.	169 mins.	156 mins.
Treadmill	119 mins.	103 mins.	91 mins.	81 mins.	70 mins.	62 mins.	57 mins.
Vacuum	305 mins.	265 mins.	234 mins.	209 mins.	180 mins.	159 mins.	148 mins.
Volleyball	267 mins.	232 mins.	205 mins.	183 mins.	158 mins.	139 mins.	129 mins.
Washing Dishes	464 mins.	403 mins.	356 mins.	319 mins.	274 mins.	242 mins.	225 mins.
Weight Lifting	356 mins.	309 mins.	273 mins.	244 mins.	210 mins.	186 mins.	172 mins.

KFC Lunch

To burn off 1 roasted Caesar salad with creamy parmesan Caesar dressing and 1 Tropicana fruit punch *(approx. 600 calories)* you would have to:

Activity	130 lbs	150 lbs	170 lbs	190 lbs	220 lbs	250 lbs	270 lbs
Aerobics, General	94 mins.	81 mins.	72 mins.	64 mins.	55 mins.	49 mins.	45 mins.
Bicycle, Stationary	87 mins.	76 mins.	67 mins.	60 mins.	51 mins.	46 mins.	42 mins.
Calisthenics *(push-ups, sit-ups, pull-ups, jumping jacks)*	76 mins.	66 mins.	58 mins.	52 mins.	45 mins.	40 mins.	37 mins.
Food Shopping	265 mins.	230 mins.	203 mins.	182 mins.	157 mins.	139 mins.	128 mins.
Gardening, General	153 mins.	132 mins.	117 mins.	105 mins.	90 mins.	80 mins.	74 mins.
Raking Lawn	142 mins.	123 mins.	109 mins.	97 mins.	84 mins.	74 mins.	69 mins.
Sex, General, Moderate	469 mins.	407 mins.	360 mins.	322 mins.	277 mins.	245 mins.	227 mins.
Shoveling Snow	102 mins.	88 mins.	78 mins.	70 mins.	60 mins.	53 mins.	49 mins.
Sweep Floors	185 mins.	160 mins.	142 mins.	127 mins.	109 mins.	97 mins.	89 mins.
Treadmill	68 mins.	59 mins.	52 mins.	47 mins.	40 mins.	35 mins.	33 mins.
Vacuum	174 mins.	151 mins.	134 mins.	120 mins.	103 mins.	91 mins.	84 mins.
Volleyball	153 mins.	132 mins.	117 mins.	105 mins.	90 mins.	80 mins.	74 mins.
Washing Dishes	244 mins.	230 mins.	203 mins.	182 mins.	157 mins.	139 mins.	128 mins.
Weight Lifting	203 mins.	176 mins.	156 mins.	140 mins.	120 mins.	106 mins.	98 mins.

KFC Dinner

To burn off 3 crispy chicken strips, potato salad, corn on the cob and 1 large Pepsi *(approx. 900 calories)* you would have to:

Activity	130 lbs	150 lbs	170 lbs	190 lbs	220 lbs	250 lbs	270 lbs
Aerobics, General	141 mins.	122 mins.	108 mins.	97 mins.	83 mins.	74 mins.	68 mins.
Bicycle, Stationary	131 mins.	113 mins.	100 mins.	90 mins.	77 mins.	68 mins.	63 mins.
Calisthenics *(push-ups, sit-ups, pull-ups, jumping jacks)*	114 mins.	99 mins.	88 mins.	78 mins.	68 mins.	60 mins.	55 mins.
Food Shopping	398 mins.	345 mins.	305 mins.	273 mins.	235 mins.	208 mins.	192 mins.
Gardening, General	229 mins.	199 mins.	175 mins.	157 mins.	135 mins.	119 mins.	111 mins.
Raking Lawn	213 mins.	185 mins.	163 mins.	146 mins.	126 mins.	111 mins.	103 mins.
Sex, General, Moderate	704 mins.	611 mins.	539 mins.	483 mins.	415 mins.	368 mins.	340 mins.
Shoveling Snow	153 mins.	132 mins.	117 mins.	105 mins.	90 mins.	80 mins.	74 mins.
Sweep Floors	277 mins.	241 mins.	213 mins.	190 mins.	164 mins.	145 mins.	134 mins.
Treadmill	102 mins.	88 mins.	78 mins.	70 mins.	60 mins.	53 mins.	49 mins.
Vacuum	262 mins.	227 mins.	200 mins.	179 mins.	154 mins.	137 mins.	126 mins.
Volleyball	229 mins.	199 mins.	175mins.	157 mins.	135 mins.	119 mins.	111 mins.
Washing Dishes	398 mins.	345 mins.	305 mins.	273 mins.	235 mins.	208 mins.	192 mins.
Weight Lifting	305 mins.	265 mins.	234 minss.	209 mins.	180 mins.	159 mins.	148 mins.

A series of books that I LOVE and cite a lot in this book is the *Eat This, Not That!* series written by the Editor-in-Chief of *Men's Health*. BUY these books and read them; they will truly open your eyes. Here are a few of my all time favorite nuggets from the book and/or *Men's Health* magazine.

The 20 WORST Foods in America

Found at www.msnbc.msn.com/id/21838237/ns/today-today_health

20: Worst fast-food chicken meal

Chicken Selects Premium Breast Strips from McDonald's *(5 pieces)* **with creamy ranch sauce**

- 830 calories 55 g fat *(4.5 g trans fat)*
- 48 g carbohydrates

The only thing premium about these strips is the caloric price you pay. Add a large fries and regular soda and this seemingly innocuous chicken meal tops out at 1,710 calories.

Change Your Chicken: 20 McNuggets have the same impact. Instead, choose Mickey D's six-piece offering with BBQ sauce and save yourself 530 calories.

19: Worst drink

Jamba Juice Chocolate Moo'd Power Smoothie *(30 fl oz)*

- 900 calories, 10 g fat
- 183 g carbs *(166 g sugar)*

Jamba Juice calls it a smoothie; we call it a milk shake. In fact, this beverage contains as much sugar as 2 pints of Ben & Jerry's butter pecan ice cream.

Turn Down the Power: Seventy-five percent of this chain's power smoothies contain in excess of 100 grams of sugar. Stick to Jamba's lower-calorie All Fruit Smoothies, which are the only menu items that contain no added sugar. And always opt for the 16-oz. small.

18: Worst supermarket meal

Pepperidge Farm Roasted Chicken Pot Pie *(whole pie)*

- 1,020 calories, 64 g fat
- 86 g carbs

The label may say this pie serves two, but who ever divided a small pot pie in half? The sad truth is, once you crack the crust, there will be no stopping, which makes this 300 calories worse than anything else you'll find in the freezer case.

Pick a Better Pie: Swanson's chicken pot pie has just 400 calories.

17: Worst 'healthy' burger

Ruby Tuesday Bella Turkey Burger

- 1,145 calories, 71 g fat
- 56 g carbs

We chose this burger for more than its calorie payload: Its name implies that it's healthy.

The Truly Healthy Choice: Skip burgers entirely *(few at Ruby Tuesday come in under 1,000 calories)*. Instead, order a 9-oz. sirloin with a side of steamed vegetables, and keep things under 1,000 calories.

16: Worst Mexican entree

Chipotle Mexican Grill Chicken Burrito

- 1,179 calories, 47 g fat
- 125 g carbs
- 2,656 milligrams *(mg)* sodium

Despite a reputation for using healthy, fresh ingredients, Chipotle's menu is limited to king-size burritos, overstuffed tacos, and gigantic salads —all of which lead to a humongous waistline.

Make Over the Menu: There are two ways to Men's Healthify a burrito at Chipotle: *(1)* 86 the rice and tortilla and request your meat, vegetables and beans served in a bowl or *(2)* bring a friend and saw the burrito in half.

15: Worst kids' meal

Macaroni Grill Double Macaroni 'n' Cheese

- 1,210 calories, 62 g fat
- 3,450 mg sodium

It's like feeding your kid 1 ½ boxes of Kraft mac 'n' cheese.

Your Best Option: The 390-calorie Grilled Chicken and Broccoli.

14: Worst sandwich

Quiznos Classic Italian *(large)*

- 1,490 calories, 85 g fat
- 4,510 mg sodium, 96 g carbs

A large homemade sandwich would more likely provide about 500 calories.

Cut the Calories: Isn't it obvious? Order a small, or save half for later.

13: Worst salad

On the Border Grande Taco Salad with Taco Beef

- 1,450 calories, 102 g fat
- 78 g carbs, 2,410 mg sodium

This isn't an anomaly: Five different On the Border salads on the menu contain more than 1,100 calories each.

The Salad for You: The Sizzling Chicken Fajita Salad supplies an acceptable 760 calories. But remember to choose a noncaloric beverage, such as water or unsweetened iced tea.

12: Worst burger

Carl's Jr. Double Six Dollar Burger

- 1,520 calories, 111 g fat

Carl's Jr. brags that its home to this enormous sandwich, but the restaurant chain also provides convenient nutrition info on its Web site—so ignorance is no excuse for eating it.

A Simple Solution: The Low Carb Six Dollar Burger has just 490 calories.

11: Worst steak

Lonestar 20 oz T-bone

- 1,540 calories, 124 g fat

Add a baked potato and Lonestar's Signature Lettuce Wedge, and this is a 2,700-calorie blowout.

Choose with Your Head: The golden rule of steak restaurants is this: Limit yourself to a 9-oz. or smaller. After all, that's more than half a pound of meat. You won't walk away hungry.

10: Worst breakfast

Bob Evans Caramel Banana Pecan Cream Stacked and Stuffed Hotcakes

- 1,540 calories, 77 g fat *(9 g trans fat)*
- 198 g carbs *(109 g sugar)*

Five Egg McMuffins yield the same caloric cost as this stack of sugar-stuffed flapjacks, which is truly a heavy breakfast, weighing in at a hefty pound and a half.

Order This Instead: A Bob Evans Western Omelet starts your day with a reasonable 654 calories and 44 grams of muscle-building protein.

9: Worst dessert

Chili's Chocolate Chip Paradise Pie with Vanilla Ice Cream

- 1,600 calories, 78 g fat
- 215 g carbs

Would you eat a Big Mac for dessert? How about three? That's the calorie equivalent of this decadent dish. Clearly, Chili's customers get their money's worth.

Don't Overdo It: If you want dessert at Chili's, order one single-serving Sweet Shot; you'll cap your after-dinner intake at 310 calories.

8: Worst Chinese entree

P.F. Chang's Pork Lo Mein

- 1,820 calories, 127 g fat
- 95 g carbs

The fat content in this dish alone provides more than 1,100 calories. And you'd have to eat almost five servings of pasta to match the number of carbohydrates it contains. Now, do you really need five servings of pasta?

Pick Another Noodle: P.F. Chang's Singapore Street Noodles will satisfy your craving with only 570 calories. Or try the Moo Goo Gai Pan or the Ginger Chicken & Broccoli, which have 660 calories each.

7: Worst chicken entree

Chili's Honey Chipotle Crispers with Chipotle Sauce

- 2,040 calories, 99 g fat
- 240 g carbs

Crispers refers to an extra-thick layer of bread crumbs that soaks up oil and adds unnecessary calories and carbs to these glorified chicken strips.

Switch Your Selection: Order the Chicken Fajita Pita: At 450 calories, 43 g protein, it's one of the healthiest entrées you'll find in a chain restaurant.

6: Worst fish entree

On the Border Dos XX Fish Tacos with Rice and Beans

- 2,100 calories, 130 g fat
- 169 g carbs, 4,750 mg sodium

Perhaps the most misleadingly named dish in America: A dozen crunchy tacos from Taco Bell will saddle you with fewer calories.

Lighten the Load: Ask for grilled fish, choose the corn tortillas instead of flour *(they're lower in calories and higher in fiber)*, and swap out the carbohydrate-loaded rice for grilled vegetables.

5: Worst pizza

Uno Chicago Grill Chicago Classic Deep Dish Pizza

- 2,310 calories, 162 g fat
- 123 g carbs, 4,470 mg sodium

Downing this personal pizza is equivalent to eating 18 slices of Domino's Crunchy Thin Crust cheese pizza.

Swap Your Slices: Switch to the Sausage Flatbread Pie and avert deep-dish disaster by nearly 1,500 calories.

4: Worst pasta

Macaroni Grill Spaghetti and Meatballs with Meat Sauce

- 2,430 calories, 128 g fat
- 207 g carbs, 5,290 mg sodium

This meal satisfies your calorie requirements for an entire day.

Downsize the Devastation: Ask for a lunch portion of this dinner dish *(or any pasta on the menu, for that matter)*, and request regular tomato sauce instead of meat sauce. You'll cut the calories in half.

3: Worst nachos

On the Border Stacked Border Nachos

- 2,740 calories, 166 g fat
- 191 g carbs, 5,280 mg sodium

2: Worst starter

Chili's Awesome Blossom

- 2,710 calories, 203 g fat
- 194 g carbs, 6,360 mg sodium

1: The worst food in America

Outback Steakhouse Aussie Cheese Fries with Ranch Dressing

- 2,900 calories, 182 g fat
- 240 g carbs

Even if you split these starters with three friends, you'll have downed a dinner's worth of calories before your entrée arrives.

Super Substitutions Front-load your meal with a protein-based dish that's not deep-fried. A high-protein starter helps diminish hunger without putting you into calorie overload. And remember: Appetizers are meant to be shared.

- At On the Border: Chicken Soft Tacos *(250 calories each)*. This entrée is as close as you'll come to a healthy starter.
- At Chili's: Garlic & Lime Grilled Shrimp. Look for this item in the sides.
- At Outback: Seared Ahi or Shrimp on the Barbie.

Dr. Sharon's Let's Get REAL Moment: Tell the truth, you KNOW that the Outback cheese fries have called your name in the past. You thought well it's just some cheese and of course I need strong bones so this is actually good for me. I am not even going to TRY to tell you what you would have to do to burn these calories; JUST SAY NO! WALK AWAY, AWAY, AWAY RUN!

America's Best Fast-Food Restaurants

The authors of ***Eat This, Not That!*** shine a light on drive-through and chain restaurants that offer healthier fare. By Dave Zinczenko and Matt Goulding, *Men's Health*

Eating out invariably raises a number of tricky questions: sit down or drive through? Burgers or pizza? Thin or stuffed crust? Choosing one over the other could mean saving hundreds of calories in a single meal, up to 50 pounds of flab in the course of a year, and countless health woes over the course of a lifetime. That's why *Eat This, Not That!* launched an investigation and put 66 major chain restaurants under the nutritional microscope—so that you and your family can continue to eat out, but do so knowing the types of insider tips and savvy strategies that can help melt fat all year long.

To separate the commendable from the deplorable:

- We calculated the total number of calories per entrée. This gave us a snapshot of how each restaurant compared in average serving size—a key indicator of unhealthy portion distortion.

- We rewarded establishments with fruit and vegetable side-dish choices, as well as offering whole-wheat bread.

- We penalized places for excessive amounts of trans fats and menus that tempt you with gut-busting desserts. Hey, if the neighborhood is crowded with shady characters, sooner or later, one of them will jump you.

What we ended up with is the *Eat This, Not That!* Restaurant Report Card, which will show you how all of the nation's largest eating establishments stack up nutritionally.

Check out those restaurants that scored a B+ or higher:

Chick-fil-A: A-

Between the breakfast and lunch menus, there are only two entrées at Chick-fil-A that break 500 calories, a rare feat in the fast-food world. What this means is that you can't possibly do too much harm—especially if you stick to the chicken. And unlike the typical fast-food chain, Chick-fil-A offers a list of sides that goes beyond breaded and fried potatoes and onions. *(Just beware the large cole slaw, which adds an extra 600 calories to your daily intake!)* That's why we dub the Atlanta-based chicken shack one of our all-time favorite fast-food restaurants.

Also, be sure to check out our exclusive list of the best and worst restaurants for kids to see why Chick-fil-A receives an even higher grade when it comes to kids' meals.

Survival strategy: The worst thing you can do is supplement your meal with a milkshake—not a single cup has fewer than 600 calories. And instead of nuggets or strips, look to the Chargrilled Chicken Sandwiches, which average only 320 calories apiece.

Subway: A-

A menu based on lean protein and vegetables is always going to score well in our book. With more than half a dozen sandwiches under 300 calories, plus a slew of soups and healthy sides to boot, Subway can satisfy even the pickiest eater without breaking the caloric bank. But, despite what Jared may want you to believe, Subway is not nutritionally infallible: Those rosy calorie counts posted on the menu boards include neither cheese nor mayo *(add 160 calories per 6-inch sub)*, and some of the toasted subs, like the Meatball Marinara, contain hefty doses of calories, saturated fat, and sodium.

Survival strategy: Cornell researchers have discovered a "health halo" at Subway, which refers to the tendency to reward yourself or your kid with chips, cookies, and large soft drinks because the entrée is healthy. Avoid the halo, and all will be well.

Jamba Juice: A-

Jamba offers a viable and tasty solution to the dearth of fresh fruits and vegetables in the American diet: Stick it all in a blender and let us slurp it up. But make this your rule: If it includes syrup or added sugar, it ceases to be a smoothie. Jamba Juice makes plenty of real-deal smoothies, but their menu is sullied with more than a few faux-fruit blends. Just make sure you choose the right one.

Survival strategy: For a perfectly guilt-free treat, opt for a Jamba Light or All Fruit Smoothie in a 16-oz. cup. And unless you're looking to put on weight for your new acting career, don't touch the Peanut Butter Moo'd, which has more sugar than an entire bag of chocolate chips!

Au Bon Pain: A-

Sure the menu has its pitfalls, but what menu doesn't? The bottom line is that Au Bon Pain combines an extensive inventory of healthy items with an unrivaled standard of nutritional transparency. Each store has an on-site nutritional kiosk to help customers find a meal to meet their expectations, and the variety of ordering options provides dozens of paths to a sensible meal.

Survival strategy: Most of the café sandwiches are in the 650-calorie range, so make a lean meal instead by combining a hot soup with one of the many low-calorie options on the Portions menu. And if you must indulge, eschew the baked goods in favor of a cup of fruit and yogurt, or serving of chocolate-covered almonds.

Boston Market: B+

With more than a dozen healthy vegetable sides and lean meats like turkey and roast sirloin on the menu, the low-cal, high-nutrient possibilities at Boston Market are endless. But with nearly a dozen calorie-packed sides and fatty meats like dark meat chicken and meat loaf, it's almost as easy to construct a lousy meal.

Survival strategy: There are three simple steps to nutritional salvation: 1) Start with turkey, sirloin, or rotisserie chicken. 2) Add two non-creamy, non-starchy vegetable sides. 3) Ignore all special items, such as pot pie and nearly all of the sandwiches.

Cici's Pizza Buffet: B+

Cici's began in Texas in 1985 and now boasts more than 600 locations, proving definitively that Americans love a good buffet. The good news for our waistlines is that the crust is moderately sized, and the pizza comes in varieties beyond simple sausage and pepperoni. But if you check your willpower at the door, you're probably better off skipping the pizza buffet entirely.

Survival strategy: It takes 20 minutes for your brain to tell your body it's full, so start with a salad and then proceed slowly to the pizza. Limit yourself to the healthier slices like the Zesty Vegetable, Alfredo, and the Olé, which is a Mexican-inspired pie with only 108 calories per slice.

McDonald's: B+

The world-famous burger baron has come a long way since the days of *Fast Food Nation*—at least, nutritionally speaking. The trans fats are mostly gone, the number of gut-wrecking calorie bombs are now fewer than ever, and the menu holds plenty of healthy options such as salads and yogurt parfaits. Don't cut loose at the counter just yet, though. Too many of the breakfast and lunch sandwiches still top the 500-calorie mark, and the dessert menu is fodder for some major belly-building.

Survival strategy: The Egg McMuffin remains one of the best ways to start your day in the fast-food world. As for the later hours, you can splurge on a Big Mac or a Quarter Pounder, but only if you skip the fries and soda, which add an average of 590 calories onto any meal.

Taco Bell: B+

Taco Bell combines two things with bad nutritional reputations: Mexican food and fast food. The result should be horrendous, yet somehow it works out so that a little prudence at the ordering window can bag you a meal with fewer than 500 calories. The potential for belly-building is still there, but the calorie bombs are generally easy to spot. And to limit the chances of a mistake, Taco Bell reengineered some of its classic items and listed them under the Fresco Menu for a savings of up to 10 g fat per item.

Survival strategy: Grilled Stuft *(Stuffed)* Burritos, anything served in a bowl, and anything prepared with multiple layers are your worst options. Instead, order any combination of two of the following: crunchy tacos, bean burritos, or anything on the Fresco menu.

Wendy's: B+

Scoring a decent meal at Wendy's is just about as easy as scoring a bad one, and that's a big compliment for a burger joint. Options such as chili and baked potatoes offer the side-order variety that's missing from less-evolved fast-food chains like Dairy Queen and Carl's Jr. Plus they offer a handful of Jr. Burgers that don't stray far over 300 calories. And for our money, the ¼-pound single is one of the best substantial burgers in the industry.

Where they err is in their recently expanded line of desserts and a lackluster selection of beverages. But you're happy just drinking water, right?

Survival strategy: The grilled chicken sandwiches and wraps don't have more than 320 calories, which is less than even a small order of french fries. Choose the chicken or a small burger and pair it with a healthy side, and then hit the door before you receive the 500-calorie penalty for giving in to your Frosty hankering.

You've seen the better choices; the authors also give us the flip side, the unhealthy restaurants. Read the article and you are faced once again with deciding. *Is it Worth It.*

America's Unhealthiest Restaurants

Going out to eat? The authors of *Eat This, Not That!* have some recommendations on places to avoid. By David Zinczenko and Matt Goulding, *Men's Health*

Here's our list of the Worst Restaurants in America. It'll help you stay on the safer side of town.

Baskin-Robbins: D+

We thought we'd see some improvements after we identified Baskin's Heath Shake as the Worst Drink on the Planet. But all they did was lower it from 2,300 to 1,900 calories, leaving an almost equally egregious drinkable disaster to set back unsuspecting sippers. It's typical of the menu there; B-R's soft serve is among the most caloric in the country; the smoothies contain more sugar than fruit; and most of what Baskin sticks into a cup winds up with more fat than a steakhouse buffet. Check out our list of the 20 Unhealthiest Drinks in America to see other liquid offenders. If you learn how to make smart choices when you sip, you can lose a few pounds a month, without giving up your favorite foods or ever dieting again.

Survival strategy: With frozen yogurt, sherbet, and no-sugar-added ice cream, Baskin's lighter menu is the one bright spot. Just be sure to ask for your ice cream in a sugar or cake cone, the waffle cone will swaddle your treat in an extra 160 calories.

Carl's Jr.: D+

Most fast-food restaurants today are making at least some attempt to offset their bulging burgers and deep-fried sides with healthier options such as lean sandwiches or yogurt parfaits. But Carl's Jr. is swimming against the nutritional tide, trying to attract those with hearty appetites and less concern about fat, salt, and calories. The lightest

item on the breakfast menu, for instance, is the Hash Brown Nuggets—but even they have 21 g fat, 5.5 of them are trans fats. *(As a rule, you should try to get 2 g or fewer of the stuff in an entire day!)* The burgers are worse, and there's not a side on the menu that hasn't been given a long, bubbling bath in their trans-fatty frying oil.

Survival strategy: Find another place to grab lunch. Failing that, you should settle on either the Charbroiled Chicken Salad with Low-Fat Balsamic Dressing or the Charbroiled BBQ Chicken Sandwich—the only sandwich on the menu with fewer than 400 calories.

Denny's: D+

Too bad the adult menu at Denny's doesn't adhere to the same standard as the kids' menu. The famous Slam breakfasts all top 800 calories and the burgers are even worse. The Double Cheeseburger is one of the worst in the country, with 116 g fat, 7 of which are trans fats. Make sure you try to avoid it whenever possible.

Survival strategy: The Fit Fare menu gathers together all the best options on the menu. Outside of that, stick to the sirloin, grilled chicken or soups. For breakfast, order a Veggie Cheese Omelet or create your own meal from à la carte options such as fruit, oatmeal, toast and eggs.

Dairy Queen: D+

Dairy Queen's taste for excess rivals that of other fast-food failures such as Carl's Jr. and Hardees. But unlike Carl's, DQ offers an avalanche of abominable ice cream creations to follow up its sodium-spiked, trans-fatty foods. Here's a look at one hypothetical meal: A Bacon Cheddar GrillBurger with onion rings and a Small Snickers Blizzard—a staggering 1,740-calorie meal with 2,640 mg sodium, 83 g fat, 2 g of which are trans fats.

Survival strategy: Play solid defense. Skip elaborate burgers, fried sides and specialty ice cream concoctions entirely. Order a Grilled Chicken Sandwich or an Original Burger, and if you must have a treat, stick to a small soft-serve or a small sundae.

Ruby Tuesday: D+

The chain earned its fame from a hearty selection of hamburgers. The problem: They average 75 g fat apiece—more than enough to exceed the USDA's recommended limit for the day. Even the veggie and turkey burgers have more than 850 calories! The chain rounds out its menu with a selection of appetizers than hover around 1,000 calories *(supposedly to be split four ways)*, a smattering of high-impact entrées like potpie and ribs, and sloppy selection of salads that's just as bad.

Survival strategy: Solace lies in the three Ss: steak, seafood, and sides. Sirloins, salmon, and shrimp all make for relatively innocuous eating, especially when paired with one of Ruby Tuesday's half-dozen healthy sides such as mashed cauliflower and baby green beans. Other than that, think Mick Jagger, and think about occasionally saying goodbye to Ruby Tuesday!

Chili's: D

From burgers to baby back ribs, Chili's serves up some of the saltiest and fattiest fare on fast-food row. In fact, with 3,810 mg of sodium and 122 g fat, Chili's Smokehouse Bacon Triple Cheese Big Mouth Burger earns the distinction as being one of the worst burgers in America. The Guiltless Grill menu is Chili's attempt to offer healthier options, but with only eight items and an average sodium count of 1,320 mg, there's meager hope for nutritional salvation.

Survival strategy: There's not too much to choose from after you omit the ribs, burgers, fajitas, chicken, and salads. You're better off with a Classic Sirloin and steamed vegetables or broccoli.

Another decent option is the Chicken Fajita Pita with Black Beans and Pico de Gallo. The appetizers are off limits—the Texas Cheese Fries with Jalapeño-Ranch Dressing has 2,070 calories, 160 g fat, and 73 grams of saturated fat!

Uno Chicago Grill: D

Uno has some serious strikes against it: The chain invented the deep-dish pizza, they encouraged gluttony with their Bigger and Better menu, and in 1997 they faced false-advertising charges for erroneously claiming that some of their pizzas were low in fat. They've cleaned up some of the more conspicuous health hazards and have increased nutritional transparency at all of their stores, but from appetizers to desserts, this menu is still riddled with belt-busting fat.

Survival strategy: First off, cast aside the bloated breadstick that Uno tries to sneak onto most plates. Next, choose flatbread over deep-dish pizzas—it could save you more than 1,000 calories. Beyond that, stick to soups or entree items served with mango salsa.

Chevy's: D

Don't let the made-fresh-daily shtick distract you; Chevy's massive portions push many of meals beyond the 1,000-calorie threshold. The Taco Trader's menu has three strikes against it: 1.) The consistently dangerous amount of fat in its entrees *(the average salad has 67 grams)*; 2.) the outrageous salt levels that make it difficult to find a meal with fewer than 2,000 mg of sodium; and 3.) the chain earns its poor score by failing to offer complete nutritional disclosure. It provides no information for its appetizers or quesadillas, for instance, and although it maintains it uses trans-fat free oils, there's no trans-fat data for the full entrees.

Survival strategy: The best items on the menu are the Homemade Tortilla Soup, with just 393 calories and a full 26 grams of protein, and the Santa Fe Chopped Salad, which has only 470 calories when you order it without cheese. If you can't resist an entrée, order it without all the fixin's—tamalito, rice, sour cream, and cheese. That should knock more than 300 calories off your meal.

On the Border: D-

On the Border is a subsidiary of Brinker International, the same parent company that owns Chili's and Romano's Macaroni Grill. It should come as no surprise then that this chain is just as threatening to your health as its corporate cohorts.

The overloaded menu offers appetizers with 120 g fat, salads with a full day's worth of sodium, and taco entrées with a horrific 960 calories—and that's the calculation without rice and beans. Border crossing is a decidedly dangerous enterprise.

Survival strategy: The Border Smart Menu highlights four items with fewer than 600 calories and 25 g fat. Those aren't great numbers, considering they average 1,800 mg of sodium apiece, but that's all you've got to work with.

Romano's Macaroni Grill: D-

For years now we've been on Romano's case to clean up the menu at his beloved Macaroni Grill. So far we've had no luck. This Italian grease spot serves some of the worst appetizers in the country, offers not one dinner entrée with fewer than 800 calories, and hosts no fewer than 60 menu items with more than 2,000 mg of sodium—almost an entire day's worth of salt! A select few menu items earn the restaurant's Sensible Fare logo—a fork with a halo over it—but unfortunately these items can still carry up to 640 calories and 25 g fat.

Survival strategy: Macaroni Grill will let you build your own dish. Ask for the marinara over a bed of the restaurant's whole-wheat penne, and then top it with grilled chicken and steamed vegetables. Just beware their salads—the Seared Sea Scallops Salad has more than 1,000 calories and 90 g fat!

Baja Fresh: D-

It's a surprise Baja Fresh's menu has yet to collapse under the weight of its own fatty fare. About a third of the items on the menu have more than 1,000 calories, and most of them are spiked with enough sodium to melt a polar icecap. Order the Shrimp Burrito Dos Manos Enchilado-Style, for instance, and you're looking at 5,130 mg sodium—that's more than 2 days' worth in one sitting!

Survival strategy: Unless you're comfortable stuffing 110 g fat into your arteries, avoid the nachos at all costs. In fact, avoid almost everything on this menu. The only safe options are the tacos, or a salad topped with salsa verde and served without the belly-busting tortilla bowl.

Applebee's, IHOP, Outback, T.G.I. Friday's: F

These titans of the restaurant industry are among the last national chains that don't offer nutritional information on their dishes. Even after years of badgering their representatives, we still hear the same old excuses: It's too pricey; it's too time-consuming, it's impossible to do accurately because their food is so fresh, or we have too much variety. Our response is simple: If nearly every other chain restaurant in the country can do it, then why can't they?

Survival strategy: Write letters, make phone calls, beg, scream, and plead for these restaurants to provide nutritional information on all of their products. Here's the contact information for each of the restaurants that refuse to fess up!

Applebee's: 888-59APPLE, or send an e-mail from this link
IHOP: 818-240-6055 *(press 1 for Guest Visit issues)*
Outback: send an e-mail from this link
T.G.I. Friday's: 800-FRIDAYS

I recommend ANY and ALL of the *Eat This, Not That!* books to ANYONE that wants to lose 1 oz. of weight or maintain their current weight. I think also on the "flip side", if you want to gain weight that you can look at these books and find out what foods have the highest calories. However, you should think HEALTHY eating and not just calories. There are instances where a 5'10 woman that weighed about 145 pounds developed heart disease. She's in her right weight range but she's not HEALTHY.

Let's end this section on a good note; I've tried to show throughout that healthy eating is a choice and that you have options even at fast food restaurants. The authors of *Eat This, Not That!* have given us more great information to devour and use to avoid an ever expanding waistline.

Fast Food Meals Under 500 Calories

Found at www.health.msn.com/nutrition.com
10 extra-value meals that'll help you save cash and calories.
By Dave Zinczenko and Matt Goulding, Men's Health

Tough times call for desperate measures: Dollar menus and extra-value meals you once dutifully shunned are now starting to look pretty good. Sure, they're bad for you, but, man, what a deal! That's the thought process fast food chains like McDonald's, Burger King, KFC, Taco Bell, and Pizza Hut are banking on—literally. All of these companies have seen sales go up *(as well as their customers' weight)* this year. Considering the dismal economy, we don't blame you for eating less-than-healthy foods to save a few bucks. But we can't just stand here and watch you order the greasiest item on the menu, either. That's why *Eat This, Not That!* has compiled this list of 10 fast food meals under 500 calories.

Less than 500 calories at Burger King

Whopper Jr. without Mayo with Garden Salad and 10-oz Minute Maid Orange Juice

- 445 calories, 12 g fat *(4.5 g saturated fat)*
- 520 mg sodium

Save 9 g fat by opting for barbecue sauce instead of mayo. At 80 calories a packet, BK's mayo is one of the worst in the fast food world. Still feeling hungry after the last bite? Order another Garden Salad. You'll still take in fewer calories than if you had consumed a small order of fries.

Less than 500 calories at Hardee's

Charbroiled BBQ Chicken Sandwich with Side Salad with Low Fat Balsamic Dressing

- 445 calories, 7 g fat *(2.5 g saturated fat)*
- 1,690 mg sodium

More Healthy Eating Advice
- Best and Worst Burgers
- America's Healthiest Supermarket Foods
- Search: Low-Calorie Diets

Barbecue sauce and a mound of fresh produce keep this meal in the safe zone. Just don't order a Carl's Jr. shake or malt, and you're good to go. Check out some of the other worst beverages in America here.

Less than 500 calories at Dunkin' Donuts

Ham, Egg & Cheese English Muffin Sandwich with English Breakfast Tea

- 350 calories, 15 g fat *(6 g saturated fat)*
- 1,040 mg sodium

English muffins have a fraction of the carbohydrates of a bagel, and none of the trans fats of the donuts and croissants. The antioxidant-rich tea is also a great way to begin your day.

Less than 500 calories at Jack in the Box

Chicken Fajita Pita with Side Salad with Low-Fat Balsamic Vinaigrette Dressing, and a 20-oz Fresh Brewed Iced Tea

- 390 calories, 13.5 g fat *(5 g saturated fat)*
- 1,650 mg sodium

Loaded with fresh veggies in a fairly harmless pita vessel, this is the healthiest entrée available at Jack's, hands down. Your biggest potential culprit here is in the salad dressing—the low-fat balsamic comes with 35 calories, but other decent-sounding options, like Asian Sesame Dressing and Lite Ranch add over 100 extra to your meal.

Less than 500 calories at KFC

3 Crispy Strips with Green Beans, 3" Corn on the Cob and a Medium Diet Pepsi

- 475 calories, 22.5 g fat *(6 g saturated fat)*
- 1,165 mg sodium

Order a side of green beans for a good source of vitamins K, A and C—key players in maintaining strong bones and reducing cancer-causing free radicals.

Less than 500 calories at McDonald's

Premium Grilled Chicken Classic Sandwich with a Side Salad with Newman's Own Low Fat Balsamic Vinaigrette, and a medium iced tea

- 480 calories, 13 g fat *(2 g saturated fat)*
- 1,945 mg sodium

Counting calories doesn't mean your meal is healthy. For example: the Grilled Chicken Classic Sandwich matches the Quarter Pounder without cheese when it comes to caloric content, but the chicken has no trans fats, while the burger does. Choose the sandwich and side salad for a good combination of protein and veggies.

Less than 500 calories at Pizza Hut

Two Slices Thin 'N Crispy Pizza *(12")* **with Quartered Ham & Pineapple, and a medium Diet Coke**

- 360 calories, 12 g fat *(5 g saturated fat)*
- 1,110 mg sodium

Regardless of which pizza chain you favor, ham and pineapple is one of the most trusted combinations you can order. Ham is the leanest meat you can put on a pie, while pineapple adds low-cal sweetness and a dose of antioxidants.

Less than 500 calories at Quiznos

Small Honey Bourbon Chicken with a Cup of Chili *(no crackers)* **and bottle of water**

- 460 calories, 11.5 g fat *(2.5 g saturated fat)*
- 1,540 mg sodium

Opt for the honey bourbon mustard sauce over mayo or creamy dressings to add flavor without guilt.

Less than 500 calories at Taco Bell

Two Fresco Soft Beef Tacos with Mexican Rice and a bottle of water

- 470 calories, 17 g fat *(6 g saturated fat)*
- 1,760 mg sodium

Order almost any menu item fresco style and the Bell boys will replace cheese and sauces with a chunky tomato salsa, cutting calories and fat by at least 25 percent. Beyond being nutritious, salsa is also cheap; check out our list of the other healthiest cheap foods you can eat.

Less than 500 calories at Wendy's

Ultimate Chicken Grill Sandwich with mandarin orange cup and small Nestea Sweetened Iced Tea

- 480 calories, 7 g fat *(1.5 g saturated fat)*
- 980 mg sodium

This is the healthiest sandwich on the menu. Don't order your chicken spicy, though: That's their cue to fry, rather than grill your bird, tacking on an extra 9.5 g fat.

SPECIAL SECTION:
Spotlight on Other Interventions
Diet Pills and Surgical Procedures

According to *Fat-Exploding the Myths* by Lisa Colles, Americans are reported to spend between $30-50 billion each year on diet and weight loss programs, products and pills; $6 billion of this is said to be spent on weight loss products and pills that don't work. Again, there is NO MAGIC BULLET, PILL, SHOT or PROCEDURE. However, prescription medications can be used as tools to help you in your weight loss efforts but lifestyle changes must be implemented or when you stop popping the pill or taking the shot— the weight will jump back on you. Additionally, you should never JUST take a pill or start a diet without working in exercise and increased activity.

Prescription Diet Pills

A Dr. Sharon Sidebar:

If you are getting a prescription drug, make sure that it is with a DOCTOR that you know and that has examined you, and not someone off the Internet who wrote you a nice spam email. This is your health and you could DIE following some foolishness and that is NOT Worth It! The diet pills below are all approved for use in the United States by the Food and Drug Administration but should be used with caution. Additionally, if you have health conditions—TELL your doctor *(especially racing heart, irregular heart beats, high blood pressure, diabetes, thyroid disease, etc.).* Do not try to find a doctor who does not know your medical history in an effort to manipulate them into prescribing you change you to a medication for weight loss.

Prescription Drug	Fast Facts	Other Information
Diethylpropion **Brand names**: Tenuate, Tenuate dospan	• Appetite suppressant. • Diethylpropion stimulates the central nervous system which increases heart rate and blood pressure and decreases appetite.	• Only Orlistat and Sibutramine are cleared by the FDA for more long term use *(up to 2 years).*
Mazindol **Brand names**: Sanorex, Mazanor	• Appetite suppressant. • Possible side effect may include: 　• An irregular heartbeat or very high blood pressure 　• Severe headache, dizziness, blurred vision, hallucinations, or confusion 　• An allergic reaction 　• Restlessness, tremor, nervousness, anxiety, or insomnia 　• Dry mouth or an unpleasant taste in your mouth, 　• Diarrhea or constipation 　• Impotence or changes in your sex drive. • May also be habit forming.	
Orlistat **Brand names**: Xenical	• Fat blocker • Works by preventing your body from breaking down and absorbing fat eaten with your meals. This unabsorbed fat is eliminated in bowel movements. • Reduces the body's ability to absorb dietary fat by about one third.	• Sold over the counter as Alli • You must follow a low-fat meal plan or you may have an accident *(excess fat leaks out onto clothes).*

Prescription Drug	Fast Facts	Other Information

Phendimetrazine
 	
Brand names: Bontril Plegine, Prelu-2, X-Trozine
	▪ Appetite suppressant.
	▪ Possible side effect may include:
	  ▪ An irregular heartbeat or very high blood pressure
	  ▪ Severe headache, dizziness, blurred vision, hallucinations, or confusion
	  ▪ An allergic reaction
	  ▪ Restlessness, tremor, nervousness, anxiety, or insomnia
	  ▪ Dry mouth or an unpleasant taste in your mouth,
	  ▪ Diarrhea or constipation
	  ▪ Impotence or changes in your sex drive.
	  ▪ May also be habit forming.	

Phentermine **Brand names**: Adipex-P, Fastin, Ionamin, Oby-trim	▪ Appetite suppressant. ▪ Previously part of the Phen-Fen combination, which resulted in lawsuits.	
Sibutramine **Brand names**: Meridia	▪ Appetite suppressant. ▪ Promote weight loss by tricking the body into believing that it is not hungry or that it is full. It decreases appetite by increasing serotonin or catecholamine—two brain chemicals that affect mood and appetite.	

Over the Counter Diet Products

There is the misperception that over the counter pills and supplements are safer than prescription and that you don't need to tell your doctor about you taking them. That is a LIE! In many cases, you may believe that one is good so two must be great and you end up overdosing on medications *(yes over the counter pills are still medications in my book)* and can end up in the hospital or worse than that in a coffin. Talk with your DOCTOR or health professional prior to beginning any of these medications.

Product Name	Fast Facts	Other Information
Alli	▪ Fat blocker ▪ Works by preventing your body from breaking down and absorbing fat eaten with your meals. This unabsorbed fat is eliminated in bowel movements.	▪ Essentially an over-the-counter version of Orlistat ▪ Eating fatty foods while taking Alli can result in accidents *(excess fat leaks out onto clothes)*.
Caffeine Pills	▪ Some studies indicate that caffeine may slightly boost weight loss or prevent weight gain. But there's no evidence that increased caffeine consumption results in significant or permanent weight loss. ▪ Ways is which caffeine can affect weight: Appetite suppression, Calorie burning via thermogenesis, and water loss by acting as a diuretic.	

Product Name	Fast Facts	Other Information
CortiSlim	• Claimed that high levels of stress increase your body's production of cortisol to the point that causes you to accumulate excess fat. • What they didn't tell you is that this occurs only when your body produces large amounts of cortisol due to a side effect of medication or due to an underlying medical condition such as Cushing's syndrome. • There's no evidence that the ingredients in these products even block cortisol or that blocking cortisol results in weight loss.	
FucoThin	• FucoThin manufacturers claim that the product speeds metabolism and burns fat. • Several studies on rodents show some weight-loss effects, however, to date, there are no clinical trials to show that fucoxanthin is safe or effective for human weight loss.	• *If you want a slim rat, this may be an option.*
Green Tea Extract	• Claims to increase calorie and fat metabolism and decrease appetite • Limited evidence to support the claim. • May contain a large amount of caffeine.	
Hoodia	• A cactus that is native to the Kalahari Desert in Africa. Natives supposedly eat it to reduce hunger during long hunts, which led to interest in hoodia as a possible weight-loss aid. • No conclusive evidence that hoodia is an effective appetite suppressant or that it contributes to significant, long-term weight loss. • Concentration of hoodia in various supplements varies.	
Hydroxycut	• Claims to remove weight via thermogenics *(increasing the body's metabolism by affecting it's heat regulation and requiring to use more energy)*. • Has been linked to liver damage and some has been recalled.	
Leptoprin Generic version: Leptopril	• One of the most expensive diet pills, though the ingredients vary little from other brands and consist mainly of caffeine. • Claims to be for serious weight loss of more than 20 pounds.	
Xenadrine	• New formula recently removed ephedrine from ingredients. • Effectiveness and intensity of ingredients is disputed. • Claims to support weight loss, increase your metabolism to burn calories, and increase energy.	

Surgical Procedures

The advances in weight loss surgery are quite remarkable. However, there are RISKS with each and every procedure. This should not be taken lightly and you must understand the risks prior to undergoing the procedure. Additionally, there are Americans who are going to other countries to get the procedures done and may or may not have good outcomes. COMMON SENSE and you must still realize that it is a lifestyle change and that there is no magic bullet or scalpel.

Procedure Name	Fast Facts	Other Information
Biliopancreatic Diversion	<ul><li>Type of Gastric Bypass Surgery.</li><li>The goal is to restrict the amount of food consumed and alter the normal digestive process to a much greater degree.</li><li>While this operation reduces the size of the stomach, the stomach pouch created is much larger than with other procedures.</li></ul>	
Ear stapling	<ul><li>Based loosely on the principles of auricular acupuncture, which involves stimulating certain points on the ear with fine needles</li><li>Small surgical staples are placed into the inner cartilage of each ear. The staples are left in place for several months.</li><li>Proponents of ear stapling for weight loss claim that the staples stimulate a pressure point that controls appetite.</li><li>Hasn't been proved effective for weight loss. And the largely unregulated practice of ear stapling can be dangerous if done in unsanitary conditions or by an untrained practitioner. In fact, puncturing ear cartilage poses a risk of serious infection and permanent disfigurement.</li></ul>	<ul><li>*Can you hear me now?*</li><li>*Dumb!*</li></ul>
Gastric Balloon	<ul><li>Inserted without incisions, the balloon would fill up space in the stomach to make a person feel full after eating less food.</li><li>Not yet available in the US.</li></ul>	
Gastric Bypass Surgery	<ul><li>Changes the anatomy of your digestive system to limit the amount of food you can eat and digest.</li><li>A small pouch is created at the top of the stomach using surgical staples or a plastic band. The smaller stomach is connected directly to the middle portion of the small intestine bypassing the rest of the stomach and the upper portion of the small intestine where most absorption occurs.</li><li>Surgery is generally considered when your BMI is 40 or higher or you have a life-threatening or disabling condition related to your weight.</li></ul>	<ul><li>Not a miracle cure. If you do not change your eating style, you will regain weight.</li></ul>
Laparoscopic Adjustable Gastric Banding	<ul><li>A purely restrictive surgical procedure in which a band is placed around the upper most part of the stomach.</li><li>Because food is regulated, most patients feel full faster. Food digestion occurs through the normal digestive process.</li></ul>	
Lipodissolve	<ul><li>Advertised as a noninvasive alternative to liposuction, this is a new injection that allegedly dissolves fat on your hips, waist, thighs and buttocks.</li><li>These injections are not approved for use in the United States, nor have they been proved safe.</li></ul>	<ul><li>Potential side effects include: infection, scarring, necrosis and liver damage</li></ul>
Liposuction	<ul><li>The removal of fat from deposits beneath the skin using a hollow stainless steel tube with the assistance of a powerful vacuum.</li></ul>	
Tummy Tuck	<ul><li>Surgical procedure that tightens abdominal muscles and gets rid of excess skin and fat.</li></ul>	

Part II: Let's Get to the Basics of Physical Fitness and Exercise

As a reminder, we began this book with the understanding that there are several factors that play a role in our weight. Remember the three basic factors that are the major players for most of us:

Fork

Sneakers

Parents

Fork = Food that we take in **Sneakers** = Our activity level including exercise **Parents** = Family and genetics

Exercise and physical activity are essential to achieving and maintaining a healthy weight. *The Worth It* model incorporates the fork and the sneaker into the lifestyle change that is necessary for us to achieve our healthy weight goal. If you notice, we've spent a lot of time looking at the number of calories in food, talking about how to shave calories and make better choices. We also need to continue to look at what it really takes to burn a calorie. All physical activity is not created equally. Exercise should be enjoyable.

If you've been walking for 3 miles four times a week in 30 minutes on the same route every day, chances are you're BORED out of your mind. If your mind is bored, so are you arms, legs, heart and the rest of your body. IS YOUR BODY BORED? Mix it UP! The issue is not if we're burning calories but rather it's about the balance of our calories burned vs. calories eaten. The problem is that we often OVERESTIMATE the number of calories that we burn and UNDERESTIMATE the number of calories that we eat and thus we're out of balance. This is supported by a study from Cornell University which demonstrated that the larger a meal is the less accurate people are at estimating its calories. When asked to guess the calorie count in a fast food meal, people underestimated by about 300 calories. On the opposite end of the spectrum; a recent study showed that overweight women who exercised one to two hours a week lost several pounds in six months without dieting. But those who exercised the most—about three hours a week—didn't lose as much as they should have, possibly because they increased the calories they consumed. "There is a great lesson here: People generally overestimate the calories they are burning with exercise, and they may reward themselves by eating more," says lead researcher Tim Church, director of preventive-medicine research at the Pennington Biomedical Research Center in Baton Rouge.

A Dr. Sharon Sidebar:
Let's take a moment to look at *The Worth It* philosophy. You're at your desk and you've exercised at lunch with a nice walk. You're feeling good and see some jelly beans on your desk. You believe that you've earned a treat by taking a stroll during lunch so you grab a few *(a.k.a. 25 or so)*. What did you just do? You basically just robbed yourself of some of your well earned calorie deficit and chances are because jelly beans have high sugar; you're going to eat more and get hungrier. Remember that you must BURN 3,500 calories more than you take in to lose just 1 pound.

Jelly Beans

A reminder to burn off 25 jelly beans *(approx. 140 calories)* you would have to:

Activity	130 lbs	150 lbs	170 lbs	190 lbs	220 lbs	250 lbs	270 lbs
Aerobics, General	22 mins.	19 mins	17 mins.	15 mins.	13 mins.	11 mins.	11 mins.
Bicycle, Stationary	20 mins.	18 mins.	16 mins.	14 mins.	12 mins.	11 mins.	10 mins.
Calisthenics *(push-ups, sit-ups, pull-ups, jumping jacks)*	18 mins.	15 mins.	14 mins.	12 mins.	10 mins.	9 mins.	9 mins.
Food Shopping	62 mins.	54 mins.	47 mins.	42 mins.	37 mins.	32 mins.	30 mins.
Gardening, General	36 mins.	31 mins.	27 mins	24 mins	21 mins.	19 mins.	17 mins.
Raking Lawn	33 mins.	29 mins.	25 mins.	23 mins	20 mins.	17 mins.	16 mins.
Sex, General, Moderate	110 mins.	95 mins.	84 mins.	75 mins.	65 mins.	57 mins.	53 mins.

Shoveling Snow	24 mins.	21 mins.	18 mins.	16 mins.	14 mins.	12 mins.	11 mins.
Sweep Floors	43 mins.	37 mins.	33 mins.	30 mins.	25 mins.	23 mins.	21 mins.
Treadmill	16 mins.	14 mins.	12 mins.	11 mins.	9 mins.	8 mins.	8 mins.
Vacuum	41 mins.	35 mins.	31 mins.	28 mins.	24 mins.	21 mins.	20 mins.
Volleyball	36 mins.	31 mins.	27 mins.	24 mins.	21 mins.	19 mins.	17 mins.
Washing Dishes	62 mins.	54 mins.	47 mins.	42 mins.	37 mins.	32 mins.	30 mins.
Weight Lifting	47 mins.	41 mins.	36 mins.	33 mins.	28 mins.	25 mins.	23 mins.

We all know that exercise is beneficial. This same research team was able to demonstrate in another study that sedentary women who started exercising said they had a lot more energy and were in better moods than when they were inactive. The more exercise they did, the better they felt, but even 10 minutes more exercise a day gave them some quality of life benefits, says Tim Church. The women felt more confident about doing everyday tasks—such as keeping up with their grandkids, climbing the stairs and carrying in the groceries—and they felt better about themselves when they were in social situations, he says. They experienced these improvements even if they didn't lose weight, he says.

A large body of research shows that regular physical activity lowers blood pressure, cholesterol and the risk of heart disease, diabetes and cancer. Indeed, we all are aware *(if we're honest)* of the benefits of exercise. The CDC spells it out for us in the segment below which is found on their website.

Physical Activity and Health

Found at www.cdc.gov/physicalactivity/everyone/health/index.html)

The Benefits of Physical Activity

Regular physical activity is one of the most important things you can do for your health. It can help:

- Control your weight
- Reduce your risk of cardiovascular disease
- Reduce your risk for type 2 diabetes and metabolic syndrome
- Reduce your risk of some cancers
- Strengthen your bones and muscles
- Improve your mental health and mood
- Improve your ability to do daily activities and prevent falls, if you're an older adult
- Increase your chances of living longer

If you're not sure about becoming active or boosting your level of physical activity because you're afraid of getting hurt, the good news is that *moderate-intensity aerobic activity*, like brisk walking, is generally *safe for most people*.

Start slowly. Cardiac events, such as a heart attack, are rare during physical activity. But the risk does go up when you suddenly become much more active than usual. For example, you can put yourself at risk if you don't usually get much physical activity and then all of a sudden do vigorous-intensity aerobic activity, like shoveling snow. That's why it's important to start slowly and gradually increase your level of activity.

If you have a chronic health condition such as arthritis, diabetes or heart disease talk with your doctor to find out if your condition limits, in any way, your ability to be active. Then, work with your doctor to come up with a physical activity plan that matches your abilities. If your condition stops you from meeting the minimum Guidelines, try to do as much as you can. What's important is that you avoid being inactive. Even 60 minutes a week of moderate-intensity aerobic activity is good for you.

The bottom line is the health benefits of physical activity far outweigh the risks of getting hurt.

If you want to know more about how physical activity improves your health, the section below gives more detail on what research studies have found.

Control Your Weight

Looking to get to or stay at a healthy weight? Both diet and physical activity play a critical role in controlling your weight. You gain weight when the calories you burn, including those burned during physical activity, are less than the calories you eat or drink. For more information see our section on balancing calories. When it comes to weight management, people vary greatly in how much physical activity they need. You may need to be more active than others to achieve or maintain a healthy weight.

To maintain your weight: Work your way up to 150 minutes of moderate-intensity aerobic activity, 75 minutes of vigorous-intensity aerobic activity, or an equivalent mix of the two each week. Strong scientific evidence shows that physical activity can help you maintain your weight over time. However, the exact amount of physical activity needed to do this is not clear since it varies greatly from person to person. It's possible that you may need to do more than the equivalent of 150 minutes of moderate-intensity activity a week to maintain your weight.

To lose weight and keep it off: You will need a high amount of physical activity unless you also adjust your diet and reduce the amount of calories you're eating and drinking. Getting to and staying at a healthy weight requires both regular physical activity and a healthy eating plan. The CDC has some great tools and information about nutrition, physical activity and weight loss. For more information, visit Healthy Weight.

Reduce Your Risk of Cardiovascular Disease

Heart disease and stroke are two of the leading causes of death in the United States. But following the Guidelines and getting at least 150 minutes a week *(2 hours and 30 minutes)* of moderate-intensity aerobic activity can put you at a lower risk for these diseases. You can reduce your risk even further with more physical activity. Regular physical activity can also lower your blood pressure and improve your cholesterol levels.

Reduce your risk of Type 2 Diabetes and Metabolic Syndrome

Regular physical activity can reduce your risk of developing type 2 diabetes and metabolic syndrome. Metabolic syndrome is a condition in which you have some combination of too much fat around the waist, high blood pressure, low HDL cholesterol, high triglycerides, or high blood sugar. Research shows that lower rates of these conditions are seen with 120 to 150 minutes *(2 hours to 2 hours and 30 minutes)* a week of at least moderate-intensity aerobic activity. And the more physical activity you do, the lower your risk will be.

Already have type 2 diabetes? Regular physical activity can help control your blood glucose levels. To find out more, visit Diabetes and Me.

Reduce Your Risk of Some Cancers

Being physically active lowers your risk for two types of cancer: colon and breast.

Research shows that:

- Physically active people have a lower risk of colon cancer than do people who are not active.

- Physically active women have a lower risk of breast cancer than do people who are not active.

Reduce your risk of endometrial and lung cancer. Although the research is not yet final, some findings suggest that your risk of endometrial cancer and lung cancer may be lower if you get regular physical activity compared to people who are not active.

Improve your quality of life. If you are a cancer survivor, research shows that getting regular physical activity not only helps give you a better quality of life, but also improves your physical fitness.

Strengthen Your Bones and Muscles

As you age, it's important to protect your bones, joints and muscles. Not only do they support your body and help you move, but keeping bones, joints and muscles healthy can help ensure that you're able to do your daily activities and be physically active. Research shows that doing aerobic, muscle-strengthening and bone-strengthening physical activity of at least a moderately-intense level can slow the loss of bone density that comes with age.

Hip fracture is a serious health condition that can have life-changing negative effects, especially if you're an older adult. But research shows that people who do 120 to 300 minutes of at least moderate-intensity aerobic activity each week have a lower risk of hip fracture.

Regular physical activity helps with arthritis and other conditions affecting the joints. If you have arthritis, research shows that doing 130 to 150 *(2 hours and 10 minutes to 2 hours and 30 minutes)* a week of moderate-intensity, low-impact aerobic activity can not only improve your ability to manage pain and do everyday tasks, but it can also make your quality of life better.

Build strong, healthy muscles. Muscle-strengthening activities can help you increase or maintain your muscle mass and strength. Slowly increasing the amount of weight and number of repetitions you do will give you even more benefits, no matter your age.

Improve Your Mental Health and Mood

Regular physical activity can help keep your thinking, learning, and judgment skills sharp as you age. It can also reduce your risk of depression and may help you sleep better. Research has shown that doing aerobic or a mix of aerobic and muscle-strengthening activities 3 to 5 times a week for 30 to 60 minutes can give you these mental health benefits. Some scientific evidence has also shown that even lower levels of physical activity can be beneficial.

Improve Your Ability to do Daily Activities and Prevent Falls

A functional limitation is a loss of the ability to do everyday activities such as climbing stairs, grocery shopping, or playing with your grandchildren.

How does this relate to physical activity? If you're a physically active middle-aged or older adult, you have a lower risk of functional limitations than people who are inactive

Already have trouble doing some of your everyday activities? Aerobic and muscle-strengthening activities can help improve your ability to do these types of tasks.

Are you an older adult who is at risk for falls? Research shows that doing balance and muscle-strengthening activities each week along with moderate-intensity aerobic activity, like brisk walking, can help reduce your risk of falling.

Increase Your Chances of Living Longer

Science shows that physical activity can reduce your risk of dying early from the leading causes of death, like heart disease and some cancers. This is remarkable in two ways:

1. Only a few lifestyle choices have as large an impact on your health as physical activity. People who are physically active for about 7 hours a week have a 40 percent lower risk of dying early than those who are active for less than 30 minutes a week.

2. You don't have to do high amounts of activity or vigorous-intensity activity to reduce your risk of premature death. You can put yourself at lower risk of dying early by doing at least 150 minutes a week of moderate-intensity aerobic activity.

Everyone can gain the health benefits of physical activity; age, ethnicity, shape or size do not matter.

Sometimes when we think of exercise, our immediate go to excuse is that we just don't have time. Well as I say all the time: *"If you have time to eat, you have time to exercise."* As a very busy person, I certainly understand that it is hard to carve out time to exercise. Other questions are related to "What should I do? Cardio/Aerobic or Lifting Weights/Strength training?" Let's look further at the types of physical activity.

Five Basic but Essential Definitions

Found at www.cdc.gov

Exercise. A subcategory of physical activity that is planned, structured, repetitive, and purposive in the sense that the improvement or maintenance of one or more components of physical fitness is the objective. "Exercise" and "exercise training" frequently are used interchangeably and generally refer to physical activity performed during leisure time with the primary purpose of improving or maintaining physical fitness, physical performance or health.

1. **Aerobic physical activity *(often referred to as cardio)*.** Activity in which the body's large muscles move in a rhythmic manner for a sustained period of time. Aerobic activity, also called endurance activity, improves fitness of the heart and lungs. Examples include walking, running, swimming, bicycling and even dancing. There are different levels and your heart beat will tell you if you're really working it or just playing. MIX it up—why not try a Zumba or kick boxing class? One of my personal favorites is spin class—now that will work ya!

2. **Muscle-strengthening activity *(strength training, resistance training, or muscular strength and endurance exercises)*.** Physical activity, including exercise that increases skeletal muscle strength, power, endurance, and mass. This includes resistance training either with equipment *(i.e., bands, etc.)* or your own body, weight lifting with free weights/dumbbells or machines. Anything that builds your strength is included in this category.

3. **Bone-strengthening activity**. Physical activity primarily designed to increase the strength of specific sites in bones that make up the skeletal system. Bone strengthening activities produce an impact or tension force on the bones that promotes bone growth and strength. Running, jumping rope, and lifting weights are examples of bone-strengthening activities and are often a combination of strength and cardio.

4. **Physical fitness**. The ability to carry out daily tasks with vigor and alertness, without undue fatigue, and with ample energy to enjoy leisure-time pursuits and respond to emergencies. Physical fitness includes a number of components consisting of heart/lung endurance *(aerobic power)*, skeletal muscle endurance, skeletal muscle strength, skeletal muscle power, flexibility and balance, speed of movement, reaction time and body composition.

The other essential question that must be answered is that of intensity and are we REALLY working out or just socializing. I want to discuss this before I dig into how much activity we really need; once again the CDC is a great resource of information.

Measuring Physical Activity Intensity

Found at www.cdc.gov/physicalactivity/everyone/measuring/index.html

Here are some ways to understand and measure the intensity of aerobic activity: relative intensity and absolute intensity.

Relative Intensity

The level of effort required by a person to do an activity. When using relative intensity, people pay attention to how physical activity affects their heart rate and breathing.

The talk test is a simple way to measure relative intensity. As a rule of thumb, if you're doing moderate-intensity activity you can talk, but not sing, during the activity. If you're doing vigorous-intensity activity, you will not be able to say more than a few words without pausing for a breath.

Absolute Intensity

The amount of energy used by the body per minute of activity. The table below lists examples of activities classified as moderate-intensity or vigorous-intensity based upon the amount of energy used by the body while doing the activity.

Moderate Intensity

- Walking briskly *(3 miles per hour or faster, but not race-walking)*

- Water aerobics

- Bicycling slower than 10 miles per hour

- Tennis *(doubles)*

- Ballroom dancing

- General gardening

Vigorous Intensity

- Race walking, jogging, or running

- Swimming laps

- Tennis *(singles)*

- Aerobic dancing

- Bicycling 10 miles per hour or faster

- Jumping rope

- Heavy gardening *(continuous digging or hoeing)*

- Hiking uphill or with a heavy backpack

A Dr. Sharon Sidebar:

Can you walk up three flights of stairs without sweating and being out of breath? If you can't—you are NOT physically fit. C'mon let's not lie to ourselves; we know when we're fit and we know when we are just PITIFUL. Most of us live in a world between the two, but it's a new day!

Another way to gauge your intensity is by looking at your target heart rate. I do encourage everyone to buy and use a heart rate monitor.

Target Heart Rate and Estimated Maximum Heart Rate

Found at www.cdc.gov/physicalactivity/everyone/measuring/heartrate.html

One way of monitoring physical activity intensity is to determine whether a person's pulse or heart rate is within the target zone during physical activity.

For moderate-intensity physical activity, a person's target heart rate should be 50 to 70% of his or her maximum heart rate. This maximum rate is based on the person's age. An estimate of a person's maximum age-related heart rate can be obtained by subtracting the person's age from 220. For example, for a 50-year-old person, the estimated maximum age-related heart rate would be calculated as 220 - 50 years = 170 beats per minute *(bpm)*. The 50% and 70% levels would be:

- 50% level: 170 x 0.50 = 85 bpm, and

- 70% level: 170 x 0.70 = 119 bpm

Thus, moderate-intensity physical activity for a 50-year-old person will require that the heart rate remains between 85 and 119 bpm during physical activity.

For vigorous-intensity physical activity, a person's target heart rate should be 70 to 85% of his or her maximum heart rate. To calculate this range, follow the same formula as used above, except change 50 and

70% to 70 and 85%. For example, for a 35-year-old person, the estimated maximum age-related heart rate would be calculated as 220 - 35 years = 185 beats per minute *(bpm)*. The 70% and 85% levels would be:

- 70% level: 185 x 0.70 = 130 bpm, and

- 85% level: 185 x 0.85 = 157 bpm

Thus, vigorous-intensity physical activity for a 35-year-old person will require that the heart rate remain between 130 and 157 bpm during physical activity.

Taking Your Heart Rate

Generally, to determine whether you are exercising within the heart rate target zone, you must stop exercising briefly to take your pulse. You can take the pulse at the neck, the wrist, or the chest. We recommend the wrist. You can feel the radial pulse on the artery of the wrist in line with the thumb. Place the tips of the index and middle fingers over the artery and press lightly. Do not use the thumb. Take a full 60-second count of the heartbeats, or take for 30 seconds and multiply by 2. Start the count on a beat, which is counted as zero. If this number falls between 85 and 119 bpm in the case of the 50-year-old person, he or she is active within the target range for moderate-intensity activity

The next the question becomes how much exercise do we really need to do? Once again, let's look to the CDC for guidance:

How much physical activity do adults need?

Found at .cdc.gov/physicalactivity/everyone/guidelines/adults.html

Physical activity is anything that gets your body moving. According to the 2008 Physical Activity Guidelines for Americans, you need to do two types of physical activity each week to improve your health—aerobic and muscle-strengthening.

A Dr. Sharon Sidebar:

While it's wonderful to exercise with friends and you often spend more time socializing. If you want to spend time with your best friend gossiping, then sit down and do that—don't pretty it up by saying that you're going to exercise together. If you have the energy, breath and desire to laugh and giggle as you stroll, then your intensity level is not high. Also, the gym is not a pick up spot or at least it shouldn't be. Go there with a plan, focus and be nice but be committed to working out and burning calories; otherwise you're wasting your time. I'm just saying, a hello is great, maybe even a how are you doing, but to delve into the last 6 months of your personal triumphs and struggles when you only have 30 minutes allotted in your day to work out is not exercise. PUSH yourself and commit to really working that body and varying your intensity.

For Important Health Benefits
Adults need at least:

2 hours and 30 minutes *(150 minutes)* of moderate-intensity aerobic activity *(i.e., brisk walking)* every week **and**

muscle-strengthening activities on 2 or more days a week that work all major muscle groups *(legs, hips, back, abdomen, chest, shoulders and arms)*.

OR

1 hour and 15 minutes *(75 minutes)* of vigorous-intensity aerobic activity *(i.e., jogging or running)* every week **and**

muscle-strengthening activities on 2 or more days a week that work all major muscle groups *(legs, hips, back, abdomen, chest, shoulders and arms)*.

OR

An equivalent mix of moderate- and vigorous-intensity aerobic activity **and**

muscle-strengthening activities on 2 or more days a week that work all major muscle groups *(legs, hips, back, abdomen, chest, shoulders and arms)*.

For Even GREATER Health Benefits
Adults should increase their activity to:

 5 hours *(300 minutes)* each week of moderate-intensity aerobic activity **and**

 muscle-strengthening activities on 2 or more days a week that work all major muscle groups *(legs, hips, back, abdomen, chest, shoulders and arms).*

OR

 2 hours and 30 minutes *(150 minutes)* each week of vigorous-intensity aerobic activity **and**

 muscle-strengthening activities on 2 or more days a week that work all major muscle groups *(legs, hips, back, abdomen, chest, shoulders and arms).*

OR

An equivalent mix of moderate- and vigorous-intensity aerobic activity **and**

muscle-strengthening activities on 2 or more days a week that work all major muscle groups *(legs, hips, back, abdomen, chest, shoulders and arms).*

More time equals more health benefits

If you go beyond 300 minutes a week of moderate-intensity activity, or 150 minutes a week of vigorous-intensity activity, you'll gain even more health benefits.

Aerobic activity—what counts?

Aerobic activity or "cardio" gets you breathing harder and your heart beating faster. From pushing a lawn mower, to taking a dance class, to biking to the store—all types of activities count. As long as you're doing them at a moderate or vigorous intensity for at least 10 minutes at a time.

Intensity is how hard your body is working during aerobic activity.

How do you know if you're doing light, moderate or vigorous intensity aerobic activities?
For most people, light daily activities such as shopping, cooking, or doing the laundry doesn't count toward the guidelines. Why? Your body isn't working hard enough to get your heart rate up.

Moderate-intensity aerobic activity means you're working hard enough to raise your heart rate and break a sweat. One way to tell is that you'll be able to talk, but not sing the words to your favorite song. Here are some examples of activities that require moderate effort:

*   Walking fast
*   Doing water aerobics
*   Riding a bike on level ground or with few hills
*   Playing doubles tennis
*   Pushing a lawn mower

Build up over time

If you want to do more vigorous-level activities, slowly replace those that take moderate effort like brisk walking, with more vigorous activities like jogging.

Vigorous-intensity aerobic activity means you're breathing hard and fast, and your heart rate has gone up quite a bit. If you're working at this level, you won't be able to say more than a few words without pausing for a breath. Here are some examples of activities that require vigorous effort:

- Jogging or running

- Swimming laps

- Riding a bike fast or on hills

- Playing singles tennis

- Playing basketball

You can do moderate- or vigorous-intensity aerobic activity, or a mix of the two each week. A rule of thumb is that 1 minute of vigorous-intensity activity is about the same as 2 minutes of moderate-intensity activity.

Some people like to do vigorous types of activity because it gives them about the same health benefits in half the time. If you haven't been very active lately, increase your activity level slowly. You need to feel comfortable doing moderate-intensity activities before you move on to more vigorous ones. The guidelines are about doing physical activity that is right for you.

Muscle-strengthening activities—what counts?

Besides aerobic activity, you need to do things to strengthen your muscles at least 2 days a week. These activities should work all the major muscle groups of your body *(legs, hips, back, chest, abdomen, shoulders and arms)*.

To gain health benefits, muscle-strengthening activities need to be done to the point where it's hard for you to do another repetition without help. A repetition is one complete movement of an activity, like lifting a weight or doing a sit-up. Try to do 8–12 repetitions per activity that count as 1 set. Try to do at least 1 set of muscle-strengthening activities, but to gain even more benefits, do 2 or 3 sets.

You can do activities that strengthen your muscles on the same or different days that you do aerobic activity, whatever works best. Just keep in mind that muscle-strengthening activities don't count toward your aerobic activity total.

There are many ways you can strengthen your muscles, whether it's at home or the gym. You may want to try the following:

- Lifting weights

- Working with resistance bands

- Doing exercises that use your body weight for resistance *(i.e., push ups, sit ups)*

- Heavy gardening *(i.e., digging, shoveling)*

- Yoga

What if you have a disability?

If you are an adult with a disability, regular physical activity can provide you with important health benefits, like a stronger heart, lungs, and muscles, improved mental health, and a better ability to do everyday tasks. It's best to talk with your health care provider before you begin a physical activity routine. Try to get advice from a professional with experience in physical activity and disability. They can tell you more about the amounts and types of physical activity that are appropriate for you and your abilities. If you are looking for additional information, visit The National Center on Physical Activity and Disability.*

Now what does the CDC say about our children? Sorry, "little Johnny's" excellent hand strength from hours of video games does not qualify him as being physically fit. Also, what kind of behavior are YOU modeling for junior? Do they ever see YOU exercise anything other than fork to mouth? Do they see you sweating and out of breath with just taking the garbage can to the curb?

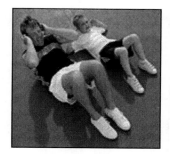

How much physical activity do children need?

Found at www.cdc.gov/physicalactivity/everyone/guidelines/children.html

Children and adolescents should do 60 minutes *(1 hour)* or more of physical activity each day.

This may sound like a lot, but don't worry! Your child may already be meeting the Physical Activity Guidelines for Americans. And, you'll soon discover all the easy and enjoyable ways to help your child meet the recommendations. Encourage your child to participate in activities that are age-appropriate, enjoyable and offer variety! Just make sure your child or adolescent is doing three types of physical activity:

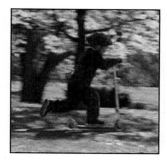

1. Aerobic Activity

Aerobic activity should make up most of your child's 60 or more minutes of physical activity each day. This can include either moderate-intensity aerobic activity, such as brisk walking, or vigorous-intensity activity, such as running. Be sure to include vigorous-intensity aerobic activity on at least 3 days per week.

2. Muscle Strengthening

Include muscle strengthening activities, such as gymnastics or push-ups, at least 3 days per week as part of your child's 60 or more minutes.

3. Bone Strengthening

Include bone strengthening activities, such as jumping rope or running, at least 3 days per week as part of your child's 60 or more minutes.

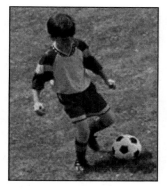

How do I know if my child's aerobic activity is moderate- or vigorous-intensity?

Here are two ways to think about moderate- and vigorous-intensity:

Want examples? Check out Aerobic, muscle- and bone-strengthening: what counts?

As a rule of thumb, on a scale of 0 to 10, where sitting is a 0 and the highest level of activity is a 10, moderate-intensity activity is a 5 or 6. When your son does moderate-intensity activity, his heart will beat faster than normal and he will breathe harder than normal. Vigorous-intensity activity is a level 7 or 8. When your son does vigorous-intensity activity, his heart will beat much faster than normal and he will breathe much harder than normal.

Another way to judge intensity is to think about the activity your child is doing and compare it to the average child. What amount of intensity would the average child use? For example, when your daughter walks to school with friends each morning, she's probably doing moderate-intensity aerobic activity. But while she is at school, when she runs, or chases others by playing tag during recess, she's probably doing vigorous-intensity activity.

What do you mean by age-appropriate activities?

Some physical activity is better-suited for children than adolescents. For example, children do not usually need formal muscle-strengthening programs, such as lifting weights. Younger children usually strengthen their muscles when they do gymnastics, play on a jungle gym or climb trees. As children grow older and become adolescents, they may start structured weight programs. For example, they may do these types of programs along with their football or basketball team practice.

Let's once again take a look at several activities and the amounts of calories burned every minute.

Number of Calories Burned Per Minute

Found at www.dietdetective.com/weightloss/BurnRateProc.do

Activity	130 lb	150 lb	170 lb	190 lb	220 lb	250 lb	270 lb	290 lb	320 lb
Aerobics, Step: 10" - 12" step	10	11	13	15	17	19	21	23	24
Aerobics, Step: 6" - 8" step	8	10	11	13	14	16	18	19	21
Aerobics: high impact	7	8	9	11	12	13	15	16	17
Aerobics: low impact	5	6	7	8	8	9	10	11	12
Aerobics: water	4	5	5	6	7	8	8	9	10
Badminton: general, social	4	5	6	7	8	8	9	10	11
Bakery: general, moderate effort	4	5	5	6	7	8	8	9	10
Basketball: playing a game	8	9	11	12	14	15	17	18	20
Basketball: shooting baskets	6	5	6	7	8	8	9	10	11
Bicycling, Stationery: moderate, 150 watts	7	8	9	11	12	13	15	16	17
Bicycling, Stationery: vigorous, 200 watts	10	12	14	16	18	20	22	24	26
Bowling	3	3	4	5	5	6	6	7	7
Boxing: punching bag	6	7	8	9	10	11	12	14	15
Calisthenics: Moderate, back exercises, going up and down from the floor	3	4	5	5	6	7	7	8	9
Calisthenics: Vigorous, jumping jacks, push-ups, sit-ups, pull-ups	8	9	11	12	14	15	17	18	20
Carpentry Work	3	4	5	5	6	7	7	8	9
Child games: moderate, hop-scotch, jacks	4	5	5	6	7	8	8	9	10
Cleaning House: general	3	3	4	5	5	6	6	7	7
Cleaning: light dusting, straightening up, taking out trash, etc.	2	3	3	4	4	5	5	6	6
Coal Mining	6	7	8	9	10	11	12	14	15
Cooking / Food Preparation	2	3	3	4	4	5	5	6	6
Custodial Work: general cleaning	3	4	5	5	6	7	7	8	9
Dancing: disco, ballroom, square, line, Irish step, polka	4	5	6	7	8	8	9	10	11
Dancing: slow, waltz, foxtrot, tango	3	3	4	5	5	6	6	7	7
Farming, bailing hay, cleaning barn	8	9	11	12	14	15	17	18	20
Farming, milking by hand	3	3	4	5	5	6	6	7	7
Fishing from boat, sitting	2	3	3	4	4	5	5	6	6
Fishing general	3	3	4	5	5	6	6	7	7
Fishing in Stream in waders	6	7	8	9	10	11	12	14	15
Food Shopping: with or without cart	2	3	3	3	4	4	5	5	6
Football or Baseball: playing catch	2	3	3	4	4	5	5	6	6

Activity	130 lb	150 lb	170 lb	190 lb	220 lb	250 lb	270 lb	290 lb	320 lb
Frisbee: general	3	3	4	5	5	6	6	7	7
Gardening: general	4	5	5	6	7	8	8	9	10
Golf: driving range, miniature	3	3	4	5	5	6	6	7	7
Gymnastics: general	4	5	5	6	7	8	8	9	10
Heavy Equip. Operator	2	3	3	4	4	5	5	6	6
Hiking: cross-country	6	7	8	9	10	11	12	14	15
Hockey: field & ice	8	9	11	12	14	15	17	18	20
Horse Grooming	6	7	8	9	10	11	12	14	15
Horseback Riding: general	4	5	5	6	7	8	8	9	10
Ice Skating: general	7	8	9	11	12	13	15	16	17
Ironing	2	3	3	3	4	4	5	5	6
Making Bed	2	2	3	3	3	4	4	5	5
Masonry	7	8	9	11	12	13	15	16	17
Masseur, standing	4	5	5	6	7	8	8	9	10
Mowing Lawn: push, power	5	6	7	8	9	10	11	12	13
Plumbing	3	4	5	5	6	7	7	8	9
Raking Lawn	4	5	6	7	7	8	9	10	11
Rock Climbing	11	12	14	16	18	21	22	24	27
Rope Jumping: general, moderate	10	11	13	15	17	19	21	23	24
Rowing, Stationery: moderate, 100 watts	7	8	9	11	12	13	15	16	17
Rowing, Stationery: vigorous, 150 watts	8	10	11	13	14	16	18	19	21
Running: on track	10	11	13	15	17	19	21	23	24
Running: stairs, up	15	17	20	23	26	28	31	34	37
Shoveling Snow: by hand	6	7	8	9	10	11	12	14	15
Sitting: light office work, meeting	1	2	2	2	3	3	3	3	4
Skateboarding	5	6	7	8	8	9	10	11	12
Ski Machine: general	7	8	9	11	12	13	15	16	17
Skiing: cross-country, light effort, general	7	8	9	11	12	13	15	16	17
Skiing: downhill, moderate effort	6	7	8	9	10	11	12	14	15
Sleeping	1	1	1	1	2	2	2	2	2
Snowmobiling	3	4	5	5	6	7	7	8	9
Soccer: general	7	8	9	11	12	13	15	16	17
Softball: pitching	6	7	8	9	10	11	12	14	15
Stretching: Mild, Yoga	2	3	3	4	4	5	5	6	6
Swimming: backstroke	7	8	9	11	12	13	15	16	17
Swimming: breaststroke	10	11	13	15	17	19	21	23	24
Swimming: butterfly	10	12	14	17	19	21	23	25	27
Swimming: general, leisurely, no laps	6	7	8	9	10	11	12	14	15
Swimming: laps, vigorous	10	11	13	15	17	19	21	23	24
Table Tennis / Ping Pong	4	5	5	6	7	8	8	9	10
Teaching aerobics	6	7	8	9	10	11	12	14	15
Tennis: general play	7	8	9	11	12	13	15	16	17
Trampoline	3	4	5	5	6	7	7	8	9
Typing: Computer, electric or manual	1	2	2	2	3	3	3	3	4

Activity	130 lb	150 lb	170 lb	190 lb	220 lb	250 lb	270 lb	290 lb	320 lb
Vacuuming	3	4	5	5	6	7	7	8	9
Volleyball: non-competitive, general play, 6 - 9 member team	3	3	4	5	5	6	6	7	7
Walking for Pleasure	3	4	5	5	6	7	7	8	9
Walking the Dog	3	3	4	5	5	6	6	7	7
Walking: work break	3	4	5	5	6	7	7	8	9
Watching TV	1	1	1	2	2	2	2	2	2
Weight Lifting: Light, free weight, nautilus or universal	3	3	4	5	5	6	6	7	7
Welding	3	3	4	5	5	6	6	7	7
Yard: watering by hand, standing/walking	1	2	2	2	3	3	3	3	4

Besides weight loss, there are numerous benefits to exercise. Whether you desire to lose or gain weight or just remain healthy; exercise should be an essential part of your life on MOST days. We know that this is true but what do we do, look at this published survey in *Health* magazine:

- 89% of Americans who agree that there's an obesity epidemic

- 26% of Americans who think exercise and fitness are not priorities

- 41% of doctors who ask their patients if they exercise

Exercise Equipment: The Good, Bad and Quacky

Equipment	Claim	Thoughts/Notes
Abdominal *(Ab)* Roller	• Curved rocker design **CLAIMS to:** • Provide support for the head and neck during your ab workout, and • Guide your spine through a natural curved movement *(this is called spinal flexion)* during your ab workout.	• *??? Okay , I'm not running to buy this one.*
Exercise Ball	• A primary benefit of exercising with an exercise ball as opposed to exercising directly on a hard flat surface is that the body responds to the instability of the ball to remain balanced, engaging many more muscles. Those muscles become stronger over time to keep balance. • Most frequently, the core body muscles—the abdominal muscles and back muscles—are the focus of exercise ball fitness programs.	• Some people recommend sitting on an exercise ball instead of a chair *(for example, an office chair)*. • This is based on the theory that the abdominal and back muscles are constantly engaged and active in order to maintain proper posture and balance on the ball. There is no scientific evidence of those benefits occurring by just sitting without additional exercises. • A personal trainer's favorite and a Dr. Sharon staple!

Equipment	Claim	Thoughts/Notes
Leg Magic	▪ Designed track and built-in Pulse Resistance Technology is designed to specifically activate and engage the muscles in your hips, buns and thighs	▪ *A question: What if you use this and the Flex Belt at the same time—how do you avoid electrocution?*
Thigh Master	▪ Made to firm and tone your inner thighs, shape and tone your stomach and abdomen, and tighten your upper arms.	
Flex Belt	▪ Electric Muscle Stimulation product ▪ Claims to deliver firmer, stronger and more toned abdominal muscles.	
The Dumbbell Phone	▪ A phone with a dumbbell attached to it. ▪ The apparent theory is to strengthen muscles by picking up the phone when you answer a call.	▪ *This is a REAL live piece of equipment. Can we say DUMB!*
Vibrating Machine	**Claims to:** ▪ Burn Excess Fat and tone and tighten your skin; ▪ Decreases cellulite and improves your body's natural collagen levels; ▪ Increase muscle strength—as much as 50% in as little as 3 weeks; ▪ Improves your blood circulation and lymphatic drainage; ▪ Builds bone density and fights osteoporosis; ▪ Increase metabolism, helping to burn fat and raise energy levels; ▪ Reduces your back and joint pain; ▪ Decrease blood pressure and cortisol levels; ▪ Dramatically increase your flexibility; ▪ Improved sense of balance and coordination; ▪ Elevates your serotonin levels *(better mood and sense of well being).*	▪ *The jury is still out with me on this one. I want to find a "vibration studio" but have not yet found one in my travels.*

Equipment	Claim	Thoughts/Notes
Resistance Bands	• Useful in performing a variety of exercises from squats to bicep-curls. • Focus should be on the stabilization of your core in order for you to maximize the benefits of the resistance bands that you use.	• Another personal trainer favorite.
Handy Trim	• Works by rotating an aluminum disc by pulling the attached twisted cord rhythmically. • Claims that this exercise showers the blood with oxygen and stimulates circulation, removes metabolites, and ultimately reduces stress levels, tones the entire upper body, firming up muscle tissue and training the large pectoral muscles and triceps.	

Your Body as Your Equipment
Strength Exercises

The Move(s)	Target Area	Other
The Crunch	• This stomach exercise will work your oblique muscles, giving you a better mobility and shape of your stomach area. • Abdominal exercises such as crunches will tone the muscle under the fat but won't flatten your stomach.	• To lose weight, you have to eat less and workout more. • Crunches come in various forms and are controversial; the bottom line is that you need to LOSE belly fat. • Don't bother just doing 100 crunches every morning and night if you're not also doing a combo of cardio and other activities.
The Plank	• Put yourself in a push-up-like position with your body resting on your toes and elbows. Keep your whole body straight like a plank. • Hold the position for a minute or as long as you can and increase as you can. Repeat this and work up to several during workout sessions.	• *I HATE this but it works. This is a great core (midsection) exercise.* • *Did I say that I HATE this?* • *I try to do planks every other day and am praying to one day not despise them.*

The Move(s)	Target Area	Other
The Push Up	• There are different forms of the push up. Traditionally the arms and legs are extended and you use your upper body to "push" you up and down. • Variation: Instead of being on the toes; you bend your knees. • Great for upper body and core strength.	• *Wonderful, great, yeah, yeah, yeah...* • *One of my current trainer's (MacArthur James of Athletic Dominance) favorites and thus the push up remains my enemy.*
Squats and Lunges	• Works the quadriceps, hamstrings and glutes *(booty)*. • Develops balance and stability. • Works large muscles, thus burns more calories. • Strengthens the knees. • Helps develop better posture. • You can do them almost anywhere. • The Squat Jump: A combination of a squat with a propelling upward. This gets the heart rate up and is a strengthening exercise.	• *The Squat Jump I'm convinced is straight from the "devil". This is yet another one of my trainer's favorites.* • *As much as I HATE to admit it; these really do work on the bottom half.*

Your Body as Your Equipment
Core Exercises

Type of Exercise	Claim	Other
Yoga	• Traditional physical and mental disciplines that originated in India. • Involves stretching, body elongation and breathing techniques. • The benefits have been well studied and research continues to mount.	• *Bikram Yoga (Hot Yoga) is a newer version of yoga. The room is heated to over 100 degrees F.* • *I've tried this and you sweat it out; hair is wrecked but you do feel refreshed after the session.*

Type of Exercise	Claim	Other
Pilates	• The program focuses on the core postural muscles which help keep the body balanced and which are essential to providing support for the spine. • In particular, Pilate's exercises teach awareness of breath and alignment of the spine, and aim to strengthen the deep torso muscles.	
Pole dancing	• This form of exercise increases upper body strength *(by using the body itself as resistance)* while toning the body as a whole.	• *Several pole and lap dancing studios have cropped up.* • *Ahhhh the additional benefits are apparent and your significant other will GLADLY pay for this.*
Capoeira	• An Afro-Brazilian art form that combines elements of martial arts, games, music and dance.	
Plyometrics	• A type of exercise training designed to produce fast, powerful movements, and improve the functions of the nervous system, generally for the purpose of improving performance in sports.	
Tae Bo	• Such programs use the motions of martial arts at a rapid pace designed to promote fitness. • Made famous by the "guru" Billy Blanks.	• *My mother swears by Tae Bo and has all the videos.*
Tai Chi	• A series of 19 movements and 1 pose that together make up a meditative form of exercise to which practitioners attribute physical and spiritual health benefits.	

Dr. Sharon's Tips for Exercise

- **Talk with your doctor and get a physical examination before you begin this journey.**

  - This is essential if you have not been active and have other medical conditions.

- **Just DO It.**

  - You WILL come to like it!

  - Stop with all of the excuses!

- **Make an appointment to exercise, plan out your week and put it on the calendar.**

  - Time management is key, but if you can't manage an appointment with yourself then what is going on with your life.

  - We have time to make our hair, nail and shopping appointments. I'm just saying....

- **Work out in the morning.**

  - That's just a Dr. Sharon tip—I try to work out twice a day *(am and pm)* but if I can get in the morning; if my day goes crazy then I've still gotten my workout in.

- **Consider a 10 minute walk after every meal—the mini walks are just as effective as longer ones.**

- **Get the family involved with group physical activities whenever possible—instead of watching a movie—swim, hide and seek, football, basketball and relays.**

  - Have you ever noticed that sometimes the ENTIRE family will be overweight? I wonder why?

- **Take the stairs, park a longer distance from the car, and walk FASTER even when shopping.**

- **KILL the excuses.**

  - I'll mess up my hair:

    - Key point: we focus on hair but what about the lumps and bumps? I want to mess up my lumps and bumps! A ponytail with some serious makeup on looks glamorous. A big booty that is still shaking when you've stopped walking looks like rolling hills. I'm just saying…

  - I don't have time. *(but you always have time to inhale a Big Mac).*

  - I'm too fat to exercise.

    - Some things don't even deserve a response. WHO cares—this is about you start slow and build yourself up. Forget who's looking at you!

  - I don't have the money to join a gym.

    - Walking outdoors or in place in your living room is FREE. There are also places like community centers, the YMCA and other facilities that have payment plans.
    - Find money in other places; like stop eating out so much.

- **Buy a Jump Rope.**

  - You can jump rope anywhere and anytime of the day and TORCH calories. I also like to jump rope between my strength training sets to get the heart rate up *(learned this from personal trainer Jennifer Boozer—hated her for it but learned it anyway).*

- **Gym Membership vs. NO is based on YOU.**

- **I belong to 2 gyms and have in the past belonged to 3. I have a gym in my home that is beautiful but I never use it. I need the motivation, the variety of activity, machines and the lack of distractions that my gyms bring to me.**

  - A great big shout out to the staff and members of Bowie Sportfit, if you live in Maryland check them out and tell them that I sent you *(ask for Gigi Nash)* and ask for a discount! I work out with my current trainer, MacArthur James, Jr. at this club. EXCELLENT spin classes with Gigi, Lo, Becky and other instructors.

  - Another shout out to Bally's Total Fitness on Central Avenue in Capital Heights Maryland. *The "Worth It" Philosophy* was born there working out with Jennifer Boozer, personal trainer. I remain at Bally's for convenience as it is closer to my office but also for 1 class—that is the Saturday KILLER class with Howard *(come get it)*—the "baddest" instructor on the planet. Ask for a discount here too—really always ask no matter where you go for a discount; what could it hurt?

- **Aim to work out for 6-7 times a week a minimum of 45-90 minutes.**

  - If you don't hit this target then you may come close; but if you aim for 2-3 times a week you may only make one day. This being said, avoid overtraining and becoming obsessive about working out *(note to self)*.

  - If you're serious about losing the weight then you have to be serious about your time commitment.

  - Get up earlier and make some adjustments in your life to find time for workouts.

  - Don't just focus on cardio or strength training; you should do both.

- **Vary your workouts; avoid burnout and your body getting used to your routine.**

  - Visit with a personal trainer, most gyms will give you at least a free session with your membership.

  - Personal trainers are EXPERTS *(or should be)* and often you need their guidance, motivation and ability to help you meet your goals.

    - Make sure that you check references and keep the trainer "in their lane". Trainers are not nutritionists and although they may be well versed in this area; sometimes you need to just focus on the exercise and body mechanics.

    - Get an evaluation BEFORE the trainer puts you on a program. Did you know that according to one study 77% of trainers put clients on a fitness program without assessing them first?

  - The question of finances comes up with the cost of gym memberships and of course with personal trainers. However, you have to decide if it's worth it to you? If it means that you purchase one less pair of shoes, six less Big Macs that you don't need or make other adjustments in your budget—that is a question that you have to answer.

  - Another good idea is to join a boot camp *(MacArthur James of Athletic Dominance is the master boot camp instructor)* which is usually less expensive than individual training sessions. Grab a friend and commit to buddy sessions with a trainer so that you can split the costs.

- **Listen to Music.**

  - Studies show that persons that listen to music actually burn more calories.

  - Also if you have your iPod on, people won't talk to you as much and distract you.

Other Exercise and Fitness Tips
I BET you don't know all of these!
(Found from a variety of sources like Shape, Fitness *and* Health *magazines as well as online site).*

- Shape magazine reported in 2006 that nearly 20 percent of women now strength train twice a week, slightly more than the 17.5 percent who pumped iron in 2004, according to research from the U.S. Centers for Disease Control and Prevention. That's great, but it also means that 80 percent of women still aren't lifting regularly. To give you a nudge—okay, a firm push—toward the dumbbells, here are three mini mantras Shape published to will help persuade you to add weights to your routine today. Take a look at them whenever you need incentive to head to the gym and do some strength training:

    a.   I'll stave off osteoporosis. Resistance training increases bone density, which can prevent age-related loss.

    b.   I'll keep my metabolism revved—muscle trumps fat for calorie burning—add more, burn more.

    c.   I'll look slimmer. Pound for pound, muscle takes fat. Boost muscle and I'll appear thinner.

- Pick up the pace. In study at the University of Alberta, people who exercised at a moderate intensity *(55 to 70 percent of their maximum heart rate)* four times a week for six months increased their fitness level by 10 percent. While those who walked 10,000 steps daily at a speed of their choice only improved by 4 percent. To boost your intensity, spend half of each walk moving at a pace that makes it tough to chat.

- Burn 100 calories FAST

    a.   Eat high-fiber cereal or an apple before you work out.

    In a study at Loughborough University in England, exercisers who had a meal that contained low-glycemic carbs *(from certain fruits as well as from whole grains)* three hours before a run were able to keep at it eight minutes longer than those who fueled up with high-glycemic carbs *(found in white-flour breads)*. Get more oomph from whole-wheat crackers, an apple, or half a cup of beans.

    b.   Plunk a few ice cubes into your water bottle.

    Researchers from England's University of Birmingham found that cyclists who sipped an icy 40°F drink were able to work out seven minutes longer than those who hydrated with a beverage at room temperature. "When your body gets too warm, your brain tells you to stop," says lead author Toby Mündel, PhD. "Cold drinks may slow this process." Whether you're biking or dancing, Mündel recommends drinking half a cup of ice water every 15 to 20 minutes.

- According to *Shape* magazine, **whether your workout includes cardio, weights or a little of both, these tips will help you get more bang from your bout.**

    - *Reorder your strength moves* begin with exercises that work smaller muscle groups—like triceps extensions and calf raises—and finish with moves for your chest, back, and legs. You'll produce less lactic acid early on, say researchers from Elon University, which will help you crank out more reps and get sculpted faster.

    - *Don't tune out when you run* You push harder and move quicker when you know how much farther you have to go, according to a study published in the *British Journal of Sports Medicine*. So amp your route and look for mile markers to cue you to sprint to the finish.

    - *Get in the game during cardio* A medicine & Science in sports & Exercise study found that people who rode stationary bikes with interactive programs torched more calories—without feeling like they were working harder—than those who pedaled on game-free rides.

- Don't forget: Exercise boosts your memory. Those of us who can never seem to find our keys are one sweaty step closer to a cure. We already know exercise can help improve memory, but the scientists behind a recent study in the *Proceedings of the National Academy of Sciences* are the first to show that working out sparks the regrowth of neurons in the part of the brain affected by age-related memory loss.

- Sore subject. Lifting dumbbells is a smart way to beat backaches, a study in *The Journal of Strength and Conditioning Research* shows. Sufferers who trained with free weights and machines for 16 weeks reduced back pain by 60 percent; those who did cardio had only a 6 percent drop being toned all over fights fatigue throughout the day, which eases soreness, experts say

- Fabulous Abs formula. Picking up your workout pace can streamline your midsection, according to researchers from the University of Virginia in Charlottesville. Women who added three 20-minutes high-intensity jogs or walks to their weekly walking routine lost an average of 2 inches from their waist over for months, whereas those who stuck with less intense strolls lost only half an inch. Scientists say stepping up your sessions may release more growth hormones, which help your body burn fat faster. Not hot on trotting? Sub any vigorous activity you enjoy to help flatten your middle in a flash.

- Run it Then eat it or Vice Versa? Planning to indulge in a decadent dinner? Hit the gym first to burn fat and afterwards for heart health.

  - Cardio stints before high-cal meals can fend off fat, researchers from the University of Michigan at Ann Arbor report. Women who worked out before overeating increased their fat-burning rate, and those who pigged out without exercising decreased theirs. Aim to sweat at a moderate intensity, researchers say.

  - Eating fatty foods can cause arteries to lose elasticity for six hours, but exercise can buffer the effect, scientists at Indiana University at Bloomington suggest. Study participants who walked for 45 minutes two hours after a fast food breakfast maintained the same healthy heart function as those who are a fat-free meal and then rested. Have a side of strides with that burger.

- Try the 20-minute rule—and make every minute count. If you can't get to the gym for as long as you'd like, interval training—bursts of intensity followed by a brief recovery period—gets results that are often just as good *(if not better)* than longer, slower-paced workouts. A study from Laval University in Quebec found that subjects who practiced internal training lost significantly more body fat than those who went slow and steady.

- Breast bonus: Overweight women who were most active in the year before being diagnosed with breast cancer were 30 percent more likely to survive than those who were inactive, a study of some 1,200 women at the University of North Carolina at Chapel Hill shows. Exercise may be a potent weapon in battling the disease.

- Physically active people have about 20 percent more pep during the day than couch potatoes, research from the University of a Georgia in Athens concludes. After adding at least 20 minutes of daily exercise—cardio or strength—study participants reported higher energy levels and less fatigue.

- Walking wonder: A better body isn't the only reason it's good to hoof it. For every 100 calories women burn daily doing moderate-intensity exercise *(e.g., 20 minutes of walking at 4 mph)*, they lowered their LDL *("bad")* cholesterol by 1.6 points and increased their HDL *("good")* cholesterol by 1 point in one year, a study in the *International Journal of Sports Medicine* reveals.

- Go the distance: It's how far, not how fast you stride that keeps you lean, a study in the *International Journal of Obesity* notes. Women who logged at least 12 miles a week-regardless of pace-maintained a healthy weight. Still, hoof it at 3.5 miles per hour or more to reap the maximum benefits to your heart as well as your hips.

- Cold warrior: Spending more time in your sneakers can stave off sickness, a report in the American Journal of Medicine suggests. During one year, women who did moderate-intensity cardio caught half as many colds as those who didn't, with the biggest sniffle-busting gain in the final three months. Your immunity builds for every week you keep up your routine, scientists speculate.

- Adding a little hustle to your cardio helps you get results faster. Exercises in a study at Yale University in New Haven, Connecticut, who worked out at 80 percent of their max burned 300 calories 10 minutes sooner than those going at 65 percent and stabilized blood sugar levels longer, preventing an energy slump.

You Normally	Instead	The Payoff
Jog at 12 mph for 36 minutes	Go only 30 minutes, but turn your run into a game: Pick up the pace for a minute, and then resume your regular speed for a minute. Continue alternating to the end.	You'll zap the same number of calories *(roughly 300*)* and amp your cardio capacity to make runs feel easier.
Ride a stationary bike at 10 mph for 40 minutes	Pedal at 15 mph while increasing your resistance two or three levels for a total of 20 minutes.	The identical calorie burn *(approximately 230)* in half the time
Swim freestyle laps for 20 minutes	Go for 10 minutes and alternate laps with the breaststroke or butterfly to work more muscles.	A stronger upper body and the same calories *(about 150)* gone
Log 25 minutes on the rowing machine at an easy 24 strokes per minutes *(spm)*	Row 11 minutes: Do one minute at an easy pace *(24 spm)*, one at medium *(26 spm)* and two at hard *(28 spm)*. Repeat; do the final three minutes at 26 spm.	You'll get the equivalent total-body workout and calorie count *(in the ballpark of 95)* in less than half the time.

- Exercise relieves constipation in people with irritable bowel syndrome *(IBS),* a study in the International Journal of Sports Medicine reports. Researchers had 28 adults with IBS attend two classes encouraging regular exercise; 28 others received no advice. Compared with the sedentary group, people in the first group increased their activity level and reported significantly fewer bouts of backup.

- Great tips from Fitness magazine:

7 easy Exercise Shortcuts

a.   Use heavier weights, do fewer reps.

b.   Work multiple muscle groups together—perform biceps curls with lunges, or shoulder presses with squats.

c.   Add 60-second cardio bursts *(jumping rope, running in place, shuffling)* between weight-lifting sets.

d.   For six-pack abs: Do all of your standing exercises on a Bosu ball *(bosu.com)*.

e.   Mix several two-minute high-speed intervals into your standard cardio routine.

f.   Alternate three to five minutes if cardio with 30 to 60 seconds of squats, lunges, sidekicks or push-ups.

g.   Perform an upper-body, a lower-body and a core exercise with no rest in between, then jump rope for one minute; repeat circuit.

9 Ways to Avoid the Ouch

a. Take a shower after working out, alternating 30 seconds cold and 60 seconds hot.

b. Get plenty of potassium *(think bananas and yogurt)*.

c. Do a two- to three-minute meditation, envisioning your body as healthy, beautiful and pain-free.

d. Roll out muscles with a foam roller for 3 to 10 minutes before and after exercising *(find one at performbetter.com)*.

e. Build recovery into your program. Do yoga or stretch on your days off.

f. Warm up and cool down before and after every workout.

g. Go swimming the day after a tough sweat session.

h. Drink lots of water.

i. Soak in the tub with two teaspoons each of baking powder and Epsom salts.

12 Sneaky Ways to Burn an Extra 250 Calories a Day

a. Keep sneakers at work and pick a place for lunch that's brisk 15-minutes walk away.

b. Fidget! A lot. One study showed that you could burn up to 350 more calories per day.

c. Shop calories per day.

d. Stand when talking on the phone.

e. Ride your bike *(or Walk)* to do errands. *(Need a backpack? We love the ones at dakine.com.)*

f. Have more sex.

g. Plant flowers.

h. Join a recreational sports team—soccer, softball, tennis.

i. Take five 10 minutes stroll breaks throughout the day.

j. Conduct meetings at the gym or on a track.

k. Do three sets of 25 push-ups, lunges and crunches before you get ready in the morning?

l. Take the stairs. Everywhere!

8 Dumbest Pieces of Advice They've Ever Heard About Exercise

a. Women shouldn't lift heavy weights—they'll bulk up.

b. Do tons of chin tucks to get rid of a double chin.

c. No pain, no gain.

d. If you take Spinning, you'll get huge thighs.

e. If you work out every day, you can eat whatever you want.

f. Wearing a plastic sweat suit will help you lose weight.

g. Doing 300 crunches a day will give you the six-pack you've always wanted.

h. Diet to lose weight first, then worry about exercising.

8 Ways to Reach an Exercise Goal

a. Assess where you are at the beginning. How much push-ups can you do? Sit-ups? How long can you run?

b. Ask yourself these questions: What's my goal? Why do I want to achieve it? When do I want to obtain it? Will I do what's required to succeed?

c. Break your big goal into four smaller ones.

d. Recruit a friend to go through the progress with you.

e. Schedule your workouts for certain times and days—just like everything else that's essential in your week.

f. Lose the all-or-nothing attitude.

g. Write your goal in a daily planner and tell it to at least two friends.

h. Put money in a jar every time you train. After every 10 to 20 workouts, but that pair of shoes you're been lusting after.

7 Best Ways to Measure Your Progress

a. Start an exercise diary. Write down what you did and how it made you feel.

b. Take a "before" picture and post it on your refrigerator, then take an "after" shot every month or so and compare.

c. Try on your skinny jeans every other Friday.

d. Do push-ups twice weekly; once weekly write down your number of reps.

e. If your energy level's up and you're sleeping better, something's working!

f. Take note of how times you can say, feel great every day.

g. Recognize how much less winded you get walking up stairs.

6 Signs Your Workout Isn't Tough Enough

a. You leave the gym without taking a shower.

b. You're reading as you exercise.

c. You feel mentally stressed afterward.

d. Your heart rate doesn't go up.

e. You haven't increased your speed or the amount of weight you're lifting in more than three months.

f. You're bored.

Let's Burn Some Calories NOW by laughing:

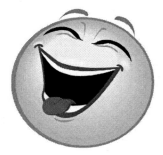

"I gave up jogging for my health when my thighs kept rubbing together and setting my pantyhose on fire."

"I'm in shape. Round is a shape."

"I don't exercise at all."

"If God had wanted me to touch my toes He would have put them up higher on my body."

"Inside me there's a thin person struggling to get out, but I can usually sedate her with four or five cupcakes."

"Every time I get the urge to exercise, I lie down till the feeling passes."

My gym teacher told me to touch my toes. I said, "I don't have that kind of relationship with my feet. Can I just wave?"

Diet Excuses

— But the doughnut was calling my name.

— But it was my birthday, so I had to eat the whole cake.

— I had to get the bitter taste out of my mouth from eating the so-called dish, so I had an ice cream.

— If you eat something and no one sees you eat it, it has no calories.

— If you drink a diet soda with a candy bar, the calories in the candy bar are canceled out by the diet soda.

— If you fatten up everyone else around you, then you look thinner.

— Cookie pieces contain no fat—the process of breaking causes fat leakage.

— Things licked off knives and spoons have no calories if you are in the process of preparing something. Examples are peanut butter on a knife making a sandwich and ice cream on a spoon making a sundae.

— Only eat things that have been broken into pieces; that way, all the calories fall out.

— Chocolate is a vegetable. How, you ask? Chocolate is derived from cacao beans. Bean = vegetable. Sugar is derived from either sugar CANE or sugar BEETS. Both are plants, which place them in the vegetable category. Thus, chocolate is a vegetable.

METABOLISM and Your Weight

A major topic of discussion regarding weight loss is metabolism. What is it? How does it work? Do I have it? How can I get it? These are questions that we may ponder in this journey to better health.

What is it?

Metabolism: The whole range of biochemical processes that occur within us *(or any living organism)*. Metabolism consists both of anabolism and catabolism *(the buildup and breakdown of substances, respectively)*. The term is commonly used to refer specifically to the breakdown of food and its transformation into energy *(from www.medicinenet.com)*.

The Dr. Sharon Quick Metabolism Definition: Your body's ability to burn calories that you eat and use every day. If your metabolism is low, this means that the calories that you eat hang around longer and contribute to weight gain. If you metabolism is high, this means that you are blessed because the calories that you eat are burned quickly and you don't gain weight as fast.

There are many factors which can affect your metabolism. There are so many myths, quick fixes, pills and remedies that all claim to increase metabolism. I will admit that I've tried a few and still drink green tea EVERY day which by some accounts increases metabolism. *(I don't really know, but there is always hope; it is a good antioxidant and I just like the taste and the fact that it has no calories)*. We must discuss metabolism and I wanted to share two very good articles with you. The information is from the experts and is sound. Some valid points are mentioned in both articles.

The Truth About Metabolism

Found at www.shape.com

Too many women are quick to blame their metabolism when those extra pounds refuse to come off. Not so fast. The idea that a low metabolic rate is always responsible for excess weight is just one of a number of misconceptions about metabolism, says researcher James Hill, PhD, director of the Center for Human Nutrition at the University of Colorado Health Sciences Center in Denver. And even if you do have a slower-than-average metabolism, it doesn't mean that you're destined to be overweight.

Because the whole subject can be so confusing, Shape went to the experts to dispel some common myths about metabolism. From pills to chili peppers to pumping iron, read on for the real scoop on what does and doesn't rev up your resting metabolic rate *(RMR)* to help you shed those extra pounds forever.

Q: We hear about metabolism all the time, but what is it exactly?

A: In simple terms, metabolism is the rate at which your body breaks down the nutrients in food to produce energy, Hill explains. A person with a fast metabolism, for example, utilizes calories more quickly, in some cases making it easier to stave off excess pounds.

Q: What are the factors that determine metabolism?

A: Body composition is the primary factor that determines your RMR, or the number of calories your body burns at rest. According to Hill, the more total fat-free mass you have *(including lean muscle, bones, organs, etc.)*, the higher your resting metabolic rate will be. That explains why the average man has a 10-20 percent higher metabolism than the average woman. Likewise, the RMR of a plus-sized woman *(whose total body mass, including both fat and fat-free mass, is significantly greater)* could be up to 50 percent higher than that of a thin woman. Heredity and hormones such as thyroid and insulin are the other important factors that dictate metabolism; though stress, calorie intake, exercise and medications also can play a role.

Q: So are we born with either a fast or a slow metabolism?

A: Yes. Studies of identical twins suggest that your baseline metabolism is determined at birth. But if you have a naturally slow metabolism, weight gain is by no means inevitable and though it may be harder to shed body fat, it's nearly always possible, says weight-loss expert Pamela Peeke, MD, MPH, an assistant professor of medicine at the University of Maryland in Baltimore. You may never burn calories as rapidly as, say, Serena Williams, but you can raise your RMR to a certain extent by exercising and building lean muscle.

Q: When I was much younger, I could eat whatever I wanted. But over the years, my metabolism seems to have slowed. What's happened?

A: If you can't eat as much as you used to without gaining weight, not enough exercise is probably the culprit. After age 30, the average woman's RMR decreases at a rate of 2-3 percent per decade, mainly due to inactivity and muscle loss, Hill says. Fortunately, some of that loss can be prevented or reversed with regular physical activity.

Q: Is it true that you can damage your metabolism by yo-yo dieting?

A: There's no conclusive evidence that yo-yo dieting does permanent harm to your metabolism, Hill says. But you will experience a temporary drop *(5-10 percent)* in RMR whenever you significantly reduce calories to lose weight.

Q: What are the best workouts for raising my metabolism?

A: Experts agree that weight training is the most effective way to build and preserve lean muscle, though most seem to concur that the influence of muscle on metabolism is rather slight. "Each pound of muscle can raise your RMR up to 15 calories per day," says researcher Gary Foster, PhD, associate professor at the University of Pennsylvania School of Medicine in Philadelphia.

In terms of cardio, a high-intensity workout that really raises your heart rate will blast the most calories and provide the biggest short-term metabolic boost, though it won't have a permanent effect on your RMR. *(A cardio workout will boost your metabolism anywhere from 20-30 percent, depending on intensity.)* After your workout, your metabolism will return to its resting level over several hours but you'll continue burning extra calories in the meantime.

Q: Can the kinds of nutrients you eat affect your metabolism?

A: Most of the scientific data shows that food choice has no significant impact on RMR. In other words, fats, proteins and carbohydrates seem to affect metabolism similarly. "The temporary metabolic increase from protein may be slightly higher, but the difference is negligible," Foster says. What does it matter how much you eat? Your metabolism is programmed to decrease whenever you slash calorie intake below what is needed to sustain your basic physiological functions, your body's way of conserving energy when food is in short supply. The more calories you cut, the lower your RMR will drop. "For example, an extremely low-calorie diet *(fewer than 800 calories a day)* could cause your metabolic rate to plunge by more than 10 percent," Foster says. The slowdown is likely to kick in within 48 hours of starting your diet. So to keep your metabolism from nose-diving, you're better off reducing calories in a healthy, moderate way. "For safe, lasting weight loss, the average woman shouldn't dip below 1,200 calories a day," Foster adds. To lose a pound of body fat a week, you need to create a deficit of 500 calories per day. The best way to do so, and avoid a major metabolic drop, is through a combination of exercise and diet *(rather than through cutting calories alone)*. For example, you could eliminate 250 calories from your diet, while adding enough activity to burn an extra 250.

Q: Can't spicy foods, such as chili peppers and curry, boost metabolism?

A: Yes, but unfortunately not enough to have an effect on weight loss. "Anything that increases your body temperature will temporarily raise your metabolic rate to a certain degree," Peeke says. But with spicy foods, the increase is so small and short-lived that it doesn't have an impact that will show on the scale.

Q: What will happen to my metabolism if I lose weight?

A: As you lose weight, your RMR will slow down because you have less body mass to support. As a result, your body requires fewer calories to sustain its vital functions. Consequently, you won't need to eat as much to feel satisfied and to fuel your exercise. If you don't further modify your eating and exercise habits, you'll eventually hit a weight-loss plateau. To get past the plateau and continue shedding pounds, if that's your goal, consume fewer calories *(without dropping too low)* or increase the intensity or duration of your workouts.

Q: What about supplements and other products that promise to elevate metabolism and melt fat?

A: Don't believe them! No pill, patch or potion can magically raise your metabolism enough to help you lose weight, Peeke says. If you want a quick metabolic boost, you're better off hitting the gym or going for a brisk walk.

Q: Can certain medications slow my metabolism?

A: Some drugs, like those used to treat depression and bipolar disorder, have been shown to lower metabolism. If you're taking a medication that causes weight gain, ask your doctor if there is an alternative drug you can try.

Make the Most of Your Metabolism

By Colette Bouchez
Found at www.webmd.com

"It's my metabolism!"

Sound familiar? If you're carrying some extra pounds *(and having a hard time losing them)*, it's tempting to put the blame on a sluggish metabolism.

But is your metabolism really the reason it's often so hard to lose weight? And, more important, is there anything you can do about it?

WebMD asked experts to explore facts and myths about metabolism; and the good news is that there are things you can do to help boost your body's calorie-burning power.

What Is Metabolism?

Your metabolism, experts say, involves a complex network of hormones and enzymes that not only convert food into fuel but also affect how efficiently you burn that fuel.

"The process of metabolism establishes the rate at which we burn our calories and, ultimately, how quickly we gain weight or how easily we lose it," says Robert Yanagisawa, MD, director of the Medically Supervised Weight Management Program at Mount Sinai Medical Center in New York.

Of course, not everyone burns calories at the same rate.

Your metabolism is influenced by your age *(metabolism naturally slows about 5% per decade after age 40)*, your sex *(men generally burn more calories at rest than women)* and proportion of lean body mass *(the more muscle you have, the higher your metabolic rate tends to be)*.

And yes, heredity makes a difference.

"Some people just burn calories at a slower rate than others," says Barrie Wolfe-Radbill, RD, a nutritionist specializing in weight loss at New York University Medical Center.

Occasionally, Yanagisawa says, a defect in the thyroid gland can slow metabolism, though this problem is relatively rare.

And here's a fact that may surprise you: the more weight you carry, the faster your metabolism is likely running.

"The simple fact is that the extra weight causes your body to work harder just to sustain itself at rest, so in most instances, the metabolism is always running a bit faster," says Molly Kimball, RD, sports and lifestyle nutritionist at the Oscher's Clinic's Elmwood Fitness Center.

That's one reason it's almost always easiest to lose weight at the start of a diet, and harder later on, Kimball says: "When you are very overweight your metabolism is already running so high that any small cut in calories will result in an immediate loss."

Then, when you lose significant amounts of body fat and muscle, your body needs fewer calories to sustain itself, she says. That helps explain why it's so easy to regain weight after you've worked to lose it.

"If two people both weigh 250 pounds, and one got there by dieting down from 350 and the other one was always at 250, the one who got there by cutting calories is going to have a slower metabolism," says Yanagisawa. "That means they will require fewer calories to maintain their weight than the person who never went beyond 250 pounds."

Revving Your Engine

Though some of the factors affecting metabolic rate can't be changed, happily, there are ways to maximize the metabolism you're born with; even when you're dieting.

Among the best ways is exercise. This includes aerobic workouts to burn more calories in the short term, and weight training to build the muscles that will boost your metabolism in the long run.

"Since muscle burns more calories than fat, even while at rest, the more muscles you have, the higher your resting metabolic rate, which means the more calories your body will be burning just to sustain you," says Kimball.

Personal fitness trainer Kelli Calabrese MS, CSCS, ACE, notes that every pound of muscle in our bodies burns 35 calories a day, while each pound of fat burns just 2 calories per day.

While 30 minutes of aerobic exercise may burn more calories than 30 minutes of weight training, Calabrese says, "in the hours following the cessation of exercise, the weight training has a longer-lasting effect on boosting metabolism."

Having extra muscle also means you can eat more and gain less.

Adds Yanagisawa: "We don't tell people to exercise while dieting only to burn calories; we also know that exercise builds muscle and that is what will help you burn more calories and maintain the weight loss you work so hard to achieve."

Some women fear they'll bulk up with weight training. But Calabrese, author of Feminine, Fit and Firm, says not to worry.

"Women don't have the hormones necessary to develop those huge muscles, so you can feel good about doing weight training," she says.

Eat More, Burn Better

Of course, the diet advice we'd all love to hear is "Eat more and lose more weight!" But what really works is "Eat more often, and you'll lose more weight." Small, but frequent, meals help keep your metabolism in high gear, and that means you'll burn more calories overall.

"When you put too many hours between meals, your metabolism actually slows down to compensate," says Kimball.

If you then eat a huge mea, at the same time your metabolism is functioning as if you're starving, your body wants to hold on to every calorie.

While this won't make much difference on an occasional basis, Kimball says, make it a way of life and it can get harder to lose or maintain weight.

Kimball's advice is borne out by the findings of a study that was presented at the 2005 annual meeting of the American College of Sports Medicine. Researchers from Georgia State University reported that when athletes ate snacks totaling about 250 calories each, three times a day, they had greater energy output then when they didn't snack.

The study also found that snacking helped the athletes eat less at each of their three regular meals. The final result was a higher metabolic rate, a lower caloric intake, and reduction in body fat.

Fat-Burning Foods?

From supermodels who douse their food with red pepper, to movie stars who swear by green tea, there's no shortage of claims for foods that are said to increase metabolism. But do any of them work?

"Actually, any food will increase your metabolism, mostly in the first hour after you eat; that's when your system is most revved," says Kimball.

Further, she says, protein generally requires about 25% more energy to digest. So, at least theoretically, a high-protein snack might rev metabolism a little more than a carb-heavy food with the same number of calories. That said, it's not clear that any food has special powers to boost metabolism significantly.

"Some studies have shown hot pepper and very spicy foods can increase metabolism by about 20% for about 30 minutes, but no one really knows if the extra burn lasts any longer than that," says Kimball.

In a small study on Japanese women published in the British Journal of Nutrition, researchers found red pepper caused the body to heat up and revved the metabolism following a meal. But the most effects were seen primarily when the red pepper was eaten with high-fat foods *(which are also higher in calories)*.

Another small study, published in the journal Medicine & Science in Sports & Exercise, reported that male athletes who added red pepper to high-carbohydrate meals boosted both their resting and active metabolic rates 30 minutes after the meal. But there was no evidence this burn power was lasting.

The same appears true for green tea, which contains a substance called EGCG *(epigallocatechin gallate)*, a powerful antioxidant that some believe can bring about the same kind of calorie-burning effect as hot pepper.

In a study of 10 men published in the American Journal of Clinical Nutrition, researchers found that 90 milligrams of EGCG and 50 milligrams of caffeine taken with meals boosted 24-hour energy expenditure by 4% *(caffeine alone did not show a similar effect)*.

But it's not clear whether this effect would be enough to boost weight loss. And that, says Radbill, is precisely the point.

"Essentially, you would have to drink so much of it in order to see even a small effect, that I don't think it's really worth it," says Radbill. "Drink green tea for other health-giving properties, but not to lose weight."

The bottom line, she says, is this: "All these foods may have a slight impact on metabolism, but the increase is still insignificant compared to what you need in order to lose weight."

Your best bet for keeping metabolism revved: Build muscles, snack on low-calorie, high-protein foods and keep moving!

Part III: The *Is It Worth It* Philosophy

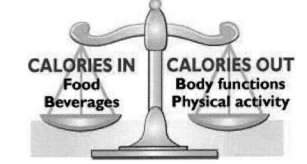

By the time you've finished this book, I hope that this scale is etched into your memory. If you learn nothing else with all that we are discussing, understand that it comes down to the math of calories in and calories out. However, you don't want to pack on empty calories with no nutritional value. The goal is to achieve a balance of healthy eating and physical activity which will carry you through a lifetime.

Let's go back to the birth of *Is it Worth It?* Remember that I was working out with my trainer Jennifer and she challenged me basically to think about what I ate and how I was going to burn it off in order to tip the scale in the right direction. In my case it was the chicken wings; I had to evaluate the *Calories In versus Calories Out* as I so desperately searched for a tipping of the scale downward as it relates to my weight.

A Dr. Sharon Sidebar: I certainly don't want you to feel that exercise is punishment. Trust me, exercise makes you feel and look good! This is not punishment; however, it is the currency that you have to use if you make a decision to eat or drink more calories than you burn in your efforts to lose weight. There are numerous benefits to exercise that I've discussed at length.

I've given you PLENTY of tools, tips and suggestions from around the globe on how to make better choices with nutrition as well as maximizing your calorie burn through physical activity. The thing to do is to put them together and begin to train your brain to think in terms of *Calories In versus Calories Out* as second nature. This means that when you're getting ready to start your day and do what we all should do, eat breakfast, that you THINK about what you're putting into your body. Not just for the moment but for the remainder of the day. You also have to THINK about your physical activity and mentally put the two on the scale. If your calories in weigh more than calories out then you need to make some new choices.

By now you've seen the tables/charts that show you how much physical activity you will need to do to burn the calories. Let's take another look at a few common beverages and food choices. Don't just glance at these charts; you know what you LOVE to eat and your own guilty pleasures. I know that when I look at these charts and see the real cost of some of my favorites, I pause and weigh my options. I really want these to sink into your memory and I've repeated them in several sections of the book.   Honestly, before you read this book, would you ever really think to add the calories from a glass of apple cider into your daily calorie counts? Would you estimated 200 calories for a 16 oz. serving? What if you were REALLY thirsty and drank more? Can you make a conscious decision how to limit the amount that you drink so that you can fill up on food and not get hungry? Is the apple cider worth paying the price of 22 minutes on a stationary bike *(170 pounds)*? What about that delicious triple strawberry shake, it's good but is it worth over 200 minutes of washing dishes? You make the call.

Apple Cider

To burn off 16 oz. of **apple cider** *(approx. 200 calories)* you would have to:

Activity	130 lbs	150 lbs	170 lbs	190 lbs	220 lbs	250 lbs	270 lbs
Aerobics, General	31 mins.	27 mins.	24 mins.	21 mins.	18 mins.	16 mins.	15 mins.
Bicycle, Stationary	29 mins.	25 mins.	22 mins.	20 mins.	17 mins.	15 mins.	14 mins.
Calisthenics *(push-ups, sit-ups, pull-ups, jumping jacks)*	25 mins.	22 mins.	19 mins.	17 mins.	15 mins.	13 mins.	12 mins.
Food Shopping	88 mins.	77 mins.	68 mins.	61 mins.	52 mins.	46 mins.	43 mins.
Gardening, General	51 mins.	44 mins.	39 mins.	35 mins.	30 mins.	27 mins.	25 mins.
Raking Lawn	47 mins.	41 mins.	36 mins.	32 mins.	28 mins.	25 mins.	23 mins.
Sex, General, Moderate	156 mins.	136 mins.	120 mins.	107 mins.	92 mins.	82 mins.	76 mins.
Shoveling Snow	34 mins.	29 mins.	26 mins.	23 mins.	20 mins.	18 mins.	16 mins.
Sweep Floors	62 mins.	53 mins.	47 mins.	42 mins.	36 mins.	32 mins.	30 mins.
Treadmill	23 mins.	20 mins.	17 mins.	16 mins.	13 mins.	12 mins.	11 mins.
Vacuum	58 mins.	50 mins.	45 mins.	40 mins.	34 mins.	30 mins.	28 mins.
Volleyball	51 mins.	44 mins.	39 mins.	35 mins.	30 mins.	27 mins.	25 mins.
Washing Dishes	88 mins.	77 mins.	68 mins.	61 mins.	52 mins.	46 mins.	43 mins.
Weight Lifting	68 mins.	59 mins.	52 mins.	47 mins.	40 mins.	35 mins.	33 mins.

Frappuccinos

To burn off one **frappuccino** with whipped cream *(approx. 600 calories)* you would have to:

Activity	130 lbs	150 lbs	170 lbs	190 lbs	220 lbs	250 lbs	270 lbs
Aerobics, General	94 mins.	81 mins.	72 mins.	64 mins.	55 mins.	49 mins.	45 mins.
Bicycle, Stationary	87 mins.	76 mins.	67 mins.	60 mins.	51 mins.	46 mins.	42 mins.
Calisthenics *(push-ups, sit-ups, pull-ups, jumping jacks)*	76 mins.	66 mins.	58 mins.	52 mins.	45 mins.	40 mins.	37 mins.
Food Shopping	265 mins.	230 mins.	203 mins.	182 mins.	157 mins.	139 mins.	128 mins.
Gardening, General	153 mins.	132 mins.	117 mins.	105 mins.	90 mins.	80 mins.	74 mins.
Raking Lawn	142 mins.	123 mins.	109 mins.	97 mins.	84 mins.	74 mins.	69 mins.
Sex, General, Moderate	469 mins.	407 mins.	360 mins.	322 mins.	277 mins.	245 mins.	227 mins.
Shoveling Snow	102 mins.	88 mins.	78 mins.	70 mins.	60 mins.	53 mins.	49 mins.
Sweep Floors	185 mins.	160 mins.	142 mins.	127 mins.	109 mins.	97 mins.	89 mins.
Treadmill	68 mins.	59 mins.	52 mins.	47 mins.	40 mins.	35 mins.	33 mins.
Vacuum	174 mins.	151 mins.	134 mins.	120 mins.	103 mins.	91 mins.	84 mins.
Volleyball	153 mins.	132 mins.	117 mins.	105 mins.	90 mins.	80 mins.	74 mins.
Washing Dishes	244 mins.	230 mins.	203 mins.	182 mins.	157 mins.	139 mins.	128 mins.
Weight Lifting	203 mins.	176 mins.	156 mins.	140 mins.	120 mins.	106 mins.	98 mins.

Champagne

To burn off a 6 oz glass of **champagne** *(approx. 165 calories)* you would have to:

Activity	130 lbs	150 lbs	170 lbs	190 lbs	220 lbs	250 lbs	270 lbs
Aerobics, General	26 mins.	22 mins.	20 mins.	18 mins.	15 mins.	13 mins.	12 mins.
Bicycle, Stationary	24 mins.	21 mins.	18 mins.	16 mins.	14 mins.	13 mins.	12 mins.
Calisthenics *(push-ups, sit-ups, pull-ups, jumping jacks)*	21 mins.	18 mins.	16 mins.	14 mins.	12 mins.	11 mins.	10 mins.
Food Shopping	73 mins.	63 mins.	56 mins.	50 mins.	43 mins.	38 mins.	35 mins.
Gardening, General	42 mins.	36 mins.	32 mins.	29 mins.	25 mins.	22 mins.	20 mins.
Raking Lawn	39 mins.	34 mins.	30 mins.	27 mins.	23 mins.	20 mins.	19 mins.
Sex, General, Moderate	129 mins.	112 mins.	99 mins.	89 mins.	76 mins.	67 mins.	62 mins.
Shoveling Snow	28 mins.	24 mins.	21 mins.	19 mins.	16 mins.	15 mins.	14 mins.
Sweep Floors	51 mins.	44 mins.	39 mins.	35 mins.	30 mins.	27 mins.	25 mins.

Treadmill	19 mins.	16 mins.	14 mins.	13 mins.	11 mins.	10 mins.	9 mins.
Vacuum	48 mins.	42 mins.	37 mins.	33 mins.	28 mins.	25 mins.	23 mins.
Volleyball	42 mins.	36 mins.	32 mins.	29 mins.	25 mins.	22 mins.	20 mins.
Washing Dishes	73 mins.	63 mins.	56 mins.	50 mins.	43 mins.	38 mins.	35 mins.
Weight Lifting	56 mins.	49 mins.	43 mins.	38 mins.	33 mins.	29 mins.	27 mins.

Frozen Strawberry Daiquiri

To burn off a **Bacardi Frozen Strawberry Daiquiri** *(8 oz) (approx. 120 calories)* you would have to:

Activity	130 lbs	150 lbs	170 lbs	190 lbs	220 lbs	250 lbs	270 lbs
Aerobics, General	19 mins.	16 mins.	14 mins.	13 mins.	11 mins.	10 mins.	9 mins.
Bicycle, Stationary	17 mins.	15 mins.	13 mins.	12 mins.	10 mins.	9 mins.	8 mins.
Calisthenics *(push-ups, sit-ups, pull-ups, jumping jacks)*	15 mins.	13 mins.	12 mins.	10 mins.	9 mins.	8 mins.	7 mins.
Food Shopping	53 mins.	46 mins.	41 mins.	36 mins.	31 mins.	28 mins.	26 mins.
Gardening, General	31 mins.	26 mins.	23 mins.	21 mins.	18 mins.	16 mins.	15 mins.
Raking Lawn	28 mins.	25 mins.	22 mins.	19 mins.	17 mins.	15 mins.	14 mins.
Sex, General, Moderate	94 mins.	81 mins.	72 mins.	64 mins.	55 mins.	49 mins.	45 mins.
Shoveling Snow	20 mins.	18 mins.	16 mins.	14 mins.	12 mins.	11 mins.	10 mins.
Sweep Floors	37 mins.	32 mins.	28 mins.	25 mins.	22 mins.	19 mins.	18 mins.
Treadmill	14 mins.	12 mins.	10 mins.	9 mins.	8 mins.	7 mins.	7 mins.
Vacuum	35 mins.	30 mins.	27 mins.	24 mins.	21 mins.	18 mins.	17 mins.
Volleyball	31 mins.	26 mins.	23 mins.	21 mins.	18 mins.	16 mins.	15 mins.
Washing Dishes	53 mins.	46 mins.	41 mins.	36 mins.	31 mins.	28 mins.	26 mins.
Weight Lifting	41 mins.	35 mins.	31 mins.	28 mins.	24 mins.	21 mins.	20 mins.

Pina Colada

To burn off one frozen **pina colada** *(8 oz) (approx. 250 calories)* you would have to:

Activity	130 lbs	150 lbs	170 lbs	190 lbs	220 lbs	250 lbs	270 lbs
Aerobics, General	39 mins.	34 mins.	30 mins.	27 mins.	23 mins.	20 mins.	19 mins.
Bicycle, Stationary	36 mins.	32 mins.	28 mins.	25 mins.	21 mins.	19 mins.	18 mins.
Calisthenics *(push-ups, sit-ups, pull-ups, jumping jacks)*	32 mins.	28 mins.	24 mins.	22 mins.	19 mins.	17 mins.	15 mins.
Food Shopping	111 mins.	96 mins.	85 mins.	76 mins.	65 mins.	58 mins.	53 mins.
Gardening, General	64 mins.	55 mins.	49 mins.	44 mins.	38 mins.	33 mins.	31 mins.
Raking Lawn	59 mins.	51 mins.	45 mins.	41 mins.	35 mins.	31 mins.	29 mins.
Sex, General, Moderate	196 mins.	170 mins.	150 mins.	134 mins.	115 mins.	102 mins.	95 mins.
Shoveling Snow	42 mins.	37 mins.	32 mins.	29 mins.	25 mins.	22 mins.	20 mins.
Sweep Floors	77 mins.	67 mins.	59 mins.	53 mins.	45 mins.	40 mins.	37 mins.
Treadmill	28 mins.	25 mins.	22 mins.	19 mins.	17 mins.	15 mins.	14 mins.
Vacuum	73 mins.	63 mins.	56 mins.	50 mins.	43 mins.	38 mins.	35 mins.
Volleyball	64 mins.	55 mins.	49 mins.	44 mins.	38 mins.	33 mins.	31 mins.
Washing Dishes	111 mins.	96 mins.	85 mins.	76 mins.	65 mins.	58 mins.	53 mins.
Weight Lifting	85 mins.	74 mins.	65 mins.	58 mins.	50 mins.	44 mins.	41 mins.

A Strawberry Triple Thick Milk Shake

To burn off 1 **strawberry triple thick milk shake** *(21 fl oz cup) (approx. 740 calories)* you would have to:

Activity	130 lbs	150 lbs	170 lbs	190 lbs	220 lbs	250 lbs	270 lbs
Aerobics, General	116 mins.	100 mins.	89 mins.	79 mins.	68 mins.	60 mins.	56 mins.
Bicycle, Stationary	108 mins.	93 mins.	82 mins.	74 mins.	63 mins.	56 mins.	52 mins.
Calisthenics *(push-ups, sit-ups, pull-ups, jumping jacks)*	94 mins.	82 mins.	72 mins.	65 mins.	56 mins.	49 mins.	45 mins.

Food Shopping	327 mins.	284 mins.	251 mins.	224 mins.	193 mins.	171 mins.	158 mins.
Gardening, General	188 mins.	163 mins.	144 mins.	129 mins.	111 mins.	98 mins.	91 mins.
Raking Lawn	175 mins.	152 mins.	134 mins.	120 mins.	103 mins.	91 mins.	85 mins.
Sex, General, Moderate	579 mins.	502 mins.	444 mins.	397 mins.	342 mins.	302 mins.	280 mins.
Shoveling Snow	125 mins.	109 mins.	96 mins.	86 mins.	74 mins.	65 mins.	61 mins.
Sweep Floors	228 mins.	198 mins.	175 mins.	156 mins.	135 mins.	119 mins.	110 mins.
Treadmill	84 mins.	73 mins.	64 mins.	57 mins.	49 mins.	44 mins.	40 mins.
Vacuum	215 mins.	187 mins.	165 mins.	148 mins.	127 mins.	112 mins.	104 mins.
Volleyball	188 mins.	163 mins.	144 mins.	129 mins.	111 mins.	98 mins.	91 mins.
Washing Dishes	327 mins.	284 mins.	251 mins.	224 mins.	193 mins.	171 mins.	158 mins.
Weight Lifting	251 mins.	218 mins.	192mins.	172 mins.	148 mins.	131 mins.	121 mins.

Candy Corn

To burn off 20 pieces of **candy corn** *(approx. 100 calories)* you would have to:

Activity	130 lbs	150 lbs	170 lbs	190 lbs	220 lbs	250 lbs	270 lbs
Aerobics, General	16 mins.	14 mins.	12 mins.	11 mins.	9 mins.	8 mins.	8 mins.
Bicycle, Stationary	15 mins.	13 mins.	11 mins.	10 mins.	9 mins.	8 mins.	7 mins.
Calisthenics *(push-ups, sit-ups, pull-ups, jumping jacks)*	13 mins.	11 mins.	10 mins.	9 mins.	8 mins.	7 mins.	6 mins.
Food Shopping	44 mins.	38 mins.	34 mins.	30 mins.	26 mins.	23 mins.	21 mins.
Gardening, General	25 mins.	22 mins.	19 mins.	17 mins.	15 mins.	13 mins.	12 mins.
Raking Lawn	24 mins.	21 mins.	18 mins.	16 mins.	14 mins.	12 mins.	11 mins.
Sex, General, Moderate	78 mins.	68 mins.	60 mins.	54 mins.	46 mins.	41 mins.	38 mins.
Shoveling Snow	17 mins.	15 mins.	13 mins.	12 mins.	10 mins.	9 mins.	8 mins.
Sweep Floors	31 mins.	27 mins.	24 mins.	21 mins.	18 mins.	16 mins.	15 mins.
Treadmill	11 mins.	10 mins.	9 mins.	8 mins.	7 mins.	6 mins.	5 mins.
Vacuum	29 mins.	25 mins.	22 mins.	20 mins.	17 mins.	15 mins.	14 mins.
Volleyball	25 mins.	22 mins.	19 mins.	17 mins.	15 mins.	13 mins.	12 mins.
Washing Dishes	44 mins.	38 mins.	34 mins.	30 mins.	26 mins.	23 mins.	21 mins.
Weight Lifting	34 mins.	29 mins.	26 mins.	23 mins.	20 mins.	18 mins.	16 mins.

Chocolate Bars

To burn off 4 bite size **chocolate bars** *(approx. 320 calories)* you would have to:

Activity	130 lbs	150 lbs	170 lbs	190 lbs	220 lbs	250 lbs	270 lbs
Aerobics, General	50 mins.	43 mins.	38 mins.	34 mins.	30 mins.	26 mins.	24 mins.
Bicycle, Stationary	46 mins.	40 mins.	36 mins.	32 mins.	27 mins.	24 mins.	22 mins.
Calisthenics *(push-ups, sit-ups, pull-ups, jumping jacks)*	41mins.	35 mins.	31mins.	28 mins.	24 mins.	21mins.	20 mins.
Food Shopping	141 mins.	123 mins.	108 mins.	97 mins.	83 mins.	74 mins.	68 mins.
Gardening, General	81 mins.	71 mins.	62 mins.	56 mins.	48 mins.	42 mins.	39 mins.
Raking Lawn	76 mins.	66 mins.	58 mins.	52 mins.	45 mins.	40 mins.	37 mins.
Sex, General, Moderate	250 mins.	217 mins.	192 mins.	172 mins.	148 mins.	131 mins.	121 mins.
Shoveling Snow	54 mins.	47 mins.	42 mins.	37 mins.	32 mins.	28 mins.	26 mins.
Sweep Floors	99 mins.	86 mins.	76 mins.	68 mins.	58 mins.	51 mins.	48 mins.
Treadmill	36 mins.	31 mins.	28 mins.	25 mins.	21 mins.	19 mins.	17 mins.
Vacuum	93 mins.	81 mins.	71 mins.	64 mins.	55 mins.	49 mins.	45 mins.
Volleyball	81 mins.	71 mins.	62 mins.	56 mins.	48 mins.	42 mins.	39 mins.
Washing Dishes	141 mins.	123 mins.	108 mins.	97 mins.	83 mins.	74 mins.	68 mins.
Weight Lifting	108 mins.	94 mins.	83 mins.	74 mins.	64 mins.	57 mins.	52 mins.

Jelly Beans

To burn off 25 **jelly beans** (approx. 140 calories) you would have to:

Activity	130 lbs	150 lbs	170 lbs	190 lbs	220 lbs	250 lbs	270 lbs
Aerobics, General	22 mins.	19 mins.	17 mins.	15 mins.	13 mins.	11 mins.	11 mins.
Bicycle, Stationary	20 mins.	18 mins.	16 mins.	14 mins.	12 mins.	11 mins.	10 mins.
Calisthenics (push-ups, sit-ups, pull-ups, jumping jacks)	18 mins.	15 mins.	14 mins.	12 mins.	10 mins.	9 mins.	9 mins.
Food Shopping	62 mins.	54 mins.	47 mins.	42 mins.	37 mins.	32 mins.	30 mins.
Gardening, General	36 mins.	31 mins.	27 mins.	24 mins.	21 mins.	19 mins.	17 mins.
Raking Lawn	33 mins.	29 mins.	25 mins.	23 mins.	20 mins.	17 mins.	16 mins.
Sex, General, Moderate	110 mins.	95 mins.	84 mins.	75 mins.	65 mins.	57 mins.	53 mins.
Shoveling Snow	24 mins.	21 mins.	18 mins.	16 mins.	14 mins.	12 mins.	11 mins.
Sweep Floors	43 mins.	37 mins.	33 mins.	30 mins.	25 mins.	23 mins.	21 mins.
Treadmill	16 mins.	14 mins.	12 mins.	11 mins.	9 mins.	8 mins.	8 mins.
Vacuum	41 mins.	35 mins.	31 mins.	28 mins.	24 mins.	21 mins.	20 mins.
Volleyball	36 mins.	31 mins.	27 mins.	24 mins.	21 mins.	19 mins.	17 mins.
Washing Dishes	62 mins.	54 mins.	47 mins.	42 mins.	37 mins.	32 mins.	30 mins.
Weight Lifting	47 mins.	41 mins.	36 mins.	33 mins.	28 mins.	25 mins.	23 mins.

Candy Apple

To burn off 1 large **candy apple** (approx. 540 calories) you would have to:

Activity	130 lbs	150 lbs	170 lbs	190 lbs	220 lbs	250 lbs	270 lbs
Aerobics, General	84 mins.	73 mins.	65 mins.	58 mins.	50 mins.	44 mins.	41 mins.
Bicycle, Stationary	78 mins.	68 mins.	60 mins.	54 mins.	46 mins.	41 mins.	38 mins.
Calisthenics (push-ups, sit-ups, pull-ups, jumping jacks)	69 mins.	60 mins.	53 mins.	47 mins.	40 mins.	36 mins.	33 mins.
Food Shopping	239 mins.	207 mins.	183 mins.	164 mins.	141 mins.	125 mins.	115 mins.
Gardening, General	137 mins.	119 mins.	105 mins.	94 mins.	81 mins.	72 mins.	66 mins.
Raking Lawn	128 mins.	111 mins.	98 mins.	88 mins.	75 mins.	67 mins.	62 mins.
Sex, General, Moderate	422 mins.	367 mins.	324 mins.	290 mins.	249 mins.	221 mins.	204 mins.
Shoveling Snow	92 mins.	79 mins.	70 mins.	63 mins.	54 mins.	48 mins.	44 mins.
Sweep Floors	166 mins.	144 mins.	128 mins.	114 mins.	98 mins.	87 mins.	80 mins.
Treadmill	61 mins.	53 mins.	47 mins.	42 mins.	36 mins.	32 mins.	30 mins.
Vacuum	157 mins.	136 mins.	120 mins.	108 mins.	93 mins.	82 mins.	76 mins.
Volleyball	137 mins.	119 mins.	105 mins.	94mins.	81 mins.	72 mins.	66 mins.
Washing Dishes	239 mins.	207 mins.	183 mins.	164 mins.	141 mins.	125 mins.	115 mins.
Weight Lifting	183 mins.	159 mins.	140 mins.	126 mins.	108 mins.	96 mins.	89 mins.

Chocolate Fudge

To burn off 1 oz **chocolate fudge** (approx. 100 calories) you would have to:

Activity	130 lbs	150 lbs	170 lbs	190 lbs	220 lbs	250 lbs	270 lbs
Aerobics, General	16 mins.	14 mins.	12 mins.	11 mins.	9 mins.	8 mins.	8 mins.
Bicycle, Stationary	15 mins.	13 mins.	11 mins.	10 mins.	9 mins.	8 mins.	7 mins.
Calisthenics (push-ups, sit-ups, pull-ups, jumping jacks)	13 mins.	11 mins.	10 mins.	9 mins.	8 mins.	7 mins.	6 mins.
Food Shopping	44 mins.	38 mins.	34 mins.	30 mins.	26 mins.	23 mins.	21 mins.
Gardening, General	25 mins.	22 mins.	19 mins.	17 mins.	15 mins.	13 mins.	12 mins.
Raking Lawn	24 mins.	21 mins.	18 mins.	16 mins.	14 mins.	12 mins.	11 mins.
Sex, General, Moderate	78 mins.	68 mins.	60 mins.	54 mins.	46 mins.	41 mins.	38 mins.
Shoveling Snow	17 mins.	15 mins.	13 mins.	12 mins.	10 mins.	9 mins.	8 mins.

Sweep Floors	31 mins.	27 mins.	24 mins.	21 mins.	18 mins.	16 mins.	15 mins.
Treadmill	11 mins.	10 mins.	9 mins.	8 mins.	7 mins.	6 mins.	5 mins.
Vacuum	29 mins.	25 mins.	22 mins.	20 mins.	17 mins.	15 mins.	14 mins.
Volleyball	25 mins.	22 mins.	19 mins.	17 mins.	15 mins.	13 mins.	12 mins.
Washing Dishes	44 mins.	38 mins.	34 mins.	30 mins.	26 mins.	23 mins.	21 mins.
Weight Lifting	34 mins.	29 mins.	26 mins.	23 mins.	20 mins.	18 mins.	16 mins.

Hot Fudge Sundae

To burn off 1 large **hot fudge sundae** (*approx. 900 calories*) you would have to:

Activity	130 lbs	150 lbs	170 lbs	190 lbs	220 lbs	250 lbs	270 lbs
Aerobics, General	141 mins.	122 mins.	108 mins.	97 mins.	83 mins.	74 mins.	68 mins.
Bicycle, Stationary	131 mins.	113 mins.	100 mins.	90 mins.	77 mins.	68 mins.	63 mins.
Calisthenics (push-ups, sit-ups, pull-ups, jumping jacks)	114 mins.	99 mins.	88 mins.	78 mins.	68 mins.	60 mins.	55 mins.
Food Shopping	398 mins.	345 mins.	305 mins.	273 mins.	235 mins.	208 mins.	192 mins.
Gardening, General	229 mins.	199 mins.	175 mins.	157 mins.	135 mins.	119 mins.	111 mins.
Raking Lawn	213 mins.	185 mins.	163 mins.	146 mins.	126 mins.	111 mins.	103 mins.
Sex, General, Moderate	704 mins.	611 mins.	539 mins.	483 mins.	415 mins.	368 mins.	340 mins.
Shoveling Snow	153 mins.	132 mins.	117 mins.	105 mins.	90 mins.	80 mins.	74 mins.
Sweep Floors	277 mins.	241 mins.	213 mins.	190 mins.	164 mins.	145 mins.	134 mins.
Treadmill	102 mins.	88 mins.	78 mins.	70 mins.	60 mins.	53 mins.	49 mins.
Vacuum	262 mins.	227 mins.	200 mins.	179 mins.	154 mins.	137 mins.	126 mins.
Volleyball	229 mins.	199 mins.	175mins.	157 mins.	135 mins.	119 mins.	111 mins.
Washing Dishes	398 mins.	345 mins.	305 mins.	273 mins.	235 mins.	208 mins.	192 mins.
Weight Lifting	305 mins.	265 mins.	234 mins.	209 mins.	180 mins.	159 mins.	148 mins.

Funnel Cake

To burn off 1 **funnel cake** (*approx. 760 calories*) you would have to:

Activity	130 lbs	150 lbs	170 lbs	190 lbs	220 lbs	250 lbs	270 lbs
Aerobics, General	119 mins.	103 mins.	91 mins.	82 mins.	70 mins.	62 mins.	58 mins.
Bicycle, Stationary	110 mins.	96 mins.	85 mins.	76 mins.	65 mins.	58 mins.	53 mins.
Calisthenics (push-ups, sit-ups, pull-ups, jumping jacks)	97 mins.	84 mins.	74 mins.	66 mins.	57 mins.	50 mins.	47 mins.
Food Shopping	336 mins.	292 mins.	257 mins.	231 mins.	198 mins.	175 mins.	163 mins.
Gardening, General	193 mins.	168 mins.	148 mins.	133 mins.	114 mins.	101 mins.	93 mins.
Raking Lawn	180 mins.	156 mins.	138 mins.	123 mins.	106 mins.	94 mins.	87 mins.
Sex, General, Moderate	595 mins.	516 mins.	456 mins.	408 mins.	351 mins.	310 mins.	288 mins.
Shoveling Snow	129 mins.	112 mins.	99 mins.	88 mins.	76 mins.	67 mins.	62 mins.
Sweep Floors	234 mins.	203 mins.	179 mins.	161 mins.	138 mins.	122 mins.	113 mins.
Treadmill	86 mins.	75 mins.	66 mins.	59 mins.	51 mins.	45 mins.	42 mins.
Vacuum	221 mins.	192 mins.	169mins.	151 mins.	130 mins.	115 mins.	107 mins.
Volleyball	193 mins.	168 mins.	148mins.	133 mins.	114 mins.	101 mins.	93 mins.
Washing Dishes	336 mins.	292 mins.	257mins.	231 mins.	198 mins.	175 mins.	163 mins.
Weight Lifting	258 mins.	224 mins.	197 mins.	177 mins.	152 mins.	135 mins.	125 mins.

Ball Park Meal

To burn off one 20 oz beer & 1 giant hot dog *(approx. 695 calories)* you would have to:

Activity	130 lbs	150 lbs	170 lbs	190 lbs	220 lbs	250 lbs	270 lbs
Aerobics, General	109 mins.	94 mins.	83 mins.	75 mins.	64 mins.	57 mins.	53 mins.
Bicycle, Stationary	101 mins.	88 mins.	77 mins.	69 mins.	60 mins.	53 mins.	49 mins.
Calisthenics *(push-ups, sit-ups, pull-ups, jumping jacks)*	88 mins.	77 mins.	68 mins.	61 mins.	52 mins.	46 mins.	43 mins.
Food Shopping	307 mins.	267 mins.	235 mins.	211 mins.	181 mins.	160 mins.	149 mins.
Gardening, General	177 mins.	153 mins.	135 mins.	121 mins.	104 mins.	92 mins.	85 mins.
Raking Lawn	164 mins.	143 mins.	126 mins.	113 mins.	97 mins.	86 mins.	79 mins.
Sex, General, Moderate	544 mins.	472 mins.	417 mins.	373 mins.	321 mins.	284 mins.	263 mins.
Shoveling Snow	118 mins.	102 mins.	90 mins.	81 mins.	70 mins.	62 mins.	57 mins.
Sweep Floors	214 mins.	186 mins.	164 mins.	147 mins.	126 mins.	112 mins.	104 mins.
Treadmill	79 mins.	68 mins.	60 mins.	54 mins.	46 mins.	41 mins.	38 mins.
Vacuum	202 mins.	175 mins.	155mins.	139 mins.	119 mins.	105 mins.	98 mins.
Volleyball	177 mins.	153 mins.	135 mins.	121 mins.	104 mins.	92 mins.	85 mins.
Washing Dishes	307 mins.	267 mins.	235 mins.	211 mins.	181 mins.	160 mins.	149 mins.
Weight Lifting	236 mins.	204 mins.	181mins.	162 mins.	139 mins.	123 mins.	114 mins.

Movie Theater Snacks

To burn off 1 large popcorn with butter 170 oz, 1 large soda and 1 box of candy *(approx. 1940 calories)* you would have to:

Activity	130 lbs	150 lbs	170 lbs	190 lbs	220 lbs	250 lbs	270 lbs
Aerobics, General	304 mins.	263 mins.	233 mins.	208 mins.	179 mins.	158 mins.	147 mins.
Bicycle, Stationary	282 mins.	245 mins.	216 mins.	193 mins.	166 mins.	147 mins.	136 mins.
Calisthenics *(push-ups, sit-ups, pull-ups, jumping jacks)*	247 mins.	214 mins.	189 mins.	169 mins.	146 mins.	129 mins.	119 mins.
Food Shopping	858 mins.	744 mins.	657 mins.	588 mins.	506 mins.	448 mins.	415 mins.
Gardening, General	493 mins.	428 mins.	378 mins.	338 mins.	291 mins.	258 mins.	239 mins.
Raking Lawn	459 mins.	398 mins.	352 mins.	315 mins.	271 mins.	240 mins.	222 mins.
Sex, General, Moderate	1518mins.	1317 mins.	1163 mins.	1041 mins.	895 mins.	792 mins.	734 mins.
Shoveling Snow	329 mins.	285 mins.	252 mins.	226 mins.	194 mins.	172 mins.	159 mins.
Sweep Floors	598 mins.	519 mins.	458 mins.	410 mins.	353 mins.	312 mins.	289 mins.
Treadmill	219 mins.	190 mins.	168 mins.	150 mins.	129 mins.	114 mins.	106 mins.
Vacuum	564 mins.	489 mins.	432 mins.	387 mins.	333 mins.	294 mins.	273 mins.
Volleyball	493 mins.	428 mins.	378 mins.	338 mins.	291 mins.	258 mins.	239 mins.
Washing Dishes	858 mins.	744 mins.	657 mins.	588 mins.	506 mins.	448 mins.	415 mins.
Weight Lifting	658 mins.	571 mins.	504mins.	451 mins.	388 mins.	343 mins.	318 mins.

Thanksgiving Dinner *(and you KNOW that you eat more than this)*

To burn off 6 oz of Turkey, ½ cup of mashed potatoes, 1 cup of stuffing, ½ cup of cranberry sauce, 1 dinner roll and 1 slice of apple pie *(approx. 1598 calories)* you would have to:

Activity	130 lbs	150 lbs	170 lbs	190 lbs	220 lbs	250 lbs	270 lbs
Aerobics, General	250 mins.	217 mins.	192 mins.	172 mins.	148 mins.	131 mins.	121 mins.
Bicycle, Stationary	232 mins.	201 mins.	178 mins.	159 mins.	137 mins.	121 mins.	112 mins.
Calisthenics *(push-ups, sit-ups, pull-ups, jumping jacks)*	203 mins.	176 mins.	156 mins.	139 mins.	120 mins.	106 mins.	98 mins.
Food Shopping	707 mins.	613 mins.	541 mins.	485 mins.	417 mins.	369 mins.	342 mins.
Gardening, General	406 mins.	352 mins.	311 mins.	279 mins.	240 mins.	212 mins.	196 mins.

Raking Lawn	378 mins.	328 mins.	290 mins.	259 mins.	223 mins.	197 mins.	183 mins.
Sex, General, Moderate	1250 mins.	1085 mins.	958 mins.	858 mins.	738 mins.	653 mins.	605 mins.
Shoveling Snow	271 mins.	235 mins.	208 mins.	186 mins.	160 mins.	141 mins.	131 mins.
Sweep Floors	492 mins.	427 mins.	377 mins.	338 mins.	291 mins.	257 mins.	238 mins.
Treadmill	181 mins.	157 mins.	138 mins.	124 mins.	107 mins.	94 mins.	87 mins.
Vacuum	464 mins.	403 mins.	356 mins.	319 mins.	274 mins.	242 mins.	225 mins.
Volleyball	406 mins.	352 mins.	311 mins.	279 mins.	240 mins.	212 mins.	196 mins.
Washing Dishes	707 mins.	613 mins.	541 mins.	485 mins.	417 mins.	369 mins.	342 mins.
Weight Lifting	542 mins.	470 mins.	415 mins.	372 mins.	320 mins.	283 mins.	262 mins.

The SAGA Begins: Let me restate that FOOD is NOT the ENEMY! You must eat to give your body the fuel that it needs to run. However, you don't need to overfill your body in one sitting but it's all about making better choices. What happens when it's breakfast time and you're hungry but didn't grab an apple, toast and/or coffee before you left for work. After all you're busy. Why not just stop at the local drive thru and pick something up. You may as well pick up lunch because you may not have time to go back out, right. Hmmmmmm, remember what YOUR daily caloric intake should be. It would be a shame to eat ¾ of it at breakfast in your car. Can we say—weight gain? High blood pressure? High cholesterol? Can we say choking arteries in the heart?

Burger King Breakfast

To burn off 1 Croissan'wich w/ Sausage, Egg & Cheese, 1 large hash brown and 1 large coffee *(approx. 900 calories)* you would have to:

Activity	130 lbs	150 lbs	170 lbs	190 lbs	220 lbs	250 lbs	270 lbs
Aerobics, General	141 mins.	122 mins.	108 mins.	97 mins.	83 mins.	74 mins.	68 mins.
Bicycle, Stationary	131 mins.	113 mins.	100 mins.	90 mins.	77 mins.	68 mins.	63 mins.
Calisthenics *(push-ups, sit-ups, pull-ups, jumping jacks)*	114 mins.	99 mins.	88 mins.	78 mins.	68 mins.	60 mins.	55 mins.
Food Shopping	398 mins.	345 mins.	305 mins.	273 mins.	235 mins.	208 mins.	192 mins.
Gardening, General	229 mins.	199 mins.	175 mins.	157 mins.	135 mins.	119 mins.	111 mins.
Raking Lawn	213 mins.	185 mins.	163 mins.	146 mins.	126 mins.	111 mins.	103 mins.
Sex, General, Moderate	704 mins.	611 mins.	539 mins.	483 mins.	415 mins.	368 mins.	340 mins.
Shoveling Snow	153 mins.	132 mins.	117 mins.	105 mins.	90 mins.	80 mins.	74 mins.
Sweep Floors	277 mins.	241 mins.	213 mins.	190 mins.	164 mins.	145 mins.	134 mins.
Treadmill	102 mins.	88 mins.	78 mins.	70 mins.	60 mins.	53 mins.	49 mins.
Vacuum	262 mins.	227 mins.	200 mins.	179 mins.	154 mins.	137 mins.	126 mins.
Volleyball	229 mins.	199 mins.	175 mins.	157 mins.	135 mins.	119 mins.	111 mins.
Washing Dishes	398 mins.	345 mins.	305 mins.	273 mins.	235 mins.	208 mins.	192 mins.
Weight Lifting	305 mins.	265 mins.	234 mins.	209 mins.	180 mins.	159 mins.	148 mins.

Burger King Lunch

To burn off 1 Double Whopper w/ Cheese, large onion rings and 1 large Coke *(approx. 1510 calories)* you would have to:

Activity	130 lbs	150 lbs	170 lbs	190 lbs	220 lbs	250 lbs	270 lbs
Aerobics, General	236 mins.	205 mins.	181 mins.	162 mins.	139 mins.	123 mins.	114 mins.
Bicycle, Stationary	219 mins.	190 mins.	168 mins.	150 mins.	129 mins.	115 mins.	106 mins.
Calisthenics *(push-ups, sit-ups, pull-ups, jumping jacks)*	192 mins.	167 mins.	336 mins.	132 mins.	113 mins.	100 mins.	93 mins.
Food Shopping	668 mins.	579 mins.	512 mins.	458 mins.	394 mins.	349 mins.	323 mins.
Gardening, General	384 mins.	333 mins.	294 mins.	263 mins.	226 mins.	200 mins.	186 mins.
Raking Lawn	357 mins.	310 mins.	274 mins.	245 mins.	211 mins.	186 mins.	173 mins.
Sex, General, Moderate	1181 mins.	1025 mins.	905 mins.	810 mins.	697 mins.	617 mins.	571 mins.

Shoveling Snow	256 mins.	222 mins.	196 mins.	176 mins.	151 mins.	134 mins.	124 mins.
Sweep Floors	465 mins.	404 mins.	357mins.	319 mins.	275 mins.	243 mins.	225 mins.
Treadmill	171 mins.	148 mins.	131 mins.	117 mins.	101 mins.	89 mins.	83 mins.
Vacuum	439 mins.	381 mins.	336 mins.	301 mins.	259 mins.	229 mins.	212 mins.
Volleyball	384 mins.	333 mins.	294 mins.	263 mins.	226 mins.	200 mins.	186 mins.
Washing Dishes	668 mins.	579 mins.	512 mins.	458 mins.	394 mins.	349 mins.	323 mins.
Weight Lifting	512 mins.	444 mins.	392 mins.	351 mins.	302 mins.	267 mins.	248 mins.

Hardees Breakfast

To burn off 1 Big Country Breakfast Platter-Country Steak *(approx. 1150 calories)* you would have to:

Activity	130 lbs	150 lbs	170 lbs	190 lbs	220 lbs	250 lbs	270 lbs
Aerobics, General	180 mins.	156 mins.	138 mins.	123 mins.	106 mins.	94 mins.	87 mins.
Bicycle, Stationary	167 mins.	145 mins.	128 mins.	115 mins.	99 mins.	87 mins.	81 mins.
Calisthenics *(push-ups, sit-ups, pull-ups, jumping jacks)*	146 mins.	127 mins.	112 mins.	100 mins.	86 mins.	76 mins.	71 mins.
Food Shopping	508 mins.	441 mins.	390 mins.	349 mins.	300 mins.	265 mins.	246 mins.
Gardening, General	292 mins.	254 mins.	224 mins.	201 mins.	172 mins.	153 mins.	141 mins.
Raking Lawn	272 mins.	236 mins.	208 mins.	187 mins.	160 mins.	142 mins.	132 mins.
Sex, General, Moderate	900 mins.	781 mins.	689 mins.	617 mins.	531 mins.	470 mins.	435 mins.
Shoveling Snow	195 mins.	169 mins.	149 mins.	134 mins.	115 mins.	102 mins.	94 mins.
Sweep Floors	354 mins.	307 mins.	272 mins.	243 mins.	209 mins.	185 mins.	171 mins.
Treadmill	130 mins.	113 mins.	100 mins.	89 mins.	77 mins.	68 mins.	63 mins.
Vacuum	334 mins.	290mins.	256 mins.	229 mins.	197 mins.	174 mins.	162 mins.
Volleyball	292 mins.	254 mins.	224 mins.	201 mins.	172 mins.	153 mins.	141 mins.
Washing Dishes	508 mins.	441 mins.	390 mins.	349 mins.	300 mins.	265 mins.	246 mins.
Weight Lifting	390 mins.	338 mins.	299 mins.	267 mins.	230 mins.	204 mins.	189 mins.

Hardees Lunch

To burn off 1 Charbroiled Chicken Club Sandwich, Crispy Curls *(Large)* and 1 large Coke *(approx. 1050 calories)* you would have to:

Activity	130 lbs	150 lbs	170 lbs	190 lbs	220 lbs	250 lbs	270 lbs
Aerobics, General	164 mins.	143 mins.	126 mins.	113 mins.	97 mins.	86 mins.	79 mins.
Bicycle, Stationary	153 mins.	132 mins.	117 mins.	105 mins.	90 mins.	80 mins.	74 mins.
Calisthenics *(push-ups, sit-ups, pull-ups, jumping jacks)*	133 mins.	116 mins.	102 mins.	92 mins.	79 mins.	70 mins.	65 mins.
Food Shopping	464 mins.	403 mins.	356 mins.	319 mins.	274 mins.	242 mins.	225 mins.
Gardening, General	267 mins.	232 mins.	205 mins.	183 mins.	158 mins.	139 mins.	129 mins.
Raking Lawn	248 mins.	215 mins.	190 mins.	170 mins.	147 mins.	130 mins.	120 mins.
Sex, General, Moderate	821 mins.	713 mins.	629 mins.	564 mins.	485 mins.	429 mins.	397 mins.
Shoveling Snow	178 mins.	154 mins.	136 mins.	122 mins.	105 mins.	93 mins.	86 mins.
Sweep Floors	324 mins.	281 mins.	248 mins.	222 mins.	191 mins.	169 mins.	156 mins.
Treadmill	119 mins.	103 mins.	91 mins.	81 mins.	70 mins.	62 mins.	57 mins.
Vacuum	305 mins.	265 mins.	234 mins.	209 mins.	180 mins.	159 mins.	148 mins.
Volleyball	267 mins.	232 mins.	205 mins.	183 mins.	158 mins.	139 mins.	129 mins.
Washing Dishes	464 mins.	403 mins.	356 mins.	319 mins.	274 mins.	242 mins.	225 mins.
Weight Lifting	356 mins.	309 mins.	273 mins.	244 mins.	210 mins.	186 mins.	172 mins.

KFC Lunch

To burn off 1 roasted Caesar salad with creamy parmesan Caesar dressing and 1 Tropicana fruit punch *(approx. 600 calories)* you would have to:

Activity	130 lbs	150 lbs	170 lbs	190 lbs	220 lbs	250 lbs	270 lbs
Aerobics, General	94 mins.	81 mins.	72 mins.	64 mins.	55 mins.	49 mins.	45 mins.
Bicycle, Stationary	87 mins.	76 mins.	67 mins.	60 mins.	51 mins.	46 mins.	42 mins.
Calisthenics *(push-ups, sit-ups, pull-ups, jumping jacks)*	76 mins.	66 mins.	58 mins.	52 mins.	45 mins.	40 mins.	37 mins.
Food Shopping	265 mins.	230 mins.	203 mins.	182 mins.	157 mins.	139 mins.	128 mins.
Gardening, General	153 mins.	132 mins.	117 mins.	105 mins.	90 mins.	80 mins.	74 mins.
Raking Lawn	142 mins.	123 mins.	109 mins.	97 mins.	84 mins.	74 mins.	69 mins.
Sex, General, Moderate	469 mins.	407 mins.	360 mins.	322 mins.	277 mins.	245 mins.	227 mins.
Shoveling Snow	102 mins.	88 mins.	78 mins.	70 mins.	60 mins.	53 mins.	49 mins.
Sweep Floors	185 mins.	160 mins.	142 mins.	127 mins.	109 mins.	97 mins.	89 mins.
Treadmill	68 mins.	59 mins.	52 mins.	47 mins.	40 mins.	35 mins.	33 mins.
Vacuum	174 mins.	151 mins.	134 mins.	120 mins.	103 mins.	91 mins.	84 mins.
Volleyball	153 mins.	132 mins.	117 mins.	105 mins.	90 mins.	80 mins.	74 mins.
Washing Dishes	244 mins.	230 mins.	203 mins.	182 mins.	157 mins.	139 mins.	128 mins.
Weight Lifting	203 mins.	176 mins.	156 mins.	140 mins.	120 mins.	106 mins.	98 mins.

McDonald's Deluxe Breakfast

To burn off scrambled eggs, hash browns, sausage, pancakes and syrup *(approx. 1120 calories)* you would have to:

Activity	130 lbs	150 lbs	170 lbs	190 lbs	220 lbs	250 lbs	270 lbs
Aerobics, General	175 mins.	152 mins.	134 mins.	120 mins.	103 mins.	91 mins.	85 mins.
Bicycle, Stationary	163 mins.	141 mins.	125 mins.	112 mins.	96 mins.	85 mins.	79 mins.
Calisthenics *(push-ups, sit-ups, pull-ups, jumping jacks)*	142 mins.	124 mins.	109 mins.	98 mins.	84 mins.	74 mins.	69 mins.
Food Shopping	495 mins.	430 mins.	379 mins.	340 mins.	292 mins.	259 mins.	239 mins.
Gardening, General	285 mins.	247 mins.	218 mins.	195 mins.	168 mins.	149 mins.	138 mins.
Raking Lawn	265 mins.	230 mins.	203 mins.	182 mins.	156 mins.	138 mins.	128 mins.
Sex, General, Moderate	876 mins.	760 mins.	671 mins.	601 mins.	517 mins.	457 mins.	424 mins.
Shoveling Snow	190 mins.	165 mins.	145 mins.	130 mins.	112 mins.	99 mins.	92 mins.
Sweep Floors	345 mins.	299 mins.	264 mins.	237 mins.	204 mins.	180 mins.	167 mins.
Treadmill	127 mins.	110 mins.	97 mins.	87 mins.	75 mins.	66 mins.	61 mins.
Vacuum	325 mins.	262 mins.	249 mins.	223 mins.	192 mins.	170 mins.	157 mins.
Volleyball	285 mins.	247 mins.	218 mins.	195 mins.	168 mins.	149 mins.	138 mins.
Washing Dishes	495 mins.	430 mins.	379 mins.	340 mins.	292 mins.	259 mins.	239 mins.
Weight Lifting	380 mins.	329 mins.	291 mins.	260 mins.	224 mins.	198 mins.	184 mins.

McDonald's Lunch

To burn off 1 McChicken sandwich, large fries and 1 large Coke *(approx. 1240 calories)* you would have to:

Activity	130 lbs	150 lbs	170 lbs	190 lbs	220 lbs	250 lbs	270 lbs
Aerobics, General	194 mins.	168 mins.	149 mins.	133 mins.	114 mins.	101 mins.	94 mins.
Bicycle, Stationary	180 mins.	156 mins.	138 mins.	124 mins.	106 mins.	94 mins.	87 mins.
Calisthenics *(push-ups, sit-ups, pull-ups, jumping jacks)*	158 mins.	137 mins.	121 mins.	108 mins.	93 mins.	82 mins.	76 mins.
Food Shopping	548 mins.	476 mins.	420 mins.	376 mins.	323 mins.	286 mins.	265 mins.
Gardening, General	315 mins.	274 mins.	242 mins.	216 mins.	186 mins.	165 mins.	152 mins.
Raking Lawn	293 mins.	254 mins.	225 mins.	201 mins.	173 mins.	153 mins.	142 mins.
Sex, General, Moderate	970 mins.	842 mins.	743 mins.	665 mins.	572 mins.	506 mins.	469 mins.
Shoveling Snow	210 mins.	182 mins.	161 mins.	144 mins.	124 mins.	110 mins.	102 mins.
Sweep Floors	382 mins.	332 mins.	293 mins.	262 mins.	225 mins.	200 mins.	185 mins.
Treadmill	140 mins.	122 mins.	107 mins.	96 mins.	83 mins.	73 mins.	68 mins.
Vacuum	360 mins.	313 mins.	276mins.	247 mins.	213 mins.	188 mins.	174 mins.
Volleyball	315 mins.	274 mins.	242mins.	216 mins.	186 mins.	165 mins.	152 mins.
Washing Dishes	548 mins.	476 mins.	420 mins.	376 mins.	323 mins.	286 mins.	265 mins.
Weight Lifting	420 mins.	365 mins.	322 mins.	288 mins.	248 mins.	219 mins.	203 mins.

Taco Bell Lunch

To burn off 1 taco, 1 burrito and 1 large Pepsi *(approx. 860 calories)* you would have to:

Activity	130 lbs	150 lbs	170 lbs	190 lbs	220 lbs	250 lbs	270 lbs
Aerobics, General	135 mins.	117 mins.	103 mins.	92 mins.	79 mins.	70 mins.	65 mins.
Bicycle, Stationary	125 mins.	108 mins.	96 mins.	86 mins.	74 mins.	65 mins.	60 mins.
Calisthenics *(push-ups, sit-ups, pull-ups, jumping jacks)*	109 mins.	95 mins.	84 mins.	75 mins.	64 mins.	57 mins.	53 mins.
Food Shopping	380 mins.	330 mins.	291 mins.	261 mins.	224 mins.	199 mins.	184 mins.
Gardening, General	219 mins.	190 mins.	168 mins.	150 mins.	129 mins.	114 mins.	106 mins.
Raking Lawn	203 mins.	176 mins.	156 mins.	140 mins.	120 mins.	106 mins.	98 mins.
Sex, General, Moderate	673 mins.	584 mins.	515 mins.	462 mins.	397 mins.	351 mins.	325 mins.
Shoveling Snow	146 mins.	126 mins.	112 mins.	100 mins.	86 mins.	76 mins.	70 mins.
Sweep Floors	265 mins.	230 mins.	203 mins.	182 mins.	156 mins.	138 mins.	128 mins.
Treadmill	97 mins.	84 mins.	74 mins.	67 mins.	57 mins.	51 mins.	47 mins.
Vacuum	250 mins.	217 mins.	191 mins.	171 mins.	147 mins.	130 mins.	121 mins.
Volleyball	219 mins.	190 mins.	168 mins.	150 mins.	129 mins.	114 mins.	106 mins.
Washing Dishes	380 mins.	330 mins.	291 mins.	261 mins.	224 mins.	199 mins.	184 mins.
Weight Lifting	292 mins.	253 mins.	223 mins.	200 mins.	172 mins.	152 mins.	141 mins.

The Saga Continues: You poor thing, you had to work late. Fortunately, your coworker volunteered to grab something for both of you. Of course, you didn't want to be choosy so he bought back a choice of dinners from KFC or Taco Bell. He's gracious enough to let you choose your poison…ooops I mean meal. At least you chose the 900 calorie KFC meal versus the 1,350 meal from Taco Bell. But if you add up everything that you've eaten and had to drink for the day—the scales are going to be moving in the totally wrong direction. Further, your cholesterol *(from the fat)* and your blood pressure *(from the salt)* are not on track. PLUS you've worked late, feel sluggish and exercise. This is a prescription for disaster, but let's be honest, how often does this happen during your week? I ask you to honestly assess your current lifestyle; look at your stomach and ask: *Is It Worth It?*

KFC Dinner

To burn off 3 crispy chicken strips, potato salad, corn on the cob and 1 large Pepsi *(approx. 900 calories)* you would have to:

Activity	130 lbs	150 lbs	170 lbs	190 lbs	220 lbs	250 lbs	270 lbs
Aerobics, General	141 mins.	122 mins.	108 mins.	97 mins.	83 mins.	74 mins.	68 mins.
Bicycle, Stationary	131 mins.	113 mins.	100 mins.	90 mins.	77 mins.	68 mins.	63 mins.
Calisthenics *(push-ups, sit-ups, pull-ups, jumping jacks)*	114 mins.	99 mins.	88 mins.	78 mins.	68 mins.	60 mins.	55 mins.
Food Shopping	398 mins.	345 mins.	305 mins.	273 mins.	235 mins.	208 mins.	192 mins.
Gardening, General	229 mins.	199 mins.	175 mins.	157 mins.	135 mins.	119 mins.	111 mins.
Raking Lawn	213 mins.	185 mins.	163 mins.	146 mins.	126 mins.	111 mins.	103 mins.
Sex, General, Moderate	704 mins.	611 mins.	539 mins.	483 mins.	415 mins.	368 mins.	340 mins.
Shoveling Snow	153 mins.	132 mins.	117 mins.	105 mins.	90 mins.	80 mins.	74 mins.
Sweep Floors	277 mins.	241 mins.	213 mins.	190 mins.	164 mins.	145 mins.	134 mins.
Treadmill	102 mins.	88 mins.	78 mins.	70 mins.	60 mins.	53 mins.	49 mins.
Vacuum	262 mins.	227 mins.	200 mins.	179 mins.	154 mins.	137 mins.	126 mins.
Volleyball	229 mins.	199 mins.	175mins.	157 mins.	135 mins.	119 mins.	111 mins.
Washing Dishes	398 mins.	345 mins.	305 mins.	273 mins.	235 mins.	208 mins.	192 mins.
Weight Lifting	305 mins.	265 mins.	234 mins.	209 mins.	180 mins.	159 mins.	148 mins.

Taco Bell Dinner

To burn off 1 double decker taco supreme, 1 beef gordita supreme, 1 cheese quesadilla and 1 large Pepsi *(approx. 1350 calories)* you would have to:

Activity	130 lbs	150 lbs	170 lbs	190 lbs	220 lbs	250 lbs	270 lbs
Aerobics, General	211 mins.	183 mins.	162 mins.	145 mins.	125 mins.	110 mins.	102 mins.
Bicycle, Stationary	196 mins.	170 mins.	150 mins.	135 mins.	116 mins.	102 mins.	95 mins.
Calisthenics *(push-ups, sit-ups, pull-ups, jumping jacks)*	172 mins.	149 mins.	131 mins.	118 mins.	101 mins.	90 mins.	83 mins.
Food Shopping	597 mins.	518 mins.	457 mins.	410 mins.	352 mins.	312 mins.	289 mins.
Gardening, General	343 mins.	298 mins.	263 mins.	235 mins.	202 mins.	179 mins.	166 mins.
Raking Lawn	319 mins.	277 mins.	245 mins.	219 mins.	188 mins.	167 mins.	154 mins.
Sex, General, Moderate	1056 mins.	916 mins.	809 mins.	725 mins.	623 mins.	551 mins.	511 mins.
Shoveling Snow	229 mins.	199 mins.	175 mins.	157 mins.	135 mins.	119 mins.	111 mins.
Sweep Floors	416 mins.	361 mins.	319mins.	285 mins.	245 mins.	217 mins.	201 mins.
Treadmill	153 mins.	132 mins.	117 mins.	105 mins.	90 mins.	80 mins.	74 mins.
Vacuum	392 mins.	340 mins.	301 mins.	269 mins.	231 mins.	205 mins.	190 mins.
Volleyball	343 mins.	298 mins.	263 mins.	235 mins.	202 mins.	179 mins.	166 mins.
Washing Dishes	597 mins.	518 mins.	457mins.	410 mins.	352 mins.	312 mins.	289 mins.
Weight Lifting	458 mins.	397 mins.	351 mins.	314 mins.	270 mins.	239 mins.	221 mins.

Home Sweet Home: You finally make it home and your partner has graciously made dinner. You only take a bite or two off of his plate; after all you did eat at the office. However, you don't want to make the same mistakes and decide to take the leftovers from dinner for lunch on tomorrow. You feel good as you put together your food, but decide not to take the garden salad, after all it will wilt. Your partner is a great cook and made all of your favorites: fried chicken, macaroni salad and there's some potato salad from the night before. You don't know which you'll prefer tomorrow so you take some of both. You'll pass on the bread; after all you're trying to lose weight. *Is It Worth It?* That's no longer the question; you've answered it—NO. I just hope that you've paid up your health insurance and your life insurance because this is a recipe for *death by fork.*

Fried Chicken

To burn off **1 chicken breast** *(approx. 510 calories)* you would have to:

Activity	130 lbs	150 lbs	170 lbs	190 lbs	220 lbs	250 lbs	270 lbs
Aerobics, General	80 mins.	69 mins.	61 mins.	55 mins.	47 mins.	42 mins.	39 mins.
Bicycle, Stationary	74 mins.	64 mins.	57 mins.	51 mins.	44 mins.	39 mins.	36 mins.
Calisthenics *(push-ups, sit-ups, pull-ups, jumping jacks)*	65 mins.	56 mins.	50 mins.	44 mins.	38 mins.	34 mins.	72 mins.
Food Shopping	225 mins.	196 mins.	173 mins.	155 mins.	133 mins.	118 mins.	109 mins.
Gardening, General	130 mins.	112 mins.	99 mins.	89 mins.	76 mins.	68 mins.	63 mins.
Raking Lawn	121 mins.	105 mins.	92 mins.	83 mins.	71 mins.	63 mins.	58 mins.
Sex, General, Moderate	399 mins.	346 mins.	306 mins.	274 mins.	235 mins.	208 mins.	193 mins.
Shoveling Snow	86 mins.	75 mins.	66 mins.	59 mins.	51 mins.	45 mins.	42 mins.
Sweep Floors	157 mins.	136 mins.	120 mins.	108 mins.	93 mins.	82 mins.	76 mins.
Treadmill	58 mins.	50 mins.	44 mins.	40 mins.	34 mins.	30 mins.	28 mins.
Vacuum	148 mins.	129 mins.	114 mins.	102 mins.	87 mins.	77 mins.	72 mins.
Volleyball	130 mins.	112 mins.	99 mins.	89 mins.	76 mins.	68 mins.	63 mins.
Washing Dishes	225 mins.	196 mins.	173mins.	155 mins.	133 mins.	118 mins.	109 mins.
Weight Lifting	173 mins.	150 mins.	132 mins.	119 mins.	102 mins.	90 mins.	84 mins.

Macaroni Salad

To burn off **1 cup of macaroni** *(approx. 700 calories)* you would have to:

Activity	130 lbs	150 lbs	170 lbs	190 lbs	220 lbs	250 lbs	270 lbs
Aerobics, General	110 mins.	95 mins.	84 mins.	75 mins.	65 mins.	57 mins.	53 mins.
Bicycle, Stationary	102 mins.	88 mins.	78 mins.	70 mins.	60 mins.	53 mins.	49 mins.
Calisthenics *(push-ups, sit-ups, pull-ups, jumping jacks)*	89 mins.	77 mins.	68 mins.	61 mins.	52 mins.	46 mins.	43 mins.
Food Shopping	310 mins.	269 mins.	237 mins.	212 mins.	183 mins.	162 mins.	150 mins.
Gardening, General	178 mins.	154 mins.	136 mins.	114 mins.	105 mins.	93 mins.	86 mins.
Raking Lawn	166 mins.	144 mins.	127 mins.	117 mins.	98 mins.	86 mins.	80 mins.
Sex, General, Moderate	548 mins.	475 mins.	420 mins.	376 mins.	323 mins.	286 mins.	265 mins.
Shoveling Snow	119 mins.	103 mins.	91 mins.	81 mins.	70 mins.	62 mins.	57 mins.
Sweep Floors	216 mins.	187 mins.	165 mins.	148 mins.	127 mins.	113 mins.	104 mins.
Treadmill	79 mins.	69 mins.	61 mins.	54 mins.	47 mins.	41 mins.	38 mins.
Vacuum	203 mins.	176 mins.	156 mins.	140 mins.	120 mins.	106 mins.	98 mins.
Volleyball	178 mins.	154 mins.	136 mins.	122 mins.	105 mins.	93 mins.	86 mins.
Washing Dishes	310 mins.	269 mins.	237mins.	212 mins.	183 mins.	162 mins.	150 mins.
Weight Lifting	237 mins.	206 mins.	182 mins.	163 mins.	140 mins.	124 mins.	115 mins.

Potato Salad

To burn off **1 cup of potato salad** *(approx. 440 calories)* you would have to:

Activity	130 lbs	150 lbs	170 lbs	190 lbs	220 lbs	250 lbs	270 lbs
Aerobics, General	69 mins.	60 mins.	53 mins.	47 mins.	41 mins.	36 mins.	33 mins.
Bicycle, Stationary	64 mins.	55 mins.	49 mins.	44 mins.	38 mins.	33 mins.	31 mins.
Calisthenics *(push-ups, sit-ups, pull-ups, jumping jacks)*	56 mins.	49 mins.	43 mins.	38 mins.	33 mins.	29 mins.	27 mins.
Food Shopping	195 mins.	169 mins.	149 mins.	133 mins.	115 mins.	102 mins.	94 mins.
Gardening, General	112 mins.	97 mins.	86 mins.	77 mins.	66 mins.	58 mins.	54 mins.
Raking Lawn	104 mins.	90 mins.	80 mins.	71 mins.	61 mins.	54 mins.	50 mins.
Sex, General, Moderate	344 mins.	299 mins.	264 mins.	236 mins.	203 mins.	180 mins.	166 mins.
Shoveling Snow	75 mins.	65 mins.	57 mins.	51 mins.	44 mins.	39 mins.	36 mins.
Sweep Floors	136 mins.	118 mins.	104 mins.	93 mins.	80 mins.	71 mins.	66 mins.
Treadmill	50 mins.	43 mins.	38 mins.	34 mins.	29 mins.	26 mins.	24 mins.
Vacuum	128 mins.	111 mins.	98 mins.	88 mins.	75 mins.	67 mins.	62 mins.
Volleyball	112 mins.	97 mins.	86 mins.	77 mins.	66 mins.	58 mins.	54 mins.
Washing Dishes	195 mins.	169 mins.	149 mins.	133 mins.	115 mins.	102 mins.	94 mins.
Weight Lifting	149 mins.	129 mins.	114 mins.	102 mins.	88 mins.	78 mins.	72 mins.

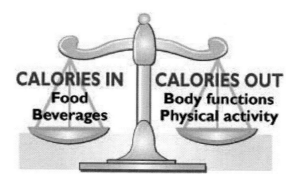

Is It Really Worth It? ARE YOU REALLY WORTH IT?

"A wise man should consider that health is the greatest of human blessings, and learn how by his own thought to derive benefit from his illnesses."
Hippocrates

Well we've read all the things that we're eating and doing wrong. You may be overwhelmed and think—*"Who cares! I can't do anything right, I gotta die of something"* and *"I'm destined to be overweight, why fight it."*

Here are three other reasons to stay on track:

1. **Your Sex Life Improves and is Safer**

    a. You can choose to eat chocolate or have an orgasm; one gives you calories and the other burns the calories, both release happy hormones or endorphins in your brain. Further, researchers at Duke University showed that even a 10% reduction in your weight results in major improvements in all areas of the study participants' sex lives, including arousal, feelings of attractiveness and enjoyment of sex. *Hmmmmmmm can we say join the gym?*

    b. A woman who has a positive self-image is more discriminating when it comes to choosing sexual partners and more likely to use condoms than a woman who is unhappy with her appearance, say University of Pennsylvania researchers. The payoff: a lower risk of STDs and unwanted pregnancies. For a quick self-esteem boost, work out. "Women at any weight who exercise report higher levels of body satisfaction than women who don't," says Ann Kearney-Cooke, PhD, author of *Change Your Mind, Change Your Body.*

c. Pushing through an extra incline mile on the treadmill or a third set of lifting does more than shape you up. It preps your brain for sex by reducing stress and releasing a cascade of feel good hormones in your body, two musts when it comes to lust. "Physical activities that get blood flowing to the thighs and buttocks are especially beneficial from an arousal standpoint," says Susan Kellogg, PhD, director of sexual medicine at the Pelvic and Sexual Health Institute of Philadelphia. Add lunges to your usual workout today, and see what happens. If you're not currently exercising, try this for motivation: Kellogg says patients consistently report an increase in sexual interest the day they start working out. Talk about instant results!

2. Your Sleep Improves

a. According to Michael Twery, PhD, director of the National Center for Sleep Disorders Research at the National Heart, Lung and Blood Institute, research studies indicate that weight loss is associated with a reduction in the severity of mild to moderate sleep apnea. Apparently, more fat around the neck means more obstruction while sleeping. Lose the fat and you're able to breathe better. A bonus for men. Some findings suggest that the benefits of weight loss may be greater for them than for women.

3. Your Salary May Improve

a. Research by John Cawley of the University of Michigan has shown that an overweight woman may earn 7% less pay than an ideal sized woman. ***This is just WRONG, but the facts speak for themselves.***

"Health is not simply the absence of sickness." *Hannah Green*

Bottom Line: Are You Worth It?

Only you can decide how valuable your health, wellness and family are to you. This is so very personal and there are so many pieces that go into this puzzle. I hate it when people judge other people based on how they look. I believe that people are beautiful in all different shapes, sizes, colors and styles. Further, beauty has so very little to do with outer looks versus who you are as a person and the inside. However, we must be honest, you personality does not walk up and say hello first—it is the visual first. This book is not about you becoming model thin (*they really need to EAT*); it is about you being as healthy as you can be and making the informed decision on how to get there.

I don't judge your methods as long as they are based on a healthy model and realistic expectations. However, when you expect a miracle in a bottle, in a doctor's office or on an operating table; I have to tell you NO! There is no magic bullet. There must be a commitment to lifestyle changes and if you don't make that commitment you may be a perfect size 8 for 2 weeks but then "blow back up" to a size 18 once you start back on the pig's feet, chicken wings, Outback cheese fries and other foods that caused you to gain weight. This INCLUDES people that undergo invasive surgeries and therapies for weight loss such as gastric bypass and banding. These procedures have risks which can be life threatening and serious. You should talk to your doctor and get a second opinion prior to undergoing these procedures. People who regain weight after gastric bypass surgery usually are consuming too many high calorie foods and beverages and not incorporating exercise into their lives. Many that regain after the invasive interventions have looked at the surgery as the cure all and forget the sneakers and lifestyle modifications. You must have the mindset that you are going to make permanent lifestyle changes and that the intervention is a TOOL and not the ANSWER.

Let me be clear, I believe that for many people these are excellent TOOLS to a healthier life just as Weight Watchers, Jenny Craig, Nutrisystem, etc., are excellent tools. There is bias against people that undergo procedures and I believe that this is just foolishness. YOU and your physician must make the decisions about your health. These interventions may be lifesaving to people, just as you having your appendix out may be lifesaving to you. My warning is to understand that even these surgical procedures require a commitment to lifestyle change. No matter what method you choose on this weight loss journey, the *Worth It* Model works.

What do we SAY that We Want?

A survey by National Women's Health Resource Center, Harris Interactive and *Fitness Magazine* found that:
YOUR Main Mission for Health:

- 76% want to eat healthier

- 71% want to exercise more

- 61% want to lose weight

- 52% want less stress

- 40% want more sleep

- 88% of those surveyed had MULTIPLE health goals

YOUR Biggest Roadblock:

- 42% No time

- 25% Too expensive

- 21% Too much effort

- 15% Me-time guilt

- 14% No game plan

- 10% No support

- Only 1% of those surveyed cited lack of willpower as a get-healthy obstacle.

Other findings:

- One half crave a better understanding of how small changes can affect your health.

- Eating better gets easier, 44% of 18-29 year olds are meeting their eat right goals, while an impressive 60% of women in their 40s are meeting them.

- 35% of persons surveyed say that knowing the nutritional breakdown of menu items would help you eat smarter.

- 37% of persons surveyed say smaller restaurant portions would help.

What are YOU willing to Trade Off for your Health?

- 66% of those surveyed are willing to spend less time working, enjoying leisure activities or tackling your to-do list.

- 15% of those surveyed are willing to give up some money.

- 25% aren't willing to sacrifice anything.

"Look to your health; and if you have it, praise God and value it next to conscience; for health is the second blessing that we mortals are capable of, blessing money can't buy." Izaak Walton

What is Your DESIRE?

"Whatever you vividly imagine, ardently desire, sincerely believe, and enthusiastically act upon must inevitably come to pass." Paul Meyer

The first step in your weight loss journey begins not with your fork, sneakers or family. It begins in your brain, in your spirit and with your desire. Notice that I didn't say commitment; I said DESIRE, do you desire to be healthy, fit and to weigh less? For many of us there is a point in time that is a moment of sheer, brutal and in your face reality that we will cope with as it relates to our weight. It is very personal and you may experience several such moments. Do you know what I'm talking about? These are a few that have been shared with me from people around the country.

- "My 9 year old son came home from school with a bruise on his arm. I was upset and asked what happened. He wouldn't tell me, even when I threatened him with no television for a week and other punishments. He was adamant that he could not tell me. I took him to school the next morning and confronted his teacher. His teacher told me that one of my son's classmates had drawn a picture of me and put underneath it half woman/half whale and my name. My son had punched the boy and he was hit back on the arm before the teacher broke it up. I looked at my son who had turned red, looked down at the ground as tears rolled down my face. My son was being teased because of me and he at the tender age of 9 didn't want to hurt my feelings by telling me. I left the school that day, went directly to Bally's and signed a year's membership. I've been working out 4 times a week for the last year and a half and have lost over sixty pounds."

- "I travel a lot for business and usually am upgraded to first/business class. The seats are larger and I can discreetly ask for a seatbelt extender. On one particular flight, the plane was full and I had to sit in coach, worse than that I was late and my aisle seat was given away. The only seat available was in the middle and as I walked sideways down the aisle I saw the man sitting in the window roll his eyes at me when he realized that I was going to be sitting next to him. Worse than that, the other guy sitting in the aisle said rather loudly, "You've gotta be kidding me!" I got to the seat and squeezed in, the arm rails dug into my sides and I asked the attendant for a seatbelt extender. She looked at the guy sitting in the aisle and winked. Once she returned she made a big production on how to put it on. I had to go to the bathroom after about an hour of the two hour trip but I refused to get up. I sat there totally humiliated and embarrassed. I wondered how I, a 41 year old educated, successful man had let myself balloon to over 400 pounds and get high blood pressure, high cholesterol and early diabetes. That was the last day that I ate any fried foods or my usual Meat Lover's large pizza and the first day that I walked for exercise. Seven months later, I'd lost over 100 pounds and I'm well on my way to a healthier life."

- "My mother was in the ICU of the hospital; she had suffered a heart attack and was dying. I visited her every day and one night the nurse said to me—you look just like your mother. You could be twins. The problem was that my mother was 69 years old and I was only 44. My reality was that my mother and I wore the same size 22/24 clothes and we both were supposed to take medications for high blood pressure and cholesterol. I looked at the nurse, who didn't mean any harm, and told her that I could not live my life like my mother. My mother passed a few days later and as I stood at her graveside, I asked her and God to help me make a change in my life for the better. You, *Dr. Sharon* spoke at our women's conference and talked about weight, health and being real; I took notes and really listened. I joined the YMCA and began walking—slowly at first but I started. I also started watching what I ate more and began to really pray for help. One night, my mother came to me in a dream and told me that I could do it. I've lost 24 pounds but I've gained confidence that I can be healthy."

- "I was unemployed and one of my best friends worked at a big name department store. She said that she would get me an interview. I had over six years of sales experience, an associate's degree in marketing and although I didn't want to go into retail again; I knew that I would get the job based on my experience and personality. I had the interview and dressed nicely in a navy suit with makeup and hair done. I thought that the interview went well and was sure that I'd get a call back. A few days later my friend came over for a visit, obviously uncomfortable. She told me that I didn't get the job and that they were still looking. I asked her why and she reluctantly told me that the department supervisor told her that I didn't *look* the part because I couldn't wear any of the designer clothes. She also told her that I would have to do a lot of walking and standing and that when I walked into her office she heard my thighs rub together and I was out of breath. That was the day that changed how I looked at my weight. I'm a very attractive woman and I've bought into the *big girls are divas too* philosophy. However, my weight now was not only a factor for my health and well being; it was affecting my ability to get a job. I've 30 pounds to lose and I'm on my way."

- "My doctor of over 14 years told me that unless I lose some weight, lowered my blood pressure and cholesterol that I probably will not live to see my 17 year old son graduate from college. He is an only child and his mother died when he was young—I'm the only parent that he has. I realized that he needed me more than I needed the ridiculous amount of food that I was eating. I've lost 36 pounds and my cholesterol has dropped over 20%, my blood pressure is in a normal range. I can't wait to see my doctor again."

- "My husband and I had been married for two years and he announced to me one day that he was moving out. We are both very active in our church and although things had been a little rocky, I didn't know that it had come to this. I asked him why and he said that he loved me as a person but that he was not sexually attracted to me and that I'd changed since we married. I pushed him for more of an explanation, even admitted that I'd gained a few pounds but so had he. He told me that it was more than a few; that I didn't look or act the same and that I was boring because all I wanted to do was sit around and eat. He said that he had to force himself to respond to me sexually but could not do that over the last few months. That night I got on the scale, something that I never do and had not done since I lost weight for my wedding. I could not believe it; I had gained over 60 pounds. I sat on the floor crying for over an hour. When I got up to wash my face, I saw for the first time how puffy it was, how my hair was looking and I took off my clothes and looked at my body. Right or wrong, I was not the woman that he had married. While I don't agree with him leaving and I'm not losing weight for him, I understand and I'm going to get myself back. It has been hard and is a struggle but I've seen my doctor and he's prescribed some medication for me and I'm seeing a nutritionist. The next step is to start working out."

- "I am a 51 year old woman and I've been overweight all my life. I am a nurse and I know better, but after years of working third shift, eating late, hardly sleeping and having 2 kids, the pounds piled on. I didn't even recognize myself anymore and the comfort of scrubs hid my weight, or so I thought. I developed diabetes and began to get blurred vision that I just attributed to old age. However, when I went to see my doctor and he told me that I may be developing kidney disease, I sat in his office and cried. My bad habits were killing me and I had to be honest, I was not just a little overweight; I weighed over 270 pounds and am just 5'7". My turning point came when I was discharging a patient from the hospital after open heart surgery. I talked to them about diet and the importance of them making lifestyle changes. This patient was not pleasant at all and we all tried to avoid him, I wasn't so lucky. He stopped me in the middle of my instructions and said, 'You need to take your own advice, you're a porker!' And started laughing, his family joined in and I smiled but was humiliated. For me, I made the decision to have gastric banding after meeting with my doctor. I have made the lifestyle changes that will carry me through the rest of my life. People think that surgery is a quick fix and that it is so easy; it really is not. I fight this battle every single day but I am happy that I'm winning."

Turning Points That Have Been Shared From Me to You

The stories that you have shared with me are so very touching and in some ways are infuriating to me. I also wanted to share two of my own turning points.

The DIVA is here!

I was a guest panelist with several other authors at a major event. I had my makeup artist meet me after having my hair done and had decided on a great designer piece to wear to the event. I wore my favorite designer jewelry, pulled out a pair of my low heeled Jimmy Choo sling backs and the matching bag. My people *(assistant and PR person)* and others told me how beautiful I looked and the discussion began. It was fun and engaging. Someone brought me some water and a tissue midway through and I really didn't think anything of it. I wondered why they came directly to me but I kept talking. Afterward we took more group shots and my assistant asked the photographer to send pictures to her. A few days later, I saw the photos and while everyone was so complementary—I looked at my thighs in one of the shots, I tell you no lie; my right thigh was the size of a toddler. I looked at my face, which I had spent money to get professionally done and in the later shots I saw that my face had become sweaty. Later, I received a clip of video that was done and was shocked to hear myself talking and breathing so hard. I had come with my game face, clothes and knowledge on but my body was not supporting my lifestyle. While I was designer down, I could not cover up that I was in poor health. *Dr. Sharon* needed a doctor, nutritionist, trainer, gym, SOMETHING!

Let the Church Say Amen

Another major moment came for me quietly but hit me like a ton of bricks. I was running late for church *(which I often do)* and I attend a large church with an expansive parking lot. If you get there late, you park in the back and you have a little hike. I had on a suit and heels and for the life of me could not find a space that was anywhere near the church. I considered for a moment parking in the handicapped space but that wouldn't be good. Well, I parked on the last row and began to walk toward the church. When I got to the sliding glass doors I got a glimpse of myself and my perfectly curled hair had started to fall, my face was sweaty, my knees hurt and I laughed a hello to security to try to play off the fact that I was out of breath. I went to the bathroom to get myself together and a member came to me and said; "Dr. Sharon, thank you so much for health awareness this year. I want you to know that I've lost 8 pounds, I'm working out and I really heard you when you talked about our health. Thank you for keeping it real." She walked out the door and I walked into a stall and held back tears. I was telling women around the world about their health, challenging us to do better and was being effective; but what about my health? What about me really keeping it real about my body. I used the excuse that I didn't have high blood pressure, diabetes or high cholesterol. I would say at forums when I talked about weight that I understood the sisters' struggle because I was in it. However, I wasn't in a struggle—I was drowning in all the fried chicken, mashed potatoes, pecan pie and other food that I wanted to eat. I was drowning and didn't find the time or the energy to work out. I was drowning a slow death that was a direct result of the fork, the sneakers and my family traditions of the south that gave me an excuse to be both a great cook and eater.

****

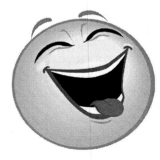

Laugh break:

A young woman having a physical exam felt very embarrassed because of a weight problem. As she removed her last bit of clothing, she said, "Doctor, I feel so ashamed and embarrassed. I guess I've really let myself go."

"Now, now," the doctor said as he began to examine her. "Don't feel that way. You really don't look that bad."

"Do you really think so?" she asked.

"Of course," replies the doctor as he held a tongue depressor in front of her face. "Now open wide and say 'MOO'!"

Let me tell you that I'm still in a struggle with my weight, pounds and pounds later. I refuse to deny the person that I was. If you look on my website you see a lot of my old pictures. They serve as reminders for me but I also love that part of my life. There's no way that I can take down a picture of me and the ever sexy Harry Belafonte; I don't care how big I was. I will reiterate that you can look great wherever you are and that it is discrimination to think that larger men or women are not sexy or attractive. However, more than your looks, we must focus on your health.

Now be ready as you begin this journey; there is a song on my iPod that I want to share with you:

HATE On Me by Jill Scott

If I could give you the world
On a silver platter
Would it even matter
You'd still be mad at me
If I can find in all this
A dozen roses
Which I would give to you
You'd still be miserable
In reality
I'm gon be who I be
And I don't feel no faults
For all the lies that you bought
You can try as you may
Break me down when I say
That it ain't up to you
Gon on do what you do

[*Chorus:*]
Hate on me hater
Now or Later
Cause I'm gonna do me
You'll be made baby
(Go head and hate)
Go head and hate on me hater
I'm not afraid of
What I got I paid for
You can hate on me...
Ooh if I gave you peaches
Out of my on garden
And I made you a peach cobbler
Would you slap me out?
Wonder if I gave you diamonds
Out of my on womb
Would you feel the love in that

Or ask why not the moon
If I gave you sanity
For the whole of humanity
Had all the solutions for the pain and pollution
No Matter Where I live
Despite the things I give
You'll always be this way
So go ahead and ...

[*Chorus x2*]
You Cannot...
Hate On me
Cause my mind is free
Feel my destiny
So Shall it Be

Why this song, well I have several on my iPod but the reality is that as you start to make changes, lose weight and be more comfortable with the inner and outer you; there may be family, friends, spouses and others that are not comfortable with your changes. In a word, they may become jealous and may try to derail you—especially if they are not making life changes OR if you've always been the fat friend. They may hate on you, I have to say that my friends and family have been absolutely wonderful to me. Now, some of them have some words when they come to my house and I don't cook four meats, eight side dishes and one vegetable and they can't find a soda. BUT for the most part they've been great. However, I've heard stories of others that are making changes and have a few little words that have been directed to me by people who really don't matter to me. You know how people do; c'mon, let me share a few of these nasty little jabs that you may encounter.

1. "She don't look healthy, she look sick."

2. "She acts like she's better than us."

3. "She's not all that, she still needs to lose more weight."

4. "She's a fanatic; it's not natural to work out that much."

5. "I wonder what she did. Did she have surgery? Did she get liposuction?"

6. "I liked her better when she was fat, now she's too stuck up."

Instead of the nastiness, what about telling the sister *(or brother)*:

1. "I'm proud of you—you look great and I know you feel better."

2. "You've inspired me to do better."

3. "Keep it up, You go Girl!"

"Learn from yesterday, life for today, hope for tomorrow." *Unknown Author*

Where Do I Start?

"Sooner or later, those who win are those who think they can." *Richard Bach*

You've already started; you're holding this book in your hands. You're getting some facts and hopefully having a reality check with yourself. These are the first steps that I recommend for anyone needing to lose weight and begin a fitness regimen:

"The past is just that, the past—learn from it and let it go. Your future is limitless; don't allow the past to shackle you." *Sharon Allison-Ottey, MD*

Dr. Sharon's Recommendations for Starting the Weight-loss Journey

1. **Contact your physician or healthcare provider and schedule a complete physical exam.**

    a. If you don't have insurance, let me tell you a secret. Physicians take cash, check or charge and they usually prefer it to billing your insurance plan. If you have to pay out of pocket—ASK FOR A DISCOUNT. There may be free or reduced payment clinics in your area if you don't have insurance or the funds to pay for your visit.

    b. Before you go for your visit:

        i. Make sure that you write down questions, give an honest assessment of things that are going on in your health and get an idea of what your daily habits are as it relates to food, exercise, sleep and general mood.

        ii. If you are currently prescribed medications and are taking over the counter meds, herbal supplements or minerals take them with you to the doctor.

        iii. If you have decided to start a specific program like Jenny Craig, Nutrisystem, the Mediterranean Diet or even are considering invasive surgery or banding; write down your questions and get their opinion.

    c. During your visit:

        i. You should expect to get your height/weight done, ask for your BMI.

        ii. You should have your blood pressure checked and there might be a need for other tests like an EKG *(heart tracing)*, bloodwork to include a check for thyroid problems, anemia, cholesterol, prostate *(men)* blood tests and other specific tests based on your medical history.

        iii. You should discuss your overall health and recommendations based on your age, race, family history and personal medical history. Tell the doctor your goals, ask what he/she thinks your ideal weight should be and any advice that they can give. You may want to ask for a referral to a nutritionist or other healthcare provider.

            1. Ask your doctor about your medications and nutritional supplements. Make sure that he/she knows that you are going to be cutting your calories and the question of vitamins should be discussed in detail.

    d. You should not leave without getting the following questions answered (*this applies to ANYTIME you or your loved one visits a healthcare professional and is called "Ask Me 3," more info can be found at www.askme3.org*)

        i. What is my main problem?

        ii. What do I need to do?

        iii. Why is it important for me to do this?

  e. After your visit:

    i. Follow your doctor's instructions and if they say that you can begin an exercise program, map out what you will do.

    ii. Wait on your lab results and don't assume that if they don't contact you that everything is all right. If you have not heard from them in about two weeks; call and ask for your results.

2. Get your MIND and SPIRIT right.

  a. Evaluate your MOTIVATION:

    i. If you are losing weight to attract a man or woman; WRONG motivation.

    ii. If you're losing weight because your wife/husband/boyfriend or friend has told you to and continues to nag and make you feel bad; WRONG motivation.

    iii. If you're losing weight because you feel that once you lose the weight you'll be perfect and that life will be rosy all your problems will go away; WRONG motivation.

  b. Search within yourself and make a list of why you desire to lose weight. Make a list of positives and negatives and be honest with yourself. Write down why you are *Worth It*.

    i. Read the *Worth It* affirmations, quotes and motivators that are provided in this book and on my website, www.drsharononline.com and come up with ones of your own.

  c. Depending on your family and social dynamics, have a discussion with those that will be directly affected by your commitment to better health.

    i. If you are a mother and responsible for meals in your house and will be making changes for the entire family, it would be nice to inform them that EVERYBODY is going to be healthier.

    ii. If you are a husband/boyfriend and have decided that you're going to join the gym and will be working out during a time that you usually spent with your partner; that will need to be discussed.

    iii. A support system (*not a nagging system*) is a good thing. However, if they become too supportive and start talking about the gumdrop that you ate and tell you you're supposed to be on a diet; this will require another conversation. I'm just saying…email me and I'll be glad to tell them to back off.

  c. Evaluate your relationship with food and exercise. From a mental and spiritual aspect you should do some soul searching. Obesity usually is not a result of pure gluttony, but often there are some emotional scars and issues that have led us here. If you are a spiritual person that believes in the power of God in your life, I advise that you pray daily about your health and the opportunity that He is giving you to make changes.

  d. Evaluate the timing in your life. This means if you are going through a major crisis that is draining you; take that into account.

    i. If you have just lost your job, your dog died, your wife left you, you found out that your three kids are not your biological children, you have four flat tires and your house is in foreclosure; now is not the exact moment to do a major overhaul of your life. You can begin to take baby steps but I imagine that you probably need to spend a few hours taking some deep breaths.

3. Choose your tool/method of action: Eating Plan

  a. Chances are you agree with me that diets don't work. It really is a lifestyle change. However, there are many tools that you can use and I refer you back to the table of popular eating plans/diets, etc. Don't, under ANY circumstances go to the fad diets that I warned you against in the beginning. The bottom line is to remember:

b. I do recommend that you start a food/exercise and emotional diary/journal. Tons of studies show that people that journal lose more weight and stick to it. There are also online programs that are FREE that you can use.

c. Set realistic goals. The goal should be to lose no more than two pounds per week. Realize that you may have peaks and valleys and certainly plateaus.

d. Purchases that you should make:

i. Buy a scale for your bathroom if you don't have one.

ii. Consider a food scale for the kitchen.

iii. Buy a calorie counter book or find a great online program.

iv. A lunch bag or container so that you can have snacks that are healthy.

4. Choose your tool/method of action: Exercise Plan

a. This does not take a lot of time, energy or money. Consider starting a walking program and start slowly if you haven't been exercising. Even if you can only do 10 minutes of walking at a slow pace, do it and in a day or two increase it by a minute or so.

b. Join a gym? Hire a trainer? Buy a DVD and an iPod? These are up to you but DO something.

c. Buy some nice workout/exercise wear. You feel better when you look better.

- **Ladies:** Don't grab the old, nasty torn up sweat pants and big 10XL T-shirt. Get yourself into a little color or pants that fit and definitely get sneakers that have support. I believe that your closet should be full of workout gear as it does motivate you. We have outfits to go to the mall in, work in, go to church in and more, why not outfits to workout in.

  a. Speaking of buying. This is truly a Dr. Sharon SUGGESTION and not mandatory. What about giving yourself some incentive? Buy a challenge skirt that is just one size smaller than you wear now—better yet pull it out of your closet because you know that you have clothes that you can't get in to.

  b. For every five pounds that I lose I believe that I need earrings, a trinket or something. Further, when I hit the double digits >10 pounds; it's on and I need an outfit. I made a deal with myself that when I hit 50, I'd buy myself a new…well I can't tell you that because I moved around the dollars and pretended that I had it for ages. *Ooops never know who's reading, but you get my point!*

- **Men:** Please don't pull out that old 1960's headband, tennis shorts and messed up T-shirt. Please don't do it and for the love of all that is HOLY don't pull out that silver sweat suit that looks like a garbage bag. If I see you on the street, I'm gonna stop and laugh in your face.

5. Set your start date and depending on the type of program *(self developed, organized weight loss center, physician supervised, medication or surgical intervention)* start your journey to a healthier you. Recognize that this is a journey and that you will have challenges and maybe setbacks but keep moving forward.

a. As a special favor to me; please email me at drsharon@sharondeniseallisonottey.com *(or just go to drsharononline.com)* and let me know that you decided you're *Worth It*! I do personally answer my email and you should make sure that you're signed up for the FREE Dr. Sharon newsletter. You never know what may come your way when you contact me—I love giveaways!

"You are so much more than even YOU have imagined or dreamed. Every day choose to live in the reality of your constant state of becoming more than you are now." *Sharon D. Allison-Ottey, MD*

Tools, Resources, Extras and Recipes

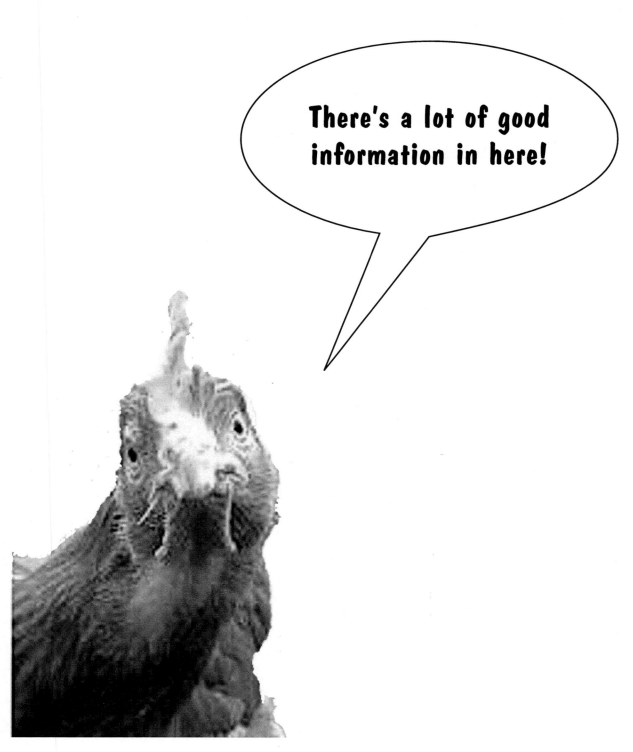

Worth It Affirmations

Affirm means: to validate, confirm, to assert and express dedication
An affirmation is simply the act of affirming.

I have written a few positive affirmations that you need to let sink in and use on your journey to health and wellness. Think about these and use them as you need to in your effort to stay on track. Often we belittle ourselves and need to be reminded of our true value.

1.   I am WORTH the extra effort that I am making to be healthier.

2.   I am WORTH all of the happiness and love that my heart can hold.

3.   I am WORTH taking an extra 15 minutes a day just to appreciate ME.

4.   I am WORTH the compliments that I give myself and receive from others every day.

5.   I am WORTH taking the time out to do something good for me, like exercise.

6.   I am WORTH saying NO when saying YES may harm me.

7.   I am WORTH getting 6-8 hours of sleep every night.

8.   I am WORTH ridding myself of bad relationships, including friendships which weigh me down.

9.   I am WORTH being valued by my employer and coworkers.

10.   I am WORTH enjoying life and exploring new things.

11.   I am WORTH NOT being verbally, mentally or physically abused by anyone.

12.   I am WORTH the love of my family and distancing myself when there is no love.

13.   I am WORTH congratulating myself on my weight loss, my healthy living and exercise goals from Day #1.

14.   I am WORTH starting over when I get off track without feeling guilty or beating myself up.

15.   I am WORTH the cute new outfits that I am going to purchase on this journey to better health and a slimmer body. *(That's a Dr. Sharon "extra"—say that a lot and out loud!)*

My Personal Affirmations

I ask that you write your own unique and personal affirmations. I also invite you to email them to me for others to use. We are all in this together!

1. _____

2. _____

3. _____

4. _____

5. _____

6. _____

7. _____

The *Is It Worth It?*   **Nutrition and Exercise Journal**   Day/Date:_____

GOALS for TODAY: _____ Calories: _____

Vitamins/Supplements? : Yes No (circle) Multivitamin Calcium Other(s): _____

Water *(write down approx. ounces then add up):* _____ Total: _____

Breakfast & Morning Snacks

Food and Drinks	Amount/ Serving	Cals.	Fat (g)	Other (carbs, etc)
Total				

Lunch   & Afternoon Snacks

Food and Drinks	Amount/ Serving	Cals.	Fat (g)	Other (carbs, etc)
Total				

Dinner& Evening Snacks

Food and Drinks	Amount/ Serving	Cals.	Fat (g)	Other (carbs, etc)
Total				

Exercise: Yes No **Aerobic/Cardio:** Yes No_____ *(mins)* Strength **Training:** Yes No *(circle)* Upper Lower Total Body

Calories In: _____ **Calories Burned:** _____   **A Worth It Day?** Yes No Why? _____
Notes *(Kudos and Areas of Improvement):*

You are WORTH being a Healthy Man

Found at www.ahrq.gov/ppip/Healthymen.htm

As a male, the most important things you can do to stay healthy are:

- Get recommended screening tests.

- Be tobacco free.

- Be physically active.

- Eat a healthy diet.

- Stay at a healthy weight.

- Take preventive medicines if you need them.

- Taking your prescribed medications as directed by your healthcare provider.

Screening Tests for Men: What You Need and When

Screening tests can find diseases early when they are easier to treat. Health experts from the U.S. Preventive Services Task Force have made recommendations, based on scientific evidence, about testing for the conditions below. Talk to your doctor about which ones apply to you and when and how often you should be tested.

- **Obesity:** Have your body mass index *(BMI)* calculated to screen for obesity. *(BMI is a measure of body fat based on height and weight.)* You can also find your own BMI with the BMI calculator from the National Heart, Lung, and Blood Institute at: www.nhlbisupport.com/bmi/.

- **High Cholesterol:** Have your cholesterol checked regularly starting at age 35. If you are younger than 35, talk to your doctor about whether to have your cholesterol checked if:

  - You have diabetes.

  - You have high blood pressure.

  - Heart disease runs in your family.

  - You smoke.

- **High Blood Pressure:** Have your blood pressure checked at least every 2 years. High blood pressure is 140/90 or higher.

- **Colorectal Cancer:** Have a test for colorectal cancer starting at age 50. Your doctor can help you decide which test is right for you. If you have a family history of colorectal cancer, you may need to be screened earlier.

- **Diabetes:** Have a test for diabetes if you have high blood pressure or high cholesterol.

- **Depression:** Your emotional health is as important as your physical health. If you have felt "down," sad, or hopeless over the last 2 weeks or have felt little interest or pleasure in doing things, you may be depressed. Talk to your doctor about being screened for depression.

- **Sexually Transmitted Infections:** Talk to your doctor to see whether you should be tested for gonorrhea, syphilis, chlamydia, or other sexually transmitted infections.

- **HIV:** Talk to your doctor about HIV screening if you:

  - Have had sex with men since 1975.

  - Have had unprotected sex with multiple partners.

  - Have used or now use injection drugs.

  - Exchange sex for money or drugs or have sex partners who do.

- Have past or present sex partners who are HIV-infected, are bisexual or use injection drugs.

- Are being treated for sexually transmitted diseases.

- Had a blood transfusion between 1978 and 1985.

- **Abdominal Aortic Aneurysm.** If you are between the ages of 65 and 75 and have ever smoked *(100 or more cigarettes during your lifetime)*, you need to be screened once for abdominal aortic aneurysm, which is an abnormally large or swollen blood vessel in your abdomen.

Daily Steps to Health

Don't Smoke. If you do smoke, talk to your doctor about quitting. Your doctor or nurse can help you. And, you can also help yourself. For tips on how to quit, go to: You Can Quit Smoking Now. http://www. smokefree.gov. To talk to someone about how to quit, call the National Quitline: 1.800.QUITNOW. For more quit-smoking resources, go to: http://www.healthfinder.gov/ and search for smoking.

Be Physically Active. Walking briskly, mowing the lawn, dancing, swimming, and bicycling are just a few examples of moderate physical activity. If you are not already physically active, start small and work up to 30 minutes or more of moderate physical activity most days of the week.

Eat a Healthy Diet. Emphasize fruits, vegetables, whole grains, and fat-free or low-fat milk and milk products; include lean meats, poultry, fish, beans, eggs and nuts; and eat foods low in saturated fats, trans fats, cholesterol, salt *(sodium)* and added sugars.

Stay at a Healthy Weight. Balance calories from foods and beverages with calories you burn off by your activities. To prevent gradual weight gain over time, make small decreases in food and beverage calories and increase physical activity.

Drink Alcohol Only in Moderation. If you drink alcohol, have no more than two drinks a day. *(A standard drink is one 12-oz. bottle of beer or wine cooler, one 5-oz. glass of wine or 1.5 oz. of 80-proof distilled spirits.)*

Should You Take Medicines to Prevent Disease?

Aspirin: Ask your doctor about taking aspirin to prevent heart disease if you are:

- Older than 45

- Younger than 45 and:

  - Have high blood pressure.

  - Have high cholesterol.

  - Have diabetes.

  - Smoke.

Immunizations: Stay up-to-date with your immunizations:

- Have a flu shot every year starting at age 50. If you are younger than 50, ask your doctor whether you need a flu shot.

- Have a pneumonia shot once after you turn 65. If you are younger, ask your doctor whether you need a pneumonia shot.

Screening Test Checklist

Take this checklist with you to your doctor's office. Write down when you have any of the tests below. Talk to your doctor about your test results and write them down here. Ask when you should have the test next. Write down the month and year. If you think of questions for the doctor, write them down and bring them to your next visit.

Test	Last Test (mo/yr)	Results	Next Test Due (mo/yr)	Questions for the Doctor
Weight (BMI)				
Cholesterol Total:				
HDL (good):				
LDL (bad):				
Blood pressure				
Colorectal cancer				
Diabetes				
Sexually transmitted diseases				
HIV infection				
Abdominal aortic aneurysm (one-time test)				

You are WORTH being a Healthy Woman

Found at www.womenshealth.gov/prevention/general

As a female, the most important things you can do to stay healthy are:
- Get recommended screening tests.
- Be tobacco free.
- Be physically active.
- Eat a healthy diet.
- Stay at a healthy weight.
- Take preventive medicines if you need them.
- Taking your prescribed medications as directed by your healthcare provider

These charts are guidelines only. Your doctor or nurse will personalize the timing of each test and immunization to meet your health care needs.

Screening tests	Ages 18–39	Ages 40–49	Ages 50–64	Ages 65 and older
General health: Full checkup, including weight and height	Discuss with your doctor or nurse.	Discuss with your doctor or nurse.	Discuss with your doctor or nurse.	Discuss with your doctor or nurse.
Thyroid (TSH) test	Discuss with your doctor or nurse.	Discuss with your doctor or nurse.	Discuss with your doctor or nurse.	Discuss with your doctor or nurse.
HIV test	Get this test at least once to find out your HIV status. Ask your doctor or nurse if and when you need the test again.	Get this test at least once to find out your HIV status. Ask your doctor or nurse if and when you need the test again.	Get this test at least once to find out your HIV status. Ask your doctor or nurse if and when you need the test again.	Discuss with your doctor or nurse.
Heart health: Blood pressure test	At least every 2 years	At least every 2 years	At least every 2 years	At least every 2 years
Cholesterol test	Start at age 20, discuss with your doctor or nurse.	Discuss with your doctor or nurse.	Discuss with your doctor or nurse.	Discuss with your doctor or nurse.
Bone health: Bone density screen		Discuss with your doctor or nurse.	Discuss with your doctor or nurse.	Get a bone mineral density test at least once. Talk to your doctor or nurse about repeat testing.
Diabetes: Blood glucose test	Discuss with your doctor or nurse.	Start at age 45, then every 3 years.	Every 3 years	Every 3 years
Breast health: Mammogram (x-ray of breast)		Discuss with your doctor or nurse.	Every 2 years. Discuss with your doctor or nurse.	Every 2 years. Discuss with your doctor or nurse.
Clinical breast exam	Discuss with your doctor or nurse.	Discuss with your doctor or nurse.	Discuss with your doctor or nurse.	Discuss with your doctor or nurse.
Reproductive health: Pap test	Every 1–3 years if you have been sexually active or are older than 21	Every 1–3 years	Every 1–3 years	Discuss with your doctor or nurse.
Pelvic Exam	Yearly beginning at age 21. Younger than 21 and sexually active, discuss with your doctor or nurse.	Yearly	Yearly	Yearly
Chlamydia test	Yearly until age 25 if sexually active. Older than age 26, get this test if you have new or multiple partners.	Get this test if you have new or multiple partners.	Get this test if you have new or multiple partners.	Get this test if you have new or multiple partners.
Sexually transmitted infection (STI) tests	Both partners should get tested for STIs, including HIV, before initiating sexual intercourse.	Both partners should get tested for STIs, including HIV, before initiating sexual intercourse.	Both partners should get tested for STIs, including HIV, before initiating sexual intercourse.	Both partners should get tested for STIs, including HIV, before initiating sexual intercourse.

Screening tests	Ages 18–39	Ages 40–49	Ages 50–64	Ages 65 and older
Mental health screening	Discuss with your doctor or nurse.	Discuss with your doctor or nurse.	Discuss with your doctor or nurse.	Discuss with your doctor or nurse.
Colorectal health: (use 1 of these 3 methods): Fecal occult blood test			Yearly	Yearly. Older than age 75, discuss with your doctor or nurse.
Flexible sigmoid-oscopy (with fecal occult blood test)			Every 5 years	Every 5 years. Older than age 75, discuss with your doctor or nurse.
Colonoscopy			Every 10 years	Every 10 years. Older than age 75, discuss with your doctor or nurse.
Eye and ear health: Complete eye exam	At least once between the ages 20–29, at least twice between the ages 30–39, or any time that you have a problem.	Get an exam at age 40, then every 2–4 years or as your doctor advises.	Every 2–4 years or as your doctor advises you	Every 1–2 years
Hearing test	Starting at age 18, then every 10 years	Every 10 years	Every 3 years	Every 3 years
Skin Health: Mole exam	Monthly mole self-exam; by a doctor or nurse as part of a routine full checkup starting at age 20.	Monthly mole self-exam; by a doctor or nurse as part of a routine full checkup.	Monthly mole self-exam; by a doctor or nurse as part of a routine full checkup.	Monthly mole self-exam; by a doctor or nurse as part of a routine full checkup.
Oral health: Dental exam	Routinely; discuss with your dentist.	Routinely; discuss with your dentist.	Routinely; discuss with your dentist.	Routinely; discuss with your dentist.
Immunizations: Influenza vaccine	Discuss with your doctor or nurse.	Discuss with your doctor or nurse.	Yearly	Yearly
Pneumococcal vaccine				One time only
Tetanus-diphtheria booster vaccine	Every 10 years	Every 10 years	Every 10 years	Every 10 years
Human papillomavirus (HPV) vaccine	Up to age 26, if not already completed vaccine series; discuss with your doctor or nurse.			
Meningococcal vaccine	Discuss with your doctor or nurse if you are a college student or military recruit.			
Herpes zoster vaccine (to prevent shingles)			Starting at age 60, one time only. Ask your doctor or nurse if it is okay for you to get it.	Starting at age 60, one time only. Ask your doctor or nurse if it is okay for you to get it.

Content last updated November 23, 2009.

American Cancer Society Guidelines for the
Early Detection of Cancer

(www.cancer.org)

The following cancer screening guidelines are recommended for those people at average risk for cancer (unless otherwise specified) and without any specific symptoms.

People who are at increased risk for certain cancers may need to follow a different screening schedule, such as starting at an earlier age or being screened more often. Those with symptoms that could be related to cancer should see their doctor right away.

Cancer-related checkup

For people aged 20 or older having periodic health exams, a cancer-related checkup should include health counseling, and depending on a person's age and gender, might include exams for cancers of the thyroid, oral cavity, skin, lymph nodes, testes, and ovaries, as well as for some non-malignant (non-cancerous) diseases.

Special tests for certain cancer sites are recommended as outlined below.

Breast cancer

- Yearly mammograms are recommended starting at age 40 and continuing for as long as a woman is in good health.

- Clinical breast exam (CBE) should be part of a periodic health exam, about every 3 years for women in their 20s and 30s and every year for women 40 and over.

- Women should know how their breasts normally feel and report any breast change promptly to their health care providers. Breast self-exam (BSE) is an option for women starting in their 20s.

- Women at high risk (greater than 20% lifetime risk) should get an MRI and a mammogram every year. Women at moderately increased risk (15% to 20% lifetime risk) should talk with their doctors about the benefits and limitations of adding MRI screening to their yearly mammogram. Yearly MRI screening is not recommended for women whose lifetime risk of breast cancer is less than 15%.

Colon and rectal cancer

Beginning at age 50, both men and women at average risk for developing colorectal cancer should use one of the screening tests below. The tests that are designed to find both early cancer and

polyps are preferred if these tests are available to you and you are willing to have one of these more invasive tests. Talk to your doctor about which test is best for you.

Tests that find polyps and cancer

- flexible sigmoidoscopy every 5 years*
- colonoscopy every 10 years
- double contrast barium enema every 5 years*
- CT colonography (virtual colonoscopy) every 5 years*

Tests that mainly find cancer

- fecal occult blood test (FOBT) every year*,**
- fecal immunochemical test (FIT) every year*,**
- stool DNA test (sDNA), interval uncertain*

A FOBT or FIT done during a digital rectal exam in the doctor's office is not adequate for screening.

People should talk to their doctor about starting colorectal cancer screening earlier and/or being screened more often if they have any of the following colorectal cancer risk factors:

- a personal history of colorectal cancer or adenomatous polyps

- a personal history of chronic inflammatory bowel disease (Crohns disease or ulcerative colitis)

- a strong family history of colorectal cancer or polyps (cancer or polyps in a first-degree relative [parent, sibling, or child] younger than 60 or in 2 or more first-degree relatives of any age)

- a known family history of hereditary colorectal cancer syndromes such as familial adenomatous polyposis (FAP) or hereditary non-polyposis colon cancer (HNPCC)

Cervical cancer

- All women should begin cervical cancer screening about 3 years after they begin having vaginal intercourse, but no later than when they are 21 years old. Screening should be done every year with the regular Pap test or every 2 years using the newer liquid-based Pap test.

---

*Colonoscopy should be done if test results are positive.

**For FOBT or FIT used as a screening test, the take-home multiple sample method should be used.

- Beginning at age 30, women who have had 3 normal Pap test results in a row may get screened every 2 to 3 years. Another reasonable option for women over 30 is to get screened every 3 years (but not more frequently) with either the conventional or liquid-based Pap test, plus the HPV DNA test. Women who have certain risk factors such as diethylstilbestrol (DES) exposure before birth, HIV infection, or a weakened immune system due to organ transplant, chemotherapy, or chronic steroid use should continue to be screened annually.

- Women 70 years of age or older who have had 3 or more normal Pap tests in a row and no abnormal Pap test results in the last 10 years may choose to stop having cervical cancer screening. Women with a history of cervical cancer, DES exposure before birth, HIV infection or a weakened immune system should continue to have screening as long as they are in good health.

- Women who have had a total hysterectomy (removal of the uterus and cervix) may also choose to stop having cervical cancer screening, unless the surgery was done as a treatment for cervical cancer or pre-cancer. Women who have had a hysterectomy without removal of the cervix should continue to follow the guidelines above.

Endometrial (uterine) cancer

The American Cancer Society recommends that at the time of menopause, all women should be informed about the risks and symptoms of endometrial cancer, and strongly encouraged to report any unexpected bleeding or spotting to their doctors. For women with or at high risk for hereditary non-polyposis colon cancer (HNPCC), annual screening should be offered for endometrial cancer with endometrial biopsy beginning at age 35.

Prostate cancer

The American Cancer Society (ACS) does not support routine testing for prostate cancer at this time. ACS does believe that health care professionals should discuss the potential benefits and limitations of prostate cancer early detection testing with men before any testing begins. This discussion should include an offer for testing with the prostate-specific antigen (PSA) blood test and digital rectal exam (DRE) yearly, beginning at age 50, to men who are at average risk of prostate cancer and have at least a 10-year life expectancy. Following this discussion, those men who favor testing should be tested. Men should actively take part in this decision by learning about prostate cancer and the pros and cons of early detection and treatment of prostate cancer.

This discussion should take place starting at age 45 for men at high risk of developing prostate cancer. This includes African American men and men who have a first-degree relative (father, brother, or son) diagnosed with prostate cancer at an early age (younger than age 65).

This discussion should take place at age 40 for men at even higher risk (those with several first-degree relatives who had prostate cancer at an early age).

If, after this discussion, a man asks his health care professional to make the decision for him, he should be tested (unless there is a specific reason not to test).

A Dr. Sharon Sidebar: If you have a family member that has been diagnosed with a specific cancer or disease, make sure that you TELL your doctor. You should discuss your risk of cancer and consider scheduling screenings earlier. If you do not have health insurance, there are programs and agencies in most states that will assist with the most common types of cancers *(prostate, breast and cervical)*. If you need assistance and don't know where to turn; contact The COSHAR Foundation *(www.cosharfoundation.org)* and our staff will try to help point you in the right direction.

YOU are the Coach of your Healthcare Team

You are the coach and the "star" player on your healthcare team. Do you deserve to be fired or do you deserve a raise? Honestly, how involved are you in your health and wellness even when you visit you physician, pharmacist, dentist or other healthcare professional? Do you prepare fore the visit or are you passive and just go through the motions? Are you WORTH taking an active part in your health? I know that you are.

I have spent my professional life pushing and empowering people to take better control of their health. The issue of health literacy is one that is bigger than being able to read. It focuses on our ability to read, understand and act on the information. Sometimes people feel "stupid" because they don't understand what the doctor is saying to them and instead of asking questions we just nod our heads. Well, let me tell you, I'm not a mechanic and when they start talking all that "stuff" about pistons, engine turnovers, whatever…I space out. However, when they start putting the dollars with the diagnosis I get involved. I'm not stupid because I don't understand the mechanic; it's just not my field. Further, if the mechanic is not good enough to explain so that I can understand in my mind he is not good enough to fix my car and certainly not get my money. I challenge you to take that same attitude to your doctor or healthcare professional. It is THEIR job to help you understand.

If you've ever heard me speak on anything even REMOTELY health related; no doubt you've heard me talk about **Ask Me 3.** I was part of this tools' development and testing and I am a huge fan because it is simple. **Ask Me 3** is a patient education program designed to promote communication between health care providers and patients in order to improve health outcomes. Whenever you visit ANY healthcare professional, you should not leave until you have the following 3 questions understood. Copy these and learn them—this is important!

ASK Me 3

1. What is my main problem?
2. What do I need to do?
3. Why is it important for me to do this?

Dr. Sharon's Tips for your Doctor's Visit

1. Write down concerns, symptoms, and questions before you go for the visit.
2. Write down or take all of your medication bottles, vitamins, herbal products and supplements with you to your visit.
3. Take a notepad with your questions/concerns and to write down the instructions that they give you.
4. ASK questions about your tests *(ask and write down what your height, weight, blood pressure, glucose, urine and any other quick tests results).*
5. If you have labs/tests done and the results are not immediately available; ask when and how you will receive the results. Write down the date in your calendar and if you have not heard back from the office, CALL them and ask for your results.
6. If you are given a follow-up appointment, KEEP IT!
7. If you are prescribed a medication, talk to your doctor about the reason that you need to take it, possible side effects and what you should expect. Get your pharmacist involved and speak with them about the medication as well.
   a. **A Dr. Sharon Sidebar:** If I put a plate of food in front of you and you didn't recognize what it was what would you do? You would *(or should)* ASK—What is this? Why on earth would you not do the same with a medication? Ask the name, dosage, what it's for and possible side effects.
8. If you have difficulty understanding what your doctor or healthcare provider tells you, feel free to ask a family member of friend that you trust to go with you to the visit.
9. Get to know the staff in the office and certainly get to know your doctor. If you feel that you can't talk to your doctor then talk to your friends and family about getting a name of another doctor that you can talk to and that you trust. It's your health and you are the "coach/captain/star player" on the team—you can fire your doctor. *(By the way, if you act a fool in the doctor's office—they can also fire you. I'm just saying.)*

Quick Tips—When Talking with Your Doctor

Found at www.ahrq.gov/CONSUMER/quicktips/doctalk.htm

The single most important way you can stay healthy is to be an active member of your own healthcare team. One way to get high-quality health care is to find and use information and take an active role in all of the decisions made about your care. This information will help you when talking with your doctor. Research has shown that patients who have good relationships with their doctors tend to be more satisfied with their care—and to have better results. Here are some tips to help you and your doctor become partners in improving your health care.

Give Information. Don't Wait to Be Asked!

- You know important things about your symptoms and your health history. Tell your doctor what you think he or she needs to know.
- It is important to tell your doctor personal information—even if it makes you feel embarrassed or uncomfortable.
- Bring a "health history" list with you, and keep it up to date. You might want to make a copy of the form for each member of your family.
- Always bring any medicines you are taking, or a list of those medicines *(include when and how often you take them)* and what strength. Talk about any allergies or reactions you have had to your medicines.
- Tell your doctor about any herbal products you use or alternative medicines or treatments you receive.
- Bring other medical information, such as x-ray films, test results, and medical records.

Get Information

- Ask questions. If you don't, your doctor may think you understand everything that was said.
- Write down your questions before your visit. List the most important ones first to make sure they get asked and answered.
- You might want to bring someone along to help you ask questions. This person can also help you understand and/or remember the answers.
- Ask your doctor to draw pictures if that might help to explain something.
- Take notes.
- Some doctors do not mind if you bring a tape recorder to help you remember things. But always ask first.
- Let your doctor know if you need more time. If there is not time that day, perhaps you can speak to a nurse or physician assistant on staff. Or, ask if you can call later to speak with someone.
- Ask if your doctor has washed his or her hands before starting to examine you. Research shows that hand washing can prevent the spread of infections. If you're uncomfortable asking this question directly, you might ask, "I've noticed that some doctors and nurses wash their hands or wear gloves before touching people. Why is that?"

Take Information Home

- Ask for written instructions.
- Your doctor also may have brochures and audio tapes and videotapes that can help you. If not, ask how you can get such materials.

Once You Leave the Doctor's Office, Follow Up

- If you have questions, call.
- If your symptoms get worse, or if you have problems with your medicine, call.
- If you had tests and do not hear from your doctor, call for your test results.
- If your doctor said you need to have certain tests, make appointments at the lab or other offices to get them done.
- If your doctor said you should see a specialist, make an appointment.

What Doctors Want You to Know
But May Not Tell You

I asked doctors from all over the country to tell me what they would tell YOU, the patient, if they could be open and honest. I promised that I would keep comments confidential upon request. Here is what they said, these are eye opening *(and sometimes funny—they chose how they would be identified)*

The Question: "If you could tell a patient ONE thing openly, honestly about their health* (clinical or not) *what would it be?"

"Stop LYING, you and I know that you're NOT exercising and that you're eating everything but the kitchen sink—it's not water weight it's FAT."   **I'm Fat too MD**

"Please don't think that the few hours you have spent on the Internet researching your subject-of-choice can compare to my knowledge based acquired through 4 years of medical school and 3 years of pediatric residency and 11 years of pediatric clinical experience." If everything you needed to know could be learned on the Internet then why do we still have medical school and licensing board exams and continuing medical education requirements so that we can work as doctors. Medical knowledge is not stagnant. Keeping up with it as well as knowing how to apply the new information to daily clinical practice is a huge responsibility and truly a full time job. I appreciate parents that are genuinely and passionately concerned about their children's well-being (since sadly, many parents are not). I also appreciate parents that come ready to discuss important and difficult issues after having done their own research so we can work together as a team to make an informed decision regarding their child's health. But research means studying all sides of the issue and getting your information from reputable sources, not just reading the anecdotal web-pages out there. Good decisions and outcomes are derived from truthful information and not based solely on emotions. Oh...and bathe* (yourself and your kids) *before your appointment. Hygiene is NOT optional!!!!!!!"*   **Dr. V, A Pediatrician**

"What part of no do you not understand, the 'N' or the 'O'. To all of my drug seekers."   **NCMD**

"Don't call and ask for a back to work slip if you've missed your last three appointments, have a balance and haven't been seen in my office in 2 years. Don't bother with the call."
                                             Doctor What Do You Think This Is?

"Take care of your parents as they get older. They took care of you and now it's your time. Be patient and don't be mean to them—what happens when your kids treat you bad."

                                                          Geriatrician

"Despite what you may think, you are the one who is in charge of your health and your health care. It is not your doctor or your mother, father, sister, brother, spouse, son or daughter. You are the one who is in control. So there are four critical things that you have to do. First, know the medications that you are currently taking and the medications that you are allergic to. Just write them down and keep them in your wallet with your driver's license. Second, know the names and telephone numbers of all of your doctors. Third, write a list of your medical problems and previous surgeries (guess where you will keep it...yes, your wallet!). *Fourth and finally, keep your health insurance and prescription cards in your wallet. So, being in control of your health is as easy as 1, 2, 3, 4."*

Susan C. Taylor, MD
Medical Director, Society Hill Dermatology, Philadelphia, PA
Founder and CEO, Rx for Brown Skin

"Healthcare reform begins with YOU. You can have access to the best care in the world but if you don't take care of your body, eat right, exercise and follow your doctor's instructions then what's the purpose. What is your health worth?"
Sharon D. Allison-Ottey, MD

"Don't give me a sob story about not having your $25 co pay when you drive a car that is newer than mine and you come into my office wearing Ferragamo shoes. It's an insult to me, my profession and my office."
Tired Doc

"Don't stop me in the grocery store or at the mall and go into details about your health. I am trying to enjoy my one or two days off and I'll smile but I really am getting pissed off; especially if I'm with my family. Respect my time."
I Have a LIFE MD

"Don't' tell me that you're taking your medications every day and following a low fat, low salt diet when I ask you if you need refills and you don't and you've gained 15 pounds. A big hint is that I only give you enough pills for 90 days and unless it's been less than that—you are NOT taking the medications every day. I'm not stupid!"
Doc that Cares

"People be careful with your partners. I had a 32 year old patient with HIV who had just given birth. When repeatedly asked if her partner knew—she said NO! I am the girlfriend. He and his wife will eventually find out! I was disgusted!!!"
OB/GYN

"A pill is a medicine, whether I prescribe it or you buy it at a health food store or from your cousin. Tell me what you are taking. I won't judge you; I'm just trying to keep you healthy."
A Doc that believes in holistic medicine but not craziness

"The EMERGENCY Dept/Room is for EMERGENCIES. Don't come with an ingrown toenail and then get mad when you have to wait for 4 hours to be seen."
ER Doc

"Please always be responsible for your own well being. Physicians are masters of helping the patient with diagnosis and decisions. The patient is ultimately in control."
Joycelyn Summey, MD

"We really are not rich and if we are it is NOT from patient care."
Primary Care MD

"Take a Bath!" **(Several MDs including Family Medicine, Internal Medicine, OB/GYN, Urologists and Colorectal Surgeons)**

"If I write a prescription or order a test and your insurance company denies it. Yell at them, not at my staff and certainly not at me. If I write it or order it—why would I deny it?"
Fed up MD

"Viagra is not the cure for being a bad lover. It doesn't make you "last longer" and it doesn't make your penis grow. You also probably don't need it before age 50 and certainly not at 25 years old with no other medical conditions. If I say no, that's really what I mean...NO."
Internist

"I don't make any more money from writing you a prescription or ordering a test. I really do have your best interest at heart. Respect me as the professional that I am and I will respect you as the patient that you are."
Family Medicine

"Take care of yourself so that you can take care of others."
Dr. H, Brooklyn, NY

"Doctors are human and we make mistakes. Just because I made a mistake or didn't diagnose you the first minute that I saw you doesn't mean that I'm a bad doctor. Don't tell everybody what I did wrong, unless you will allow me to tell them what YOU did wrong or the details of your history. We're both human, I try my best and I'm darned good at what I do."
Human MD

"Just because you read it on the internet doesn't make it right. We can talk about it and I'll give you my opinion and reasons for your treatment. I invite you to get a second opinion—from a DOCTOR not your keyboard."
Internist

"I am not nor will I ever be sexually attracted to you. Do not come on to me in my office and don't always ask for a breast or pelvic exam—you don't need them every six months!"
Gay Male Ob/Gyn

"Don't starve yourself the day before you come to the office in an effort to try get your sugar/glucose level down. The hemoglobin A1C tells me what you've been doing for the last 3 months. It's not about getting the number right for me—it's about your health."
Diabetes Doc

"Be on time for your appointment; don't assume that I'm going to be late. On the other hand, if I'm running late it is usually because I am giving more care to someone in need. I'm not just watching television. If you understand that then when it's your time maybe the next person will understand. I am committed to my patients, not the clock on the wall."
I Do Care, MD

"I've seen and heard it all; you're not going to shock me and I'm not judging you. Tell me the truth and let's handle it."
Truth Works MD

"Every day I begin with prayer in my office for you. Every night I end my day in prayer for you and your families. I would hope that you would remember me in your prayers. I believe that being a physician is a calling from God and although I may not openly talk about it—I ask for His guidance. Some Doctors are Christians too."
Just an Instrument MD

"You get what you pay for, if you get the cheapest insurance policy from your job or wherever; you coverage is going to be limited. Spend time understanding your insurance coverage and remember that I am YOUR doctor and will do what's right for you—not for your insurance company. Sometimes you will need to invest more in your health."
Concerned Doc

"Raise your kids' right so they don't tear up my office. You may think that "Little Johnny's" temper tantrum is cute but it's not; he's in training to be a terrorist."
Pediatrician

"Get your priorities right. You have no problem paying for Botox but when I tell you that you need to have a biopsy on a mole you want to know how much your insurance will cover and if it's necessary. Seriously you need to think about it."
Dermatologist with a Conscious

"Wear a seatbelt EVERY time you get in the car and don't drive drunk or even a little "tipsy"
Emergency Dept. MD

"If you don't cancel your hotel reservation, you will get charged for the night's stay. Why complain when I have signs all over telling you that there is a fee for a missed appointment? Just call and tell us you're not coming in time and if you don't—PAY THE FEE."
Psychiatrist

"No matter what your husband says you CAN"T get gonorrhea from a toilet seat. He's lying and you're stupid to believe him."
I Love My Job MD

"Pay me without me having to send you over to the collections department. If your insurance company or whomever sends you a check for your care then PAY ME. You pay everyone else, why not the office that takes care of your health? If you can't pay it all, pay SOMETHING and don't get mad when my staff asks for the money. This office does not run off of "love", we have to pay rent, staff, water, lights, other bills and my kids need to eat too."

Broke MD

"You are what you eat, "Junk In equals Junk Out" for you and your kids."

Family Doc

"Don't ask for a month's samples when you have insurance coverage and small co pay. I really try to help patients who don't have insurance and/or can't afford to buy their medications. The drug companies are also not giving out as many."

Caring MD

"Being mean and nasty to my staff gets you no where. Respect them, tell me if there's a problem but don't treat them like dirt. They are your direct connection to me."

Dr. K

"Don't threaten me with a lawsuit when I don't do what you ask me to do. I am not a vending machine; I am a professional and will give you the best care that I can. This is not a drive thru restaurant wherein you study the menu at home and then come in demanding prescriptions, tests or whatever. Let's have a discussion and just like you decide what you will do; I will decide what I professionally think is right. If you can't agree with that PLEASE find another doctor."

Internal Medicine

"Don't ask me if your husband or wife is cheating. Ask them and no I can't give you a copy of their medical records without their consent."

Chicago Doc

"I really do care about YOU, my patient. But I need for you to care about me as a professional. I do have a life outside of medicine and although I am on call after hours it really is for urgent issues. Don't call me to talk about a cold at 11pm when you could have come into the office that day or wait until the morning. It really is inconsiderate."

Family Medicine

"A Thank YOU would be nice."

Unappreciated MD

Dr. Sharon's Recommended Websites
for Credible Health/Wellness Information

Centers for Disease Control
www.cdc.gov

WebMD
www.webmd.com

Nutrition.gov
www.nutrition.gov

Drug Information MEDLINEplus
www.nlm.nih.gov/medlineplus/druginformation.html

SafeMedication.com
www.safemedication.com

Center for Drug Evaluation and Research—U.S. FDA
www.fda.gov/cder/drug/default.htm

Office of Dietary Supplements (National Institutes of Medicine)
http://dietary-supplements.info.nih.gov/index.aspx

National Institute for Mental Health
www.nimh.nih.gov/publicat/index.cfm

National Heart, Lung and Blood Institute
www.nhlbi.nih.gov/health/public/heart/obesity/lose-wt/patmats.htm

National Stroke Association
www.stroke.org

The Office on Women's Health—U.S. Department of Health and Human Services
www.4woman.gov/owh

Mayo Clinic
www.mayoclinic.com

Familydoctor.org—American Academy of Family Physicians
www.familydoctor.org

HealthWeb.org (National Library of Medicine)
www.healthweb.org

Live Well, Live Long—AOA and CDC
www.asaging.org.cdc

National Center for Complementary and Alternative Medicine
www.nccam.nih.gov

National Institute of Diabetes & Digestive & Kidney Diseases
www.niddk.nih.gov

Recipes

Appetizers & Snacks

Baked Seasoned Potato Chips

Ingredients:

- 2 teaspoons canola oil
- 1 large russet potato *(or 2 medium size)*, about 10 oz.
- Canola cooking spray
- ½ teaspoon seasoned salt

Preparation:

1. Preheat the oven to 400 degrees. Brush canola oil over the bottom of a nonstick jellyroll pan.

2. Using a large, sharp, non-serrated knife, cut the potato into very thin slices *(about 1/16 inch thick)*.

3. Immediately lay the potato slices flat onto the prepared pan *(they should completely cover the bottom of the pan)*. Spray the tops with canola cooking spray and sprinkle with the seasoned salt.

4. Bake for about 22-25 minutes, watching carefully. Remove the chips that have browned and crisped and continue to cook the remaining chips until they become nice and crisp, too—about 5 minutes more.

Yield: 3 servings

Nutritional Information: Per serving: 137 calories, 3 g protein, 25 g carbohydrate, 3 g fat, 0.2 g saturated fat, 0 mg cholesterol, 2.5 g fiber, 239 mg sodium. Calories from fat: 20%.

Recipe Source: medicinenet.com

BBQ Sausage Bites

Ingredients:

- 1 cup BBQ sauce
- 16 oz. reduced fat sausage of your choice

Preparation:

1. Turn slow cooker on HIGH and pour the BBQ sauce into the crock of your slow cooker.

2. If using large link sausage *(like Hillshire Farms Turkey Polska Kielbasa)*, slice into ⅓-inch thick slices. If using smaller link sausage, cut into 1-inch long segments. Stir the sausage pieces into the BBW sauce in the slow cooker and heat about 45 minutes or until sausage and sauce is good and hot.

3. Reduce heat to LOW for the party and keep it on low until the sausage bites are all gone. Serve the turkey bites with toothpicks if desired.

Yield: Makes 8 servings

Nutritional Information: Per serving: 90 calories, 5 g protein, 2 g carbohydrate, 5 g fat, 2 g saturated fat, 35 mg cholesterol, 0 g fiber, 510 mg sodium. Calories from fat: 50 percent.

Recipe Source: medicinenet.com

Better-for-You Buffalo Wings

Ingredients:

- 2 teaspoons seasoned salt
- 2 teaspoons chili powder
- 2 teaspoons garlic powder
- 1 teaspoon freshly ground pepper
- 2 tablespoons flour
- 2 ½ pounds *(about 28)* wing drumettes *(look for skinless drumettes if available)*
- ¼ cup nonalcoholic or light beer *(chicken broth or wine can also be used)*
- light blue cheese dressing *(optional)*

Preparation:

1. In a small mixing bowl, stir together the seasoned salt, chili powder, garlic powder, pepper, and flour. Remove and discard the skin from the wings *(if you weren't able to find skinless drumettes)*. Dip each wing into the seasoning mixture, pressing the mixture onto the chicken to coat well.

2. Generously coat a large nonstick skillet with canola cooking spray and place over medium-high heat. Add the chicken wings *(cooking in batches if necessary)* and cook for about 4 minutes, or until the bottoms are browned.

3. Flip with prongs and cook for about 4 minutes more.

4. Reduce the heat to medium-low and add the beer. Cover the pan and cook for about 5 minutes. If the wings aren't cooked through, turn them over and cook for a few minutes more.

5. Remove from the heat and serve hot with light blue cheese dressing if desired *(not included in nutrition information below)*.

Yield: Makes 7 servings *(4 wing drumettes per serving)*

Nutritional Information: per serving: 174 calories, 29 g protein, 2 g carbohydrate, 4.5 g fat, 1.2 g saturated fat, 73 mg cholesterol, 539 mg sodium. Calories from fat: 23 percent.

Recipe Source: medicinenet.com

Crab Stuffed Mushrooms

Ingredients:

- 3 tablespoons light or regular mayonnaise
- 3 tablespoons fat free sour cream
- 3 tablespoons Italian seasoned dry bread crumbs *(panko crumbs can be substituted)*
- 3 tablespoons shredded Parmesan cheese
- 1 teaspoon finely chopped garlic
- 1 can *(6 ½ oz.)* crabmeat *(or 1 cup fresh crabmeat)*, rinsed and drained well
- Dash or two Tabasco
- Black pepper to taste
- 18 medium sized mushrooms, stems removed

Preparation:

1. Preheat slow cooker to high heat.
2. Meanwhile, in small bowl, combine mayonnaise, fat free sour cream, bread crumbs, Parmesan cheese and garlic. Fold in the crabmeat. Add Tabasco and black pepper to taste.
3. Spoon heaping teaspoons full of crab filling into mushroom caps.
4. Arrange mushroom caps *(crab side up)* in the bottom of the preheated slow cooker. Add cover and cook on HIGH for about 2 hours. Reduce heat to LOW and serve the crab-stuffed mushrooms from the slow cooker if desired.

Yield: Makes 9 servings *(2 mushrooms per serving)*

Nutritional Information: Per serving: 59 calories, 5 g protein, 4 g carbohydrate, 2.5 g fat, .6 g saturated fat, 16 mg cholesterol, .5 g fiber, 177 mg sodium. Calories from fat: 38 percent.

Recipe Source: medicinenet.com

Festive Deviled Eggs Recipe

Ingredients:

- 6 large, hard-cooked eggs, cooled and peeled *(use higher omega-eggs 3 if available; you'll only use half of the yolks)*
- ¼ cup cleaned and shredded crab *(or finely chopped lean ham)*
- 2 tablespoons finely chopped red pepper
- 2 teaspoons finely chopped green onion *(mostly the green part)*
- 2 tablespoons light mayonnaise *(or low-fat or fat-free, if you prefer)*
- 2 teaspoons Dijon mustard
- Smidgen ground nutmeg
- ½ teaspoon parsley flakes
- Black pepper to taste *(or Mrs. Dash Lemon Pepper)*

Preparation:

1. Cut eggs in half lengthwise and remove the yolks. Place half the yolks in a medium bowl and mash with fork *(throw the other half away)*.
2. Add the crab, red pepper, green onion, mayonnaise, mustard, nutmeg, and parsley to the yolks and blend well with a fork. Add pepper to taste.
3. Spoon mixture evening among the 12 egg white halves.

Yield: 6 servings *(2 deviled egg halves per serving)*

Nutritional Information: Per serving: 70 calories, 6 g protein, 1 g carbohydrate, 4.5 g fat, 1 g saturated fat, 111 mg cholesterol, 0.1 g fiber, 151 mg sodium. Calories from fat: 58%

Recipe Source: medicinenet.com

Breakfast

(Although I believe breakfast can be eaten anytime of the day)

Banana Oat Breakfast Cookie

	Per Serving
Calories	300
Total Fat	9g
Saturated Fat	2g
Cholesterol	56mg
Sodium	755mg
Total Carbohydrate	46g
Dietary Fiber	6g
Sugars	--
Protein	12g
Calcium	--

Makes: 12 breakfast cookies

Prep: 20 minutes

Bake: 14 minutes per batch

Ingredients:

- Nonstick cooking spray
- 1 large banana, mashed *(½ cup)*
- ½ cup chunky natural peanut butter *(unsalted and unsweetened)* or regular chunky peanut butter
- ½ cup honey
- 1 teaspoon vanilla
- 1 cup rolled oats
- ½ cup whole wheat flour
- ¼ cup nonfat dry milk powder
- 2 teaspoons ground cinnamon
- ¼ teaspoon baking soda
- 1 cup dried cranberries or raisins

Preparation:

Preheat oven to 350 degrees F. Lightly coat two cookie sheets with cooking spray; set aside. In a large bowl, stir together banana, peanut butter, honey, and vanilla. In a small bowl, combine oats, flour, milk powder, cinnamon, and baking soda. Stir the oat mixture into the banana mixture until combined. Stir in dried cranberries.

Using a ¼-cup measure, drop mounds of dough 3 inches apart on prepared baking sheets. With a thin metal or small plastic spatula dipped in water, flatten and spread each mound of dough to a 2 ¾-inch round, about ½-inch thick. Once baked, each cookie will be about 3-½ to 4 inches in diameter.

Bake, one sheet at a time, for 14 to 16 minutes or until browned. Transfer to wire racks to cool completely. Store in an airtight container or resealable plastic bag for up to 3 days or freeze for up to 2 months; thaw before serving.

Recipe Source: my.hearthealthyonline.com

Buttermilk Belgian Waffles for Two

This is a great basic recipe for waffle batter. You can stir all sorts of ingredients, like dried blueberries or cranberries, flaked coconut, and toasted pecans.

Ingredients:

- 1 cup Bisquick® Heart Smart Baking Mix
- 2 teaspoons canola oil
- 2 tablespoons egg substitute or beaten egg
- ¾ cup low-fat buttermilk

Optional stir-ins:

- ⅛ cup dried blueberries or cranberries OR
- 2 tablespoons shredded dried coconut + 2 tablespoons toasted pecan pieces OR
- 2 tablespoons mini semisweet chocolate chips OR
- ⅛ cup raisins soaked overnight in 2 tablespoons dark rum *(drain raisins well before adding to waffle mix)*

Preparation:

1. Start preheating a Belgian waffle iron.
2. Add baking mix, canola oil, egg mixture, and buttermilk to a small mixing bowl and beat on low or stir by hand until blended. Add stir-ins now, if desired.
3. When the waffle iron is ready, give it a quick spray with canola cooking spray and pour half the batter onto the center of the iron. Close lid and cook according to manufacturer's instructions *(about 3 minutes or until steaming stops)*. Remove waffle and repeat with remaining waffle batter.

Yield: 2 Belgian waffles *(each round waffle is about 7 inches in diameter)*

Nutritional Information: Per waffle *(using egg substitute)*: 295 calories, 10 g protein, 45 g carbohydrate, 9 g fat, 1 g saturated fat, 3 mg Cholesterol, 1.5 g fiber, 760 mg sodium. Calories from fat: 27%.

Recipe Source: www.medicinenet.com

Egg Mock-Muffin Sandwich

Ingredients:

- 2 English muffins, toasted
- 1 large egg
- ¼ cup egg substitute
- 2 slices Canadian bacon
- 2 empty tuna cans *(or similar cans)*, washed and label removed
- 2 slices less-fat American or cheddar cheese slices
- Freshly ground pepper
- Canola cooking spray

Preparation:

1. Coat half of a 9" or 10" nonstick frying pan with canola cooking spray and heat over medium heat. In a small bowl, beat the egg with egg substitute with a fork or whisk and set aside.

2. Place Canadian bacon in the pan, over the sprayed area. Spray the inside of the tuna cans with canola cooking spray, and set on the non-spayed side of the frying pan to start heating. When bottom side of the bacon is light brown, flip over and cook other side until light brown. Remove bacon from pan and set aside.

3. Pour ¼ cup of the egg mixture into each tuna can. Sprinkle with freshly ground pepper to taste. When the surface of the egg begins to firm, cut around the inside of the cans with a butter knife to free the edges. Turn the eggs over with a cake fork and cook for 1 minute more. Remove eggs from can.

4. To assemble each sandwich, layer an English muffin bottom with a slice of cheese, then an egg patty, a piece of Canadian bacon, and the muffin top.

Yield: 2 sandwiches

Nutritional Information: Per sandwich: 283 calories, 22 g protein, 27 g carbohydrate, 9 g fat, 3.9 g saturated fat, 2 g fiber, 808 mg sodium. Calories from fat: 30%.

Recipe Source: www.medicinenet.com

Hash Brown Breakfast Sandwich

A fun and tasty breakfast can be yours in 10 minutes from start to finish.

Ingredients:

- 2 squares frozen shredded hash brown potatoes, made with no added fat
- Canola cooking spray
- 1 slice cheese, any type you like, cut in half
- 1 large egg *(use higher omega-3 brand if available)*, beaten with 1 teaspoon water *(or use ¼ cup egg substitute)*
- Pepper or salt-free seasoning blend *(like Mrs. Dash)* to taste
- Salt to taste, if desired
- 1 medium tomato, sliced *(or substitute a sliced avocado)*

Preparation:

1. Place hash brown squares on a microwave-safe plate and thaw in microwave on HIGH for about 90 seconds. Start heating a nonstick frying pan over medium-high heat.

2. When hash browns are out of the microwave, spray an area in the hot pan with canola cooking spray. Lay one of the hash brown squares on top. Repeat with remaining square. Spray tops of the hash browns with canola cooking spray. Sprinkle the tops with pepper or seasoning blend to taste and salt to taste, if desired. When underside is nicely brown *(about 3 minutes)*, flip hash browns over and brown other side *(about 2 minutes more)*.

3. Remove hash browns to serving plate and top with a piece of the cheese. Coat the still-hot frying pan with canola spray and pour in the beaten egg or egg substitute. Let it naturally form a circle shape in the pan. Top with black pepper or salt-free seasoning blend, as desired. When the underside is nicely browned *(about 2 minutes)*, flip the egg circle over and cook the other side about 1 minute more. Cut the egg circle in half and fold each half over. Add each egg piece on top of the cheese topped hash brown squares.

4. Top with tomato or avocado slices.

Yield: 1 serving

Nutritional Information: Per serving *(using egg substitute and tomato)*: 256 calories, 16 g protein, 33 g carbohydrate, 7 g fat, 4 g saturated fat, 21 mg cholesterol, 3.5 g fiber, 255 mg sodium. Calories from fat: 25%.

Recipe Source: www.medicinenet.com

Huevos Rancheros

	Per serving
Calories	360g
Fat	19g
Sat.	6g
Mono.	9.5g
Poly.	2g
Cholesterol	228mg
Sodium	430mg
Carbohydrate	33g
Fiber	7g
Protein	16g

Cook Time: 15 min

Level: Easy

Yield: 4 servings

Ingredients:

- 2 small tomatoes
- 1 small onion
- 1 medium jalapeno pepper, chopped
- 2 cloves garlic; 1 chopped, 1 smashed
- ½ teaspoon hot sauce
- 1 teaspoon ground cumin
- Kosher salt and freshly ground pepper
- 2 tablespoons plus 2 teaspoons extra-virgin olive oil
- 1 15.5-oz. can black beans, drained and rinsed
- 4 large eggs
- 4 6-inch corn tortillas, warmed
- ½ cup crumbled feta cheese
- ¼ cup chopped fresh cilantro

Preparation:

1. Prepare the salsa: Set a grater in a large bowl; grate the tomatoes and onion into the bowl. Add the jalapeno, chopped garlic, hot sauce, cumin and salt and pepper to taste. Heat a medium skillet over low heat and add 2 teaspoons olive oil. Fry the salsa in the oil until it thickens slightly, 3 minutes. Remove to a bowl and set aside.

2. Add the beans to the same pan along with the smashed garlic, ½ cup warm water and a pinch of salt; cook over low heat until warmed through, smashing slightly with a fork.

3. Meanwhile, heat the remaining 2 tablespoons oil in another skillet. Fry the eggs sunny-side up; season with pepper.

4. Place 1 warm tortilla on each plate. Divide the beans among them, and then top with a fried

egg, some salsa and cheese. Sprinkle with cilantro and serve with the remaining salsa.

Recipe Source: foodnetwork.com

I Love You Toast

Ingredients:

- 4 pieces of bread *(100% whole wheat or Iron Kids® Bread)*
- ¼ cup light cream cheese
- About ½ cup fresh or frozen blueberries
- ¼ cup light strawberry or raspberry jam

Preparation:

1. Toast bread slices to desired doneness. *(Young kids will need a grown-up to watch the toaster).*

2. Spread about 1 tablespoon of light cream cheese over the entire top of each piece of toast using a plastic knife.

3. Make a heart in the center of the toast, using about ⅛ cup of fresh or frozen blueberries for the outside of the heart, on each piece of toast.

4. Spoon jam into the middle of the heart *(about 1 tablespoon per toast).*

Yield: 4 servings

Nutritional Information: Per slice: 162 calories, 5 g protein, 27.5 g carbohydrate, 4 g fat *(2 g saturated fat)*, 7.5 mg cholesterol, 3 g fiber, 253 mg sodium. Calories from fat: 22%

Recipe Source: www.medicinenet.com

	Per Serving
Calories	300
Total Fat	9g
Saturated Fat	2g
Cholesterol	56mg
Sodium	755mg
Total Carbohydrate	46g
Dietary Fiber	6g
Sugars	--
Protein	12g
Calcium	--

Low-Fat French Toast

Serves: 4

Yield: 4 servings

Total Time: 23 min

Oven Temp: 200

Ingredients:

2 large egg whites

1 large egg

¾ cup low-fat *(1%)* milk

¼ teaspoon vanilla extract

Salt

2 teaspoons margarine or butter

8 slices firm whole wheat bread

Maple syrup *(optional)*

Fresh blackberries, raspberries and blueberries *(optional)*

Preparation:

1. Preheat oven to 200 degrees F. In pie plate, with whisk, beat egg whites, egg, milk, vanilla and ½ teaspoon salt until blended. In 12-inch nonstick skillet, melt 1 teaspoon margarine on medium.

2. Dip bread slices, 1 at a time, in egg mixture, pressing bread lightly to coat both sides well. Place 3 or 4 slices in skillet, and cook 6 to 8 minutes or until lightly browned on both sides.

3. Transfer French toast to cookie sheet; keep warm in oven. Repeat with remaining margarine, bread slices and egg mixture. Serve French toast with maple syrup and berries if you like.

Recipe Source: Good Housekeeping

Spinach Quiche

This recipe uses the prepared pie crusts found in the freezer section of your supermarket. You can find some alternative brands with more fiber and less saturated fat at stores like Whole Foods. Since prepared pie crusts are usually high in fat, we're keeping the filling nice and light.

Ingredients:

- ½ package *(9-10 oz.)* frozen, chopped spinach, thawed and drained
- 2 scallions or green onions *(white and part of the green)*, chopped
- 3 oz. flavored feta cheese *(such as roasted bell pepper & garlic)*, crumbled
- 1 cup shredded, reduced-fat sharp cheddar cheese
- Pepper to taste
- ½ teaspoon garlic powder *(add more if desired)*
- 9-inch unbaked deep-dish pie crust, partially thawed
- 2 large eggs *(use higher omega-3 type, if available)*
- ½ cup egg substitute
- 1 cup fat-free half-and-half *(or substitute low-fat milk)*

Preparation:

1. Preheat oven to 375 degrees. In a medium bowl, toss together spinach, green onions, feta, cheddar, pepper to taste and garlic powder.

2. Spoon mixture evenly into the pie crust.

3. Add eggs, egg substitute, and fat-free half-and-half to large mixing bowl, and beat on medium speed until combined. Pour into the pie crust, letting the spinach mixture combine nicely with the egg mixture.

4. Bake until center of quiche is cooked throughout *(about 50-55 minutes)*. Let stand 5 minutes before serving.

Yield: 8 servings

Nutritional Information: Per serving: 228 calories, 13 g protein, 15 g carbohydrate, 12 g fat *(5 g saturated fat)*, 70 mg cholesterol, 2 g fiber, 388 mg sodium. Calories from fat: 50%.

Recipe Source: www.medicinenet.com

Sweet Potato Pancakes

Ingredients:

- 6 cups peeled and finely shredded sweet potatoes
- 1 cup finely shredded onions
- 1 teaspoon no-salt herb blend
- 1 ⅔ cup unbleached flour
- ⅓ cup chopped fresh flat-leaf parsley
- 2 cups finely shredded zucchini
- ¼ cup lemon juice
- 1 ½ cups egg substitute
- 6 teaspoons canola oil, divided

Preparation:

1. In a large bowl, mix the sweet potatoes, zucchini, onions, lemon juice, herb blend, egg, flour and parsley.

2. In a large no-stick frying pan or griddle over medium-high heat, warm 2 teaspoons of the oil. Drop a large tablespoon of the batter into the pan and spread it with a spatula to form a thin pancake. Add more batter to fill the pan without crowding the pancakes.

3. Cook for about 2 minutes per side, or until golden and crispy.

4. Remove from the pan and keep warm. Repeat, adding the remaining 4 teaspoons of oil as needed, until all the batter has been used.

Yield: 8 servings

Nutritional Information: Per serving: Calories 294, Fat 4 g, Calories from Fat 12%, Cholesterol 0 mg, Fiber 6 g, Sodium 80 mg.

Recipe Source: www.medicinenet.com

Whole-Wheat Pancakes with Nutty Topping

	Per Serving
Calories	510
Total Fat	19g
Sat Fat	3g
Mono Fat	4.5g
Poly Fat	6g
Protein	21g
Carbs	68g
Fiber	7g
Cholesterol	110mg
Sodium	680mg

Cook Time: 24 min

Level: Easy

Yield: 4 servings, serving size: 3 pancakes and ¼ cup topping

Ingredients:

For the Topping:

- ¼ cup sliced almonds
- ¼ cup hulled *(green)* pumpkin seeds
- ¼ cup sunflower seeds
- 1 tablespoon sesame seeds *(preferably unhulled)*
- ¼ cup toasted wheat germ
- ¼ cup real maple syrup, plus more for serving
- Pinch salt

For the Pancakes:

- 1 medium apple, such as Golden Delicious, cored and diced *(about 2 cups)*
- ¾ cup whole-wheat flour
- ¾ cup all-purpose flour
- 2 teaspoons baking powder
- ½ teaspoon baking soda
- ¼ teaspoon salt
- 2 large eggs
- 1 cup 1 percent lowfat buttermilk
- ¾ cup lowfat milk
- 2 teaspoons honey
- Nonstick cooking spray

Preparation:

1. Make the topping: In a large skillet, toast the almonds and pumpkin seeds over medium-high heat, stirring, for about 1 minute. Add the sunflower seeds and cook, stirring, for 1 minute more. Add the sesame seeds to the pan. Cover and cook, shaking the pan, until the seeds are

toasted, about 30 seconds more. Transfer the toasted nuts and seeds to a medium sized bowl. Add the wheat germ. Stir in the syrup and a pinch of salt and set aside.

2. Make the pancakes: Put the apple in a microwave-proof bowl, tightly cover with plastic wrap and microwave on high until softened, about 2 minutes. Set aside.

3. In a large bowl, whisk the flours, baking powder, baking soda and salt. In a small bowl, whisk together the eggs, buttermilk, ½ cup of the milk and honey. Slowly whisk the egg mixture into the dry ingredients, stirring until just combined. If the batter seems too thick, add as much of the remaining ¼ cup milk as necessary.

4. Spray a large non-stick griddle with cooking spray and heat over medium heat. Spoon about ¼ cup batter per pancake into the pan and top each pancake with a heaping tablespoon of the cooked apple. Flip when the pancake tops are covered with bubbles and the edges look cooked, about 2 minutes. Cook until the pancakes are golden brown and cooked through, an additional 1 to 2 minutes. Serve immediately or transfer the cooked pancakes to an ovenproof dish and keep warm in a preheated 250 degree F oven while making the rest. To serve, arrange 3 pancakes per plate and sprinkle each serving with ¼ cup of the topping. Serve with additional maple syrup.

Recipe Source: foodnetwork.com

. . . .

Sandwiches, Side Dishes, Soups/ Stews Salads & Vegetables

All-American Light Potato Salad

The great thing about this recipe is you don't have to boil the potatoes!

Ingredients:

- 4 russet potatoes with skin *(large pink or white potatoes can be substituted)*
- ¼ cup light mayonnaise
- ¼ cup fat-free sour cream
- 1 tablespoon honey mustard *(add 1 more tablespoon, if desired)*
- ¼ teaspoon black pepper
- ½ teaspoon salt *(optional)*
- ½ cup diced or chopped celery
- ⅓ cup diced or chopped red bell pepper

- ⅓ cup chopped green onions
- 1 tablespoon fresh chopped parsley *(regular or Italian)*
- ½ teaspoon paprika *(optional)*

Preparation:

1. Wash the outside of potatoes well, then cut into 1-inch cubes. Add potato pieces to a large, microwave-safe vegetable-cooker container. Cover and cook on HIGH for about 6 minutes. Stir potatoes, cover cooker, and cook on HIGH until potatoes are just tender *(about 4-6 minutes more)*.

2. While potatoes are cooling, add mayonnaise, sour cream, honey mustard, pepper and salt *(if desired)* to large bowl. Whisk to combine.

3. Stir in cooled potatoes, celery, bell pepper, green onions and parsley. Cover and chill until ready to serve *(at least an hour)*. Sprinkle a dash or two of paprika over the top before serving, if desired.

Yield: About 6 cups of salad *(eight ¾-cup servings)*

Nutritional Information: Per serving: 148 calories, 3 g protein, 29 g carbohydrate, 2.3 g fat, 0.3 g saturated fat, 0 mg cholesterol, 3 g fiber, 89 mg sodium *(216 mg if the salt is added)*. Calories from fat: 14%.

Recipe Source: medicinenet.com

BBQ Chicken Chicago-Style Pizza Bagels

This recipe is simple when you buy rotisserie chicken from the grocery store and use bottled BBQ sauce, already shredded cheese and seasoned canned tomatoes.

Ingredients:

- 4 whole-wheat bagels, cut in half
- 2 cups shredded boneless chicken breast, skinless
- ½ cup BBQ sauce *(your favorite)*
- 3 tablespoons chopped red onions
- ½ cup chopped fresh cilantro, lightly packed
- 1 ½ cups shredded part skim mozzarella
- 1 cup canned Italian Style diced tomatoes

Preparation:

1. Preheat oven to 400 degrees. Line a jelly-roll pan with foil if desired. Place bagel halves on the lined pan.

2. In medium bowl combine the chicken, barbeque sauce, red onions, fresh cilantro,

tossing to blend well.

3. Top each bagel half with ¼ cup of the chicken mixture, then sprinkle 3 tablespoons cheese over each half. Spoon ⅛ cup of the diced canned tomatoes on top of each bagel half.

4. Bake in center of oven for 10-12 minutes or until cheese is melted and the bagel is nice and hot. Cut each bagel half in half or serve as is!

Yield: Makes 8 servings *(a half bagel)*

Nutritional Information: Per serving 225 calories, 20 g protein, 24 g carbohydrate, 5.3 g fat, 2.7 g saturated fat, 41 mg cholesterol, 3.5 g fiber, 469 mg sodium *(depending on the BBQ sauce used)*. Calories from fat: 21 percent.

Recipe Source: medicinenet.com

Bean and Vegetable Stew

Prep Time: 15 minutes

Cook Time: 45 minutes

Ingredients:

	Per Serving
Calories	278
Calories from Fat	28
Total Fat	3g *(sat 0.4g)*
Cholesterol	10mg
Sodium	289mg
Carbohydrate	49g
Fiber	12.6g
Protein	13.5g

- 1 tbsp olive oil
- 1 large onion, finely chopped
- 2 garlic cloves, crushed
- 2 large carrots, chopped
- 2 celery stalks, sliced
- 2 small red potatoes, peeled and cubed
- 1 small yellow pepper, chopped
- 1 cup sliced cremini mushrooms
- 1 tsp cumin
- 1 tbsp chili powder
- 1 ½ cups fat-free, low sodium chicken or vegetable broth
- 1 15-oz. can crushed tomatoes
- 1 15-oz. can reduced sodium black beans, rinsed and drained
- 1 15-oz. can white beans, rinsed and drained
- 1 zucchini, sliced

Preparation:

1. In a large Dutch oven, heat oil over a medium heat. Cook onion, garlic, carrots, celery, potato cubes and yellow pepper until onion has softened, about 3-4 minutes. Stir in mushrooms, cumin and chili powder. Add broth and tomatoes. Bring to a boil, then cover and simmer for 20 minutes. Stir in beans and sliced zucchini. Cook uncovered for 10 minutes. Serve over rice or with some crusty whole grain bread for a filling supper.

Yield: Serves 6-8

Recipe Source: foodnetwork.com

Better Burger with Green Olives

Cook Time: 10 min

Level: Easy

Yield: 4 servings

Ingredients:

- 1 pound lean ground turkey or beef *(at least 90 percent lean)*
- ½ cup coarsely chopped pitted green olives *(2 oz.)*
- 2 tablespoons finely chopped fresh flat-leaf parsley
- ½ teaspoon ground cumin
- ¼ teaspoon freshly ground pepper
- Cooking spray

Preparation:

1. Combine the turkey or beef, olives, parsley, cumin, and pepper in a mixing bowl and mix until well incorporated. Shape into 4 burgers.

2. Spray a grill pan with cooking spray and preheat over a medium-high heat or prepare an outdoor grill. Cook for about 5 minutes on each side, until cooked through.

3. Serving suggestion: Serve on whole-wheat buns, garnished with slices of tomato and lettuce, with ketchup and mustard on the side. Serving size 1 burger

Recipe Source: foodnetwork.com

(Turkey)

	Per Serving:
Calories	145
Total Fat	4 g *(Sat Fat 0 g, Mono Fat 1.5 g, Poly Fat 0.5 g)*
Protein	28 g; Carb 1.5 g
Fiber	0 g
Cholesterol	45 mg
Sodium	305 mg

(Beef)

	Per Serving:
Calories	155
Total Fat	7 g *(Sat Fat 1.5 g, Mono Fat 3.5 g, Poly Fat 1 g)*
Protein	22 g
Carb	1 g
Fiber	0 g
Cholesterol	60 mg
Sodium	305 mg

Broccoli Soup

Ingredients:

- 1 ½ cups chopped broccoli *(or 10-oz. pkg. frozen broccoli)*
- ¼ cup diced celery
- ¼ cup chopped onion
- 1 cup low-sodium chicken broth
- 2 cups nonfat milk
- 2 tablespoons cornstarch
- ¼ teaspoon salt
- Dash pepper
- Dash ground thyme
- ¼ cup grated Swiss cheese

Preparation:

1. Place vegetables and broth in saucepan.
2. Bring to boil, reduce heat, cover and cook until vegetables are tender *(about 8 minutes)*.
3. Mix milk, cornstarch, salt, pepper and thyme; add to cooked vegetables.
4. Cook, stirring constantly, until soup is lightly thickened and mixture just begins to boil.
5. Remove from heat. Add cheese and stir until melted.

Yield: 4 servings. *(1 cup each)*

Nutritional Information: Per serving: calories 115, cholesterol 10 mg, sodium 255 mg, fat 3 g, calories from fat 24%.

Recipe Source: medicinenet.com

Crab Quesadillas

Ingredients:

- ¾ teaspoon garlic, minced
- ¼ cup chopped green onions, white and part green
- 1 jalapeno pepper, stemmed, seeded, and finely diced
- ½ pound crabmeat, washed, drained well, shredded into bite-size pieces
- 2 teaspoons light mayonnaise
- 2 tablespoons fat-free sour cream
- 4 teaspoons minced fresh cilantro
- 4 whole-wheat tortillas
- ¾ cup shredded, reduced-fat Monterey Jack cheese
- Garnish *(optional)*: salsa, fat-free sour cream, avocado

Preparation:

1. Combine garlic, green onion, jalapeno, crabmeat, light mayo, sour cream, and cilantro in a medium-size bowl.
2. Place 1 tortilla on a microwave-safe plate and sprinkle a heaping ⅛-cup measure of cheese over the top of the tortilla. Spoon ⅓ cup of crab mixture evenly over half of the tortilla.
3. Microwave on HIGH for 2-3 minutes or until cheese is melted. Remove from microwave and fold the half without the crab over to make a quesadilla.
4. Repeat steps 2 and 3 with remaining tortillas, cheese and crab mixture.
5. If desired, brown and crisp quesadillas by heating in a nonstick frying pan over medium heat for 1 minute per side. Serve each quesadilla with desired optional garnishes such as salsa, fat-free sour cream or avocado.

Yield: 4 servings

Nutritional Information: Per serving: 246 calories, 19 g protein, 25 g carbohydrate, 8 g fat, 3 g saturated fat, 71 mg cholesterol, 6 g fiber, 608 mg sodium. Calories from fat: 29 percent.

Recipe Source: medicinenet.com

Lean & Mean Chili

This dish has quite a few interesting ingredients. The flavors come together to make a delicious chili.

Ingredients:

- 1 tablespoon canola oil
- 1 large onion, chopped
- 1 tablespoon minced or chopped garlic
- 1.3 to 1.4 pounds beef round tip pieces, trimmed of visible fat
- 1 28-oz. can diced tomatoes in tomato puree
- 1 12-oz. bottle or can of nonalcoholic or light beer

- ⅔ cup strong coffee *(decaf or regular)*
- ⅓ cup light pancake syrup
- 2 tablespoons chili powder *(or add more to taste)*
- 1 teaspoon cumin seeds
- 1 tablespoon unsweetened cocoa powder
- 1 teaspoon dried oregano
- ½ teaspoon cayenne pepper
- ½ teaspoon ground coriander *(or add more to taste)*
- 2 15-oz. cans red kidney beans, drained
- **Garnish** *(optional)*
- ½ cup shredded, reduced-fat sharp cheddar cheese
- ½ cup chopped green onion

Preparation:

1. Heat canola oil in a large, nonstick saucepan over medium-high heat. Add onions, garlic, and beef pieces and saute for about 10 minutes, or until meat is well browned.

2. Stir in the tomatoes, beer, coffee, and pancake syrup. Then stir in the seasonings *(chili powder, cumin, cocoa, oregano, cayenne pepper and coriander)*. Stir in the beans. Cover pot, reduce heat to low and simmer for about an hour.

3. Top each serving with a sprinkle of reduced-fat sharp cheddar cheese and fresh chopped green onion, if desired.

Yield: 8 servings

Nutritional Information: Per serving: 275 calories, 25 g protein, 28 g carbohydrate, 6 g fat *(1.6 g saturated fat)*, 43 mg cholesterol, 8.5 g fiber, 239 mg sodium *(if lower sodium canned beans are used)*. Calories from fat: 20%.

Recipe Source: medicinenet.com

Light New England Clam Chowder

Ingredients:

- 3 medium to large red potatoes, cubed
- ½ cup chopped or sliced celery *(about 2 large stalks)*
- 1 medium onion, chopped
- ¼ cup flour
- 4 cups whole milk *(low-fat milk can also be used)*
- 2 tablespoons whipped butter or less-fat margarine
- 1 teaspoon salt *(optional)*
- 1 teaspoon sugar
- 1 cup chopped clams *(2, 6.5-oz. cans chopped clams, drained)*
- 10 drops Tabasco sauce
- ¼ cup shredded Parmesan cheese
- Freshly ground pepper to taste

Preparation:

1. Add potatoes, celery, and onion to a large, nonstick saucepan and add just enough water to cover. Bring to a boil and cook until tender *(about 15 minutes)*.

2. While vegetables are boiling, add flour and ¼ cup milk to a 2-cup measure and stir to make a paste. Stir in another ¼ cup of milk. Melt butter or margarine in a medium, nonstick saucepan over medium heat. Stir in the flour and milk mixture, then slowly whisk in the remaining 3 ½ cups milk. Stir in the salt, if desired, and the sugar and continue cooking and stirring until soup is nicely thickened *(about 5 minutes)*.

3. Add the milk mixture to the potato mixture in large saucepan and stir in the clams and Tabasco sauce. Cover saucepan and simmer for 15 minutes.

4. Stir in Parmesan and pepper to taste.

Yield: 8 servings

Nutritional Information: Per serving: 240 calories, 13 g protein, 31 g carbohydrate, 7.5 g fat, 4.5 g saturated fat, 39 mg cholesterol, 2.5 g fiber, 181 mg sodium. Calories from fat: 28%.

Recipe Source: medicinenet.com

Easy, Super Nutritious and Low-Calorie Gazpacho

Ingredients:

- 1 64-oz container low-sodium tomato juice
- 1 64-oz container spicy *(or not)* vegetable juice
- 2 12-oz cans low-sodium beef broth
- 1 tablespoon Worcestershire sauce
- 2 tablespoon balsamic vinegar
- Juice of 2 fresh lemons and 1 fresh lime
- 1 bunch scallions, finely chopped
- 2 red bell peppers, finely chopped

- 4 tomatoes, finely chopped
- 3 large seedless cucumbers, finely chopped
- 1 or 2 jalapeno peppers, finely chopped
- **Optional**: Avocado and light sour cream for garnish

Preparation:

1. Chop all vegetables by hand or pulse in a food processor.
2. Mix all ingredients together except garnish and chill several hours.
3. Serve cold with or without a little chopped avocado and a tablespoon of light sour cream as a garnish.

Yield: 12 servings

Nutritional Information: Per serving: 100 calories, 4.5 g protein, 18.5 g carbohydrate, 0.6 g fat, 0.1 g saturated fat, 2.8 g fiber, 512 mg sodium.

Recipe Source: medicinenet.com

Eggplant Parmesan

	Per serving:
Calories 274	274
Fat 6g	6g
Calories from Fat	20%
Protein	18g
Carbohydrates	35g
Cholesterol	20mg
Fiber 8g, Sodium	427mg

Ingredients:

- 2 egg whites
- 2 ½ lbs eggplant, peeled and cut crosswise into ¼"-thick slices
- ½ cup plain dried bread crumbs
- Olive oil spray
- 1 cup tomatoes, chopped with their juice
- ¼ cup chopped fresh basil or 1 tsp dried
- ½ tsp black pepper
- 1 cup shredded part-skim mozzarella cheese *(about 4 oz)*
- ¼ cup grated Parmesan cheese
- 4 cloves garlic
- ½ cup onion, chopped

Preparation:

1. Preheat the oven to 400°F. Line baking sheet with foil. Spray foil with nonstick cooking spray. In a shallow dish, beat the egg whites and 2 tbsp of water until foamy. Dip eggplant into egg whites, then into bread crumbs, pressing crumbs into eggplant.
2. Place eggplant on prepared baking sheet and spray oil over eggplant slices. Bake 30 minutes, turning eggplant over after 20 minutes, until golden brown and cooked through.
3. Sauté the onions and garlic with oil spray. In a medium bowl, stir together tomatoes and their juice, basil, salt, pepper, garlic and onions.
4. Spoon 3 tbsp of tomato mixture into bottom of 9" square glass baking dish. Place half of eggplant over sauce; spoon half of remaining tomato mixture over eggplant; and sprinkle half of mozzarella on top. Repeat with remaining eggplant, tomato mixture and mozzarella.
5. Sprinkle Parmesan on top and bake for 20 minutes, or until eggplant is piping hot and sauce is bubbly.

Serves: 4

Recipe Source: foodnetwork.com

Low Fat Fish Chowder

Prep Time: 10 minutes
Cook Time: 25 minutes

	Per Serving
Calories	285
Calories from Fat	40
Total Fat	4.4g *(sat 0.6g)*
cholesterol	70mg
Sodium	168mg
Carbohydrate	29
Fiber	4.7g
Protein	32.2g

Ingredients:

- 2 tsp canola oil
- 1 large leek, cleaned, trimmed and sliced
- 4 medium red potatoes, skin on, quartered
- 1 cup sliced mushrooms
- 1 cup fat-free, low sodium chicken broth
- ½ cup nonfat milk
- 2 tsp herbs for fish blend
- 1 tsp freshly ground black pepper
- 20 oz. sole or flounder fillets, cut into pieces
- 1 cup broccoli florets
- ¼ cup fresh parsley, chopped

Preparation:

1. Heat oil in a Dutch oven and gently sauté leeks until softened. Add potatoes and mushrooms and sauté for 2-3 minutes. Add chicken broth, milk, herbs and pepper. Partially cover and simmer for 10-12 minutes, until potatoes start become tender. Add fish, broccoli and parsley. Cook on low heat for 5 minutes, until fish begins to flake. Serves 4-6.

Recipe Source: lowfatcooking.about.com

Farmer's Market Pasta Salad

Feel free to add or substitute ingredients to incorporate the items you find this weekend at your farmer's market.

Ingredients:

- About 8 cups cooked, drained, whole wheat blend pasta *(rotini or penne)*
- ½ cup pesto *(fresh or frozen pesto from the supermarket)*
- 2 large ripe tomatoes, diced
- 1 cup finely diced bell pepper *(use yellow, red, or orange for a color contrast)*
- 3 cups lightly cooked and cooled, in-season veggies *(zucchini or carrot slices, broccoli or cauliflower florets, green beans, or whatever veggie looks good)*
- ¼ cup toasted pine nuts* *(optional)*

Preparation:

1. Add pasta to large serving bowl along with the pesto, diced tomato, bell pepper, and in-season vegetables. Toss to blend well.
2. Sprinkle the toasted pine nuts over the top if desired and serve. If not serving immediately, cover well and keep refrigerated until needed.
3. To toast pine nuts, just add to small nonstick frying pan and cook over medium-low heat, stirring often, until they are lightly brown.

Yield: 6 servings

Nutritional Information: Per serving: 370 calories, 16 g protein, 58 g carbohydrate, 11 g fat, 2.5 g saturated fat, 6 mg cholesterol, 6-10 g fiber *(depending on whether your pasta is partial or full whole wheat)*, 171 mg sodium. Calories from fat: 25%.

Recipe Source: medicinenet.com

French-Style Ham & Cheese Sandwich

Ingredients:

- 1 teaspoon extra virgin olive oil
- 1 medium sweet onion, thinly sliced *(red or white onion can be substituted)*
- 2 teaspoons light pancake syrup *(optional)*
- 4 slices of your bread of choice *(sourdough, French, whole grain, or even a white or wheat flour tortilla)*
- 3 oz. thinly sliced extra lean ham *(honey ham, maple, or other flavor)*
- 2 tablespoons whipped light cream cheese *(light cream cheese can be substituted)*
- ½ cup shredded Gruyere cheese, firmly packed

Preparation:

1. Add olive oil to medium nonstick frying pan and begin to heat over medium-high heat. Add onion and saute, stirring often, until onion is nicely browned and caramelized *(about 4 minutes)*. Drizzle pancake syrup *(if desired)* over the top and stir into the onions. Set aside to cool.
2. Toast bread slices if desired. Top two of the slices with the ham slices and spread the caramelized onions over the ham. Then spread a tablespoon of the cream cheese over the remaining two slices. Sprinkle shredded Gruyere cheese evenly over the top of the cream cheese.
3. Place all four slices until the toaster oven broiler *(or regular broiler)* and broil, watching carefully, until the Gruyere cheese is starting to bubble *(about 3-4 minutes)*. Place the slices with the cheese over the slices with the ham and onions. Cut each sandwich on the diagonal and serve!

Yield: Makes 2 sandwiches

Nutritional Information: Per sandwich *(using whole wheat bread)*: 377 calories, 25 g protein, 32 g carbohydrate, 15.5 g fat, 7 g saturated fat, 60 mg cholesterol, 4 g fiber, 997 mg sodium. Calories from fat: 37 percent.

Recipe Source: medicinenet.com

Greek-Style Mushrooms

Ingredients:

- 2 cups mushrooms
- 4 tablespoons lemon juice
- 1 tablespoon corriander
- ½ tablespoon ground pepper
- 1 bay leaf
- 1 tablespoon parsley
- 1 dash red chili pepper or paprika

Preparation:

1. Pour 1 cup of water in a pan. Add 1 tablespoon of lemon juice, bay leaf, coriander and pepper. Bring to a boil, lower heat and simmer for 10 minutes.
2. Clean and rinse the mushrooms then cut into thin slices. Add them to pan, boil again for one minute and remove from heat.
3. Add parsley, red chili pepper or paprika, mix gently and let cool.
4. When serving, strain the mushroom mixture and then place them in a dish and sprinkle with the remaining 3 tablespoons of lemon juice *(Note: other vegetables may also be prepared Greek-style: thinly sliced leeks, carrots or turnip sticks, cauliflower, thinly sliced cucumbers or artichoke hearts).*

Yield: 4 servings

Nutritional Information: Per serving: 35 calories, 2.3 protein, 6 g carbohydrate, 0.4 g fat, 24.8 mg vitamin C, 43.6 mg calcium. Calories from fat: 10%.

Recipe Source: medicinenet.com

Green Bean Casserole

Ingredients:

- 1 tablespoon butter or canola margarine
- 1 cup fat-free or light sour cream
- 2 tablespoons Wondra® quick-mixing flour *(regular flour can also be used)*
- 1 teaspoon salt
- 1 teaspoon granulated sugar
- ½ cup chopped onion
- 16 oz. bag of frozen French-style green beans *(if you want to use canned, use 3 cans, 14.5-oz. each, drained)*
- 1 cup shredded, reduced-fat cheddar cheese
- ½ cup crumbled Reduced Fat Ritz® crackers *(or similar)*, about 10 crackers
- Canola cooking spray

Preparation:

1. Preheat oven to 350°F. Coat a 9x9-inch baking dish with canola cooking spray.
2. Melt 1 tablespoon of butter in 2 cup glass measure in microwave. Stir in 2 tablespoons of the sour cream and the flour. Add remaining sour cream, salt, and sugar, and stir until well blended.
3. In large bowl, blend the sour cream mixture with the green beans and half of the cheddar cheese and spread mixture into prepared baking dish.
4. Spread remaining cheese over the top and top with the cracker crumbs. Spray the cracker topping lightly with canola cooking spray.
5. Bake for 30-35 minutes or until the top is golden and sauce is bubbly.

Yield: 9 side servings

Nutritional Information: Per serving: 115 calories, 6 g protein, 13.5 g carbohydrate, 4 g fat *(2.2 g saturated fat, 1.1 g monounsaturated fat, 0.1 g polyunsaturated fat)*, 10 mg cholesterol, 1.5 g fiber, 368 mg sodium. Calories from fat: 31%.

Recipe Source: medicinenet.com

Halfway Homemade Chicken Noodle Soup

You can throw all the ingredients *(except green onions)* in a slow cooker and cook on HIGH for a couple of hours or bring to a gentle boil in a saucepan over the stove, cover the saucepan and simmer for an hour.

Ingredients:

- 2 Ready to Serve cans *(about 14 oz. each)* of chicken noodle soup
- 1 ½ cups shredded or cubed boneless, skinless roasted or grilled chicken breast
- 1 cup shelled frozen edamame
- ½ cup chopped carrots
- 2 tablespoons chopped green onions

Preparation:

1. Add all of the ingredients, except the green onions, to a slow cooker. Set the slow cooker on HIGH, cover, and let simmer for around 2 hours. If you would rather use the stove, add the ingredients to a medium saucepan, bring to a gentle boil, and reduce heat to a simmer. Cover the saucepan and simmer for about an hour.
2. Ladle soup into individual bowls and sprinkle green onions over the top.

Yield: 4 servings

Nutritional Information: per serving: 280 calories, 18 g protein, 32 g carbohydrate, 8.5 g fat, 2 g saturated fat, 2 g monounsaturated fat, 3 g polyunsaturated fat, 65 mg cholesterol, 4 g fiber, 440 mg sodium. Calories from fat: 28 percent

Recipe Source: medicinenet.com

Macaroni and Cheese

Cook Time: 15 minutes

	Per 1 Cup Serving
Calories	314
Calories from Fat	51
Total Fat	5.7g *(sat 3.1g)*
Cholesterol	18mg
Sodium	258mg
Carbohydrate	49.6
Fiber	1.5g
Protein	16.2g

Ingredients:

- 12 oz. uncooked elbow macaroni or other short
- tube pasta
- 2 ½ tbsp flour
- 2 cups nonfat milk
- 1 ¼ cups reduced-fat extra-sharp cheddar, grated
- 1 tsp Dijon mustard
- Freshly ground black pepper

Preparation:

Cook pasta according to the instructions on the package. While pasta is cooking, place flour in a medium saucepan and gradually whisk in milk. Heat the milk and flour on medium and bring to a boil, stirring constantly to prevent lumps. Reduce heat and allow to simmer until the milk begins to thicken. Stir in cheese and mustard, and stir until cheese melts. Toss drained pasta and sauce in a large bowl. Add freshly ground black pepper and serve immediately. Serves 4-6.

Recipe Source: foodnetwork.com

Pan Fried Cabbage

Cabbage is the better half of the famous Irish duo, 'Corned Beef and Cabbage'. This is a flavorful recipe for just the cabbage that you can make easily in a large, nonstick frying pan.

Ingredients:

- 3 slices Louis Rich® Turkey Bacon
- ¼ cup chopped onion
- ½ head of cabbage, cut into 4 wedges
- 1 cup low-sodium beef or chicken broth
- ½ teaspoon sugar or Splenda®
- Pepper to taste
- 1 ½ teaspoon rice wine vinegar or cider vinegar

Preparation:

1. Add turkey bacon strips to a large nonstick frying pan and cook over medium heat until crisp. Remove strips to a paper towel to cool. Crumble the bacon and set aside.

2. Add the onions to the pan with any turkey bacon drippings *(there won't be much)*, and cook over medium heat until lightly browned *(four minutes)*.

3. Add cabbage, broth, and sugar to the frying pan with onions. Cover pan and cook for five minutes, stirring occasionally. Remove cover and cook until cabbage wilts and broth is almost evaporated *(about five minutes more)*, stirring occasionally.

4. Stir in turkey bacon pieces and vinegar. Serve immediately.

Yield: 3 servings

Nutritional Information: Per serving: 78 calories, 5 g protein, 7.5 g carbohydrate, 3.4 g fat *(0.9 g saturated fat, 1.3 g monounsaturated fat, 0.9 g polyunsaturated fat)*, 12 mg cholesterol, 2.2 g fiber, 225 mg sodium. Calories from fat: 38%.

Recipe Source: medicinenet.com

Perfect Pita Pizza

Ingredients:

- 1 large pita bread *(use whole-grain if available)*
- ⅛ cup low-fat ricotta cheese
- ⅛ cup bottled pizza sauce or marinara sauce
- ¼ cup shredded part-skim mozzarella cheese
- **Favorite pizza toppings:**
- sliced mushrooms, less-fat pepperoni or light salami, chopped green pepper or green onions, chopped red onion, pineapple chunks and lean ham, etc.

Preparation:

1. Preheat oven to 450 degrees. Place pita, rounded side down, on a baking sheet.

2. Spread ricotta cheese over the pita *(leaving a crust-like edge around the pita)*. Spoon the pizza sauce over the cheese and add desired toppings. Sprinkle mozzarella over the top and bake for 6-8 minutes *(watch carefully so it doesn't burn)*.

Yield: 1 serving

Nutritional Information: Per serving *(using whole-wheat pita and not including extra toppings)*: 256 calories, 16 g protein, 29.5 g carbohydrate, 8.8 g fat, 4.7 g saturated fat, 24 mg cholesterol, 4 g fiber, 492 mg sodium. Calories from fat: 30%.

Recipe Source: medicinenet.com

Peppered Steak Sandwiches with Caramelized Onions and Light Horseradish Sauce

Ingredients:

- 3 1-inch-thick filet mignon steaks *(beef tenderloin steaks)*, about 1 ¼ pound total*
- 2 teaspoons canola oil, divided use
- Freshly ground salt and pepper
- 1 large sweet onion *(or 2 small ones)*, cut in half and thinly sliced
- 2 cups sliced crimini mushrooms *(or use sliced regular mushrooms, or chopped portabellas)*
- ½ cup water or low-sodium beef broth
- 2 ½ tablespoons light mayonnaise
- 2 teaspoons white *(or creamed)* horseradish
- 4 French, sourdough, or submarine rolls *(part whole-wheat, if available)*

*Note: If the filet mignon is 1 ½ inch thick, have your butcher cut in half lengthwise to make ¾-inch steaks *(these will cook a little more quickly)*.

Preparation:

1. Add a teaspoon of canola oil to a medium nonstick frying pan or skillet, and let it get nice and hot over medium- high heat. Meanwhile, salt and pepper both sides of each steak *(heavier on the pepper than the salt)*. Add steaks to the pan, and cook to desired doneness *(about 5-6 minutes per side for medium-well)*. Use a fork to remove steaks to a plate *(keep the steak juices in the pan for use later)*.

2. Add the remaining teaspoon of oil to a large, nonstick skillet and saute the onion slices over medium-high heat until golden *(about 5 minutes)*. Add the mushroom slices, ½ cup broth or water, and all the juices from the steak pan. Continue to cook the onions and mushrooms, stirring often, for about 5 minutes. Remove from heat.

3. Put light mayonnaise and horseradish in a custard cup and stir to blend well.

4. Place the bottoms of your sandwich rolls on a serving plate. Spread horseradish sauce on top of each. Top each with steak slices and the onion/mushroom mixture, then place tops on the sandwiches.

Yield: 4 sandwiches

Nutritional Information: Per sandwich: 393 calories, 30 g protein, 33 g carbohydrate, 15 g fat *(4 g saturated fat, 5.2 g monounsaturated fat, 1.5 g polyunsaturated fat)*, 70 mg cholesterol, 3 g fiber, 430 mg sodium. Calories from fat: 36%.

Recipe Source: medicinenet.com

Pecan & Gorgonzola Greens Salad

Ingredients:

- 4 cups escarole, washed, patted dry, and torn into bite-size pieces
- 4 cups baby arugula, washed and patted dry
- 1 head fennel bulb, thinly sliced
- ¼ cup pecan pieces, toasted
- ¼ cup Gorgonzola cheese, crumbled
- ¼ cup dried cranberries
- 4 tablespoons light bottled balsamic vinaigrette *(with more on the table in case someone would like to add more)*

Preparation:

1. In 4 bowls, arrange in each, a mixture of the escarole, arugula and endive slices. Top each with pecans, Gorgonzola, and cranberries.

2. Drizzle a tablespoon over each bowl and serve!

Yield: 4 servings

Nutritional Information: Per serving: 160 calories, 5 g protein, 18 g carbohydrate, 9 g fat, 1.8 g saturated fat, 6 mg cholesterol, 4.5 g fiber, 272 mg sodium. Calories from fat: 47%.

Recipe Source: medicinenet.com

Pesto Pasta Salad

Ingredients:

- 12 oz. pasta of choice, dried *(rotelle, penne, etc.)*
- ⅓ cup pine nuts
- 1 cup fresh basil, rinsed and well drained
- 2 cups chopped vine-ripened tomatoes or quartered cherry tomatoes
- 2 jars *(6 oz. each)* artichoke hearts *(water packed or marinated)*, rinsed and drained
- 7 oz. container Armanino® Pesto Sauce *(in frozen food section of your supermarket)* or 14 tablespoons of another pesto made with olive oil or canola oil, thawed
- 3 tablespoons grated parmesan cheese

Preparation:

1. Boil water in large saucepan. Add pasta and continue to boil until pasta is tender *(according to directions on package)*, about 10-12 minutes, then drain well in colander.
2. While noodles are boiling, toast pine nuts in 400°F oven *(use 300°F if using a toaster oven)* until light brown, watching carefully *(about 3-5 minutes)*. Cool and add to serving bowl.
3. Coarsely chop fresh basil; add to serving bowl. Chop tomatoes and artichoke hearts and add to serving bowl.
4. Add drained noodles to serving bowl. Add pesto sauce and parmesan cheese and toss well. Store in refrigerator until needed.

Yield: 10 servings *(about 1 cup per serving)*

Nutritional Information: Per serving: 245 calories, 9 g protein, 32 g carbohydrate, 9.5 g fat *(1.8 g saturated fat)*, 5 mg cholesterol, 3.5 g fiber, 168 mg sodium. Calories from fat: 35%.

Recipe Source: The HRT-free Cookbook

Quick Vegetable Bean Salad

One serving of this quick salad gives you a dose of alpha- and beta-carotene, folic acid, vitamin C, fiber and plant omega-3 fatty acids from the canola oil. If you want to make this more of a meal and you want to add fish omega-3 fatty acids and some protein into the picture, stir in a can of albacore tuna.

Ingredients:

- 3 cups baby carrots, diced, or thinly sliced carrots
- 3 cups broccoli florets cut into bite-sized pieces
- 15 oz. can kidney beans, drained and rinsed well
- ½ cup finely chopped mild onion *(use less if desired)*
- ½ cup ⅓-less-fat bottled vinaigrette made with canola or olive oil *(I use Seven Seas® ⅓ less fat Red Wine Vinaigrette with canola)*
- 6 oz. can albacore tuna canned in water *(optional)*

Preparation:

1. Add carrot pieces to microwave-safe covered dish with ¼ cup water and cook on HIGH about 3-5 minutes *(or until just barely tender)*. Drain well and add to medium-sized serving bowl.
2. Add broccoli pieces to microwave-safe covered dish with ¼ cup water and cook on HIGH about 3-5 minutes *(or until just barely tender)*. Drain well and add to medium-sized serving bowl.
3. Add beans, chopped onion, and vinaigrette *(and tuna if desired)* to serving bowl and toss well to blend.

Yield: 8 servings

Nutritional Information: Per serving: 110 calories, 5 g protein, 19 g carbohydrate, 2.5 g fat *(0 g saturated fat)*, 0 mg cholesterol, 7 g fiber, 310 mg sodium, 1568 RE Carotenes/vitamin A *(196% RDA)*, 70 mcg folic acid *(39% RDA)*, 51 mg vitamin C *(86% RDA)*. Calories from fat: 20%.

Recipe Source: medicinenet.com

Simple Tomato & Herb Salad

This dish is simple because it uses a bottled salad dressing. The rest of the chopping and slicing goes quickly. It's all about featuring the garden fresh or vine-ripened tomato in all of its glory.

Ingredients:

- 2 ½ pounds *(about 6 medium)* garden fresh or vine-ripened tomatoes
- ½ cup thinly sliced red onion, separated into rings
- 2 shallots, sliced thin
- 6 tablespoons lite or reduced fat Italian-style salad dressing *(your choice)*
- ⅓ cup minced mixed fresh herbs such as basil, parsley, and tarragon

Preparation:

1. Core tomatoes and cut them into ½-inch thick slices. Arrange tomato slices in a deep serving

dish *(a 9 x 11-inch dish works well)*, and scatter onion and shallots over them.

2. Drizzle the bottled salad dressing evenly over the salad. Cover the dish and chill for 20-30 minutes.

3. Sprinkle herb mixture over the top and serve.

Yield: 6 servings

Nutritional Information: Per serving: 72 calories, 2 g protein, 12 g carbohydrate, 3 g fat, .6 g saturated fat, 1 g monounsaturated fat, 1 g polyunsaturated fat, 0 mg cholesterol, 2.5 g fiber, 243 mg sodium. Calories from fat: 35%.

Recipe Source: medicinenet.com

Teriyaki Portobello Mushroom Burger with Garlic Mayonnaise

Ingredients:

- 2 portobello mushrooms *(about 3 ½ inches wide)*, cleaned and stems removed
- 2 tablespoons bottled teriyaki sauce
- 2 large thin slices or of reduced-fat Monterey Jack cheese *(about 1-2 oz.)*
- 2 multigrain or whole-wheat hamburger buns
- 2 leaves of lettuce
- 4 tomato slices

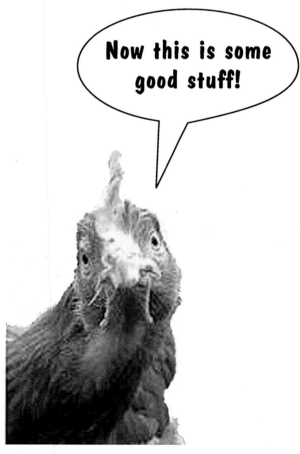

Now this is some good stuff!

Garlic Mayonnaise:

1 tablespoon light mayonnaise

½ teaspoon minced garlic

¼-½ teaspoon lemon juice

a few drops Worcestershire sauce for an extra kick *(optional)*

ground pepper and seasoning salt to taste

Preparation:

1. Heat the coals or grill. Spread teriyaki sauce over the mushrooms and marinate while the coals are getting ready.

2. Grill the mushrooms about 6 inches from the heat until tender *(about 4-5 minutes a side)*.

3. Add the cheese on top and continue to grill briefly to melt cheese.

4. Assemble burgers by placing the lettuce leaf and tomato on the bottom bun then top with the cheese-topped mushroom. Spread the top bun lightly with half of the garlic mayonnaise and place on top of the mushroom *(the lettuce keeps the bottom bun from getting soggy from some of the mushroom juice)*.

Yield: 2 burgers

Nutritional Information: Per burger: 268 calories, 14 g protein, 32 g carbohydrate, 9.5 g fat *(3.4 g saturated fat, 2.5 g monounsaturated fat, 0.8 g polyunsaturated fat)*, 11 mg cholesterol, 5 g fiber, 410 mg sodium *(not including seasoning salt)*. Calories from fat: 32%.

Recipe Source: medicinenet.com

The Broccoli and Everything Salad

Ingredients:

- 3 cups raw broccoli, chopped
- 1 cup seedless raisins
- 2 strips lean Canadian bacon
- ½ cup red onion, chopped

Vegetable Dressing

- ¼ cup low calorie mayonnaise
- ½ cup plain nonfat yogurt
- ¼ cup sugar
- ½ teaspoon vinegar

Preparation:

1. In large bowl, combine chopped broccoli, raisins, cooked diced bacon, and raw chopped onions.

2. Combine dressing ingredients and stir well.

3. Add dressing to combined ingredients, and stir to coat evenly.

Yield: 4 servings

Nutritional Information: Per serving: calories 268; fat 6 g, calories from fat 19%, cholesterol 10.2 g, fiber 3 g, sodium 303 mg.

Recipe Source: medicinenet.com

Tuna and Pasta Salad

Prep Time: 10 minutes

Cook Time: 10 minutes

	Per Serving
Calories	444
Calories from Fat	125
Total Fat	13.9g *(sat 2.1g)*
Cholesterol	36mg
Sodium	355mg
Carbohydrate	52.1g
Fiber	3.6g
Protein	27.7g

Ingredients:

- 8-oz. fusilli pasta
- 2 6-oz. cans water-packed tuna, drained
- 4 scallions, chopped
- 1 small red bell pepper, sliced
- 1 small mango, peeled and cubed
- 2 tbsp fresh parsley, chopped
- Handful of fresh basil leaves
- 2 tbsp white wine vinegar
- 3 tbsp olive oil
- 1 garlic clove, crushed
- 1 tsp Dijon mustard
- pinch salt and black pepper

Preparation:

1. Boil pasta according to instructions on package. Drain and rinse with cold water. Place cooled pasta in a large bowl and add tuna, scallions, bell pepper, mango, parsley and basil.

2. For the dressing, whisk oil, vinegar, garlic, mustard, salt and pepper together in a small bowl. Add dressing to salad and toss well to coat. Garnish with some extra basil and serve chilled on 4 plates.

Recipe Source: lowfatcooking.about.com

Tropical Fruit Salad

Bring a taste of the tropics to your fruit salad with this recipe.

Ingredients:

- 20-oz. can pineapple chunks canned in juice
- 2 kiwi, peeled, halved and sliced
- 2 cups strawberries, quartered
- 1 large banana, sliced
- 1 papaya or mango, peeled and cubed *(or substitute an 11-oz. can of mandarin oranges, drained)*
- ½ teaspoon finely grated lime zest or peel
- 2 tablespoons lime juice
- 1 ½ tablespoons honey
- ⅓ cup unsweetened or sweetened shredded coconut *(optional)*

Preparation:

1. Drain pineapple chunks, and reserve ¼ cup of the pineapple juice.

2. Add pineapple chunks, kiwi, strawberries, banana, and papaya or mango to large serving bowl.

3. Put ¼ cup pineapple juice, lime peel, lime juice and honey in a 2-cup measure and whisk together until nicely blended. Drizzle over the salad, and toss to coat the fruits well. Sprinkle coconut over the top before serving, if desired.

Yield: About 7 cups

Nutritional Information: Per cup: 101 calories, 1.2 g protein, 25 g carbohydrate, 0.6 g fat, 0 g saturated fat, 0 mg cholesterol, 3 g fiber, 4 mg sodium. Calories from fat: 5%.

Recipe Source: medicinenet.com

Waldorf Salad

Ingredients:

- ¼ cup light mayonnaise
- ¼ cup light or regular plain yogurt or fat-free sour cream
- 2 teaspoons sugar
- ¾ teaspoon lemon juice
- 3 apples, peeled, cored and chopped *(about 3 cups)*
- 1 cup thinly sliced celery
- ⅓ cup walnut pieces *(or coarsely chopped walnuts)*
- ⅓ cup dried fruit like raisins, cherries or cranberries *(optional)*

Preparation:

1. Add mayonnaise, yogurt or sour cream, sugar and lemon juice to serving bowl and whisk well to blend.

2. Add apple pieces, celery, walnuts and dried fruit if desired and toss everything together. Cover and chill in refrigerator until ready to serve.

Yield: About 4 ½ cups *(9, ½-cup servings)*

Nutritional Information: Per serving: 90 calories, 2 g protein, 11 g carbohydrate, 4.5 g fat,0 .6 g saturated fat, 0 mg cholesterol, 1.3 g fiber, 66 mg sodium. Calories from fat: 45%.

Recipe Source: medicinenet.com

Zucchini Parmesan Crisps

Per Serving: *(serving size, ½ cup)*	
Calories	105
Total Fat	6g
Sat Fat	2g
Mono Fat	2g
Poly Fat	0g
Protein	5g
Carb	5g
Fiber	1.5g
Cholesterol	1mg
Sodium	22mg

Cook Time: 30 min

Level: Easy

Yield: 4 servings, serving size ½ cup

Ingredients:

- Cooking spray
- 2 medium zucchini *(about 1 pound total)*
- 1 tablespoon olive oil
- ¼ cup freshly grated Parmesan *(¾-oz.)*
- ¼ cup plain dry bread crumbs
- ⅛ teaspoon salt
- Freshly ground black pepper

Preparation:

1. Preheat the oven to 450 degrees F. Coat a baking sheet with cooking spray.

2. Slice the zucchini into ¼-inch thick rounds. In a medium bowl, toss the zucchini with the oil. In a small bowl, combine the Parmesan, bread crumbs, salt, and a few turns of pepper. Dip each round into the Parmesan mixture, coating it evenly on both sides, pressing the coating on to stick, and place in a single layer on the prepared baking sheet.

3. Bake the zucchini rounds until browned and crisp, 25 to 30 minutes. Remove with spatula. Serve immediately.

Recipe Source: foodnetwork.com

• •

Main Dishes/Entrees Poultry

Finger-Lickin' Oven-Fried Chicken

Marinate skinless chicken pieces in buttermilk and coat with a seasoned flour mixture, then spray with canola cooking spray, and bake in the oven, followed with a quick turn under the broiler. This chicken is great cold, too!

Ingredients:

- 1 whole chicken, cut into pieces
- 1 cup low-fat buttermilk
- 1 cup unbleached white flour
- ½ teaspoon ground chipotle pepper *(cayenne red pepper can be substituted—increase to 1 teaspoon if extra 'heat' is desired)*
- ¼ teaspoon ground cumin
- 1 teaspoon salt
- ½ teaspoon white pepper
- Canola cooking spray

Preparation:

1. Remove skin from chicken pieces and discard. Combine chicken pieces and buttermilk in a gallon-sized zip-top bag. Refrigerate sealed bag in a medium-size bowl for several hours or overnight.

2. Preheat oven to 450°F. Add flour, chipotle pepper, cumin, salt, and white pepper to a new gallon-sized, zip-top bag or medium-size shallow bowl. Stir with fork to blend ingredients well.

3. Remove a piece of chicken from buttermilk and gently shake off excess buttermilk. Immediately dip chicken into flour mixture; coat well. Holding chicken piece over a plate, spray top and bottom well with canola cooking spray. Dip chicken piece into flour mixture a second time and spray again with canola cooking spray. Place chicken bone-side down onto a cookie sheet.

4. Repeat with remaining pieces of chicken.

5. Bake until chicken is cooked throughout and coating is golden brown *(about 25-30 minutes)*. Switch the oven to broil, and broil the chicken 6 inches from the heat for a minute or two *(until outside of chicken is*

nicely browned), watching very carefully so as not to burn.

Yield: 4 servings

Nutritional Information: Per serving: 261 calories, 32 g protein, 13 g carbohydrate, 8 g fat *(2 g saturated fat, 3.2 g monounsaturated fat, 1.9 g polyunsaturated fat)*, 92 mg cholesterol, 0.5 g fiber, 365 mg sodium, 2 mg iron, 35 mg calcium.

Recipe Source: Fry Light, Fry Right!, Black Dog & Leventhal

Baked Chicken Teriyaki

	Per Serving:
Calories	296
Calories from Fat	62
Total	Fat 6.9g *(sat 1.7g)*
Cholesterol	141mg
Sodium	878mg
Carbohydrate	21.5g
Fiber	2.3g
Protein	36.9g

Prep Time: 15 minutes

Cook Time: 45 minutes

Ingredients:

- 8 chicken thighs
- ½ cup teriyaki marinade
- 2 tsp of fresh grated ginger
- 1 tbsp clear honey
- 4 chopped scallions
- 2 medium red peppers, quartered and seeded
- 3 small zucchini, cut into quarters lengthwise

Preparation:

1. Preheat the oven to 400 degrees.
2. Place chicken thighs in a roasting tin in a single layer.
3. Combine teriyaki marinade with ginger, honey and scallions. Pour over chicken; turn the pieces to coat them evenly.
4. Bake chicken for 25 minutes, turning once halfway through. Add vegetables, coating them in the marinade.
5. Bake for another 15-20 minutes until chicken and vegetables are tender.

Serves 4

Recipe Source: lowfatcooking.about.com

Glazed Lemon Chicken

	Per Serving:
Calories	262
Calories from Fat	20
Total Fat	2.2g *(sat 0.6g)*
Cholesterol	98mg
Sodium	113mg
Carbohydrate	20.8
Fiber	1.3g
Protein	39.8g

Cook Time: 25 minutes

Ingredients:

- 4 skinless boneless chicken breast halves
- 4 tbsp honey
- Juice and zest of 1 large lemon
- 1 garlic clove, crushed
- 1 tbsp Dijon mustard
- 1 tsp freshly ground black pepper

Preparation:

1. Combine honey, lemon juice and zest, garlic, mustard and black pepper in a glass dish. Place chicken breasts in marinade, coating both sides with mixture. Cover and marinate for at least 2 hours, preferably longer.
2. Preheat oven to 400 degrees. Place chicken breasts in a baking dish and spoon marinade over them. Roast for 25 minutes. Serve with a wild rice blend and steamed vegetables.

Serves 4.

Recipe Source: lowfatcooking.about.com

Healthy Fried Chicken Recipe

Serves: 4

Total Time: 45 min

Prep Time: 10 min

Cook Time: 35 min

Ingredients:

- 1 ½ cups buttermilk
- ½ teaspoon ground red pepper *(cayenne)*
- ¾ teaspoon salt
- 1 *(3-pound)* cut-up chicken, skin removed from all pieces except wings
- 1 ½ cups panko *(Japanese-style)* bread crumbs
- 1 teaspoon(s) grated fresh lemon peel

Preparation:

1. In large self-sealing plastic bag, place buttermilk, ground red pepper, and ¾ teaspoon salt; add chicken pieces, turning to coat. Seal bag, pressing out excess air. Refrigerate chicken at least 1 hour or preferably overnight, turning bag over once.

2. Preheat oven to 425 degrees F. Spray 15 ½" by 10 ½" jelly-roll pan with nonstick spray. In large bowl, combine panko and lemon peel.

3. Remove chicken from marinade, shaking off excess. Discard marinade. Add chicken pieces, a few at a time, to panko mixture, turning to coat. Place chicken in prepared pan.

4. Bake 30 to 35 minutes or until coating is crisp and juices run clear when thickest part of chicken is pierced with tip of knife. For browner coating, after chicken is cooked, turn oven to broil. Broil chicken 5 to 6 inches from source of heat 1 to 2 minutes or until golden.

Recipe Source: Good Housekeeping

Roasted Garlic & Chicken *(Foil Wrapped)*

	Per Serving
Calories	305
Total Fat	9g
Saturated Fat	3g
Cholesterol	101mg
Sodium	370mg
Total Carbohydrate	16g
Dietary Fiber	1g
Sugars	--
Protein	36g
Calcium	

Ingredients:

- Canola or olive oil nonstick cooking spray
- 2 chicken breasts, boneless, skinless
- Black pepper to taste
- Seasoning salt to taste *(optional)*
- 2 teaspoons olive oil
- 6 garlic cloves, peeled
- ½ onion, sliced thin
- 1 ½ medium sized carrots *(or 1 large)*, sliced thin
- 1 medium potato, peeled and sliced thin *(sweet potato can be substituted)*
- 1 tomato, sliced
- 1 teaspoon dried chervil or any other herb du jour *(herb of choice)*
- 2 tablespoons dry white wine, champagne, apple juice, or chicken broth

Preparation:

1. Preheat oven to 350 degrees. Place a 2 ½ foot long piece of foil in a 9"x13" baking pan. Coat top of foil with nonstick cooking spray.

2. Lay chicken breasts in middle of foil. Sprinkle tops with pepper and seasoning salt to taste if desired. Add olive oil to small cup. Peel garlic cloves and dip in oil. Drop 3 garlic cloves evenly over each chicken breast.

3. Lay onion slices over the chicken. Then spread carrots over the onion and potato slices over the carrots. Top with tomato slices.

4. Sprinkle top with chervil. Drizzle remaining olive oil over the top, then drizzle with wine.

5. Fold foil over to wrap chicken and vegetable mixture up well. Bake for 1 hour. Cut into center of chicken to make sure chicken is cooked throughout. To double this recipe, make two foil wrapped chicken and vegetable packages. They will both fit in the 9"x13" baking pan. They will still bake for 1 hour. To serve, make sure every portion has a chicken breast and a sampling of the various vegetables. Drizzle some of the juices over the top.

Yield: 2 servings

Nutritional Information: Per serving: 321 calories, 31 g protein, 33 g carbohydrate, 6.5 g fat, 68 mg cholesterol, 4 g fiber, 110 mg sodium *(seasoning salt is optional)*. Calories from fat: 19%.

Recipe Source: medicinenet.com

Turkey Fettuccini Alfredo

Ingredients:

- 2 to 2 ½ cups roasted turkey breast, cut into strips *(skinless)*
- ¼ cup light cream cheese
- 1 ½ cups fat-free half-and-half or whole milk, divided
- 1 tablespoon Wondra quick-mixing flour
- 1 tablespoon butter *(or no/low-trans fat margarine)*
- 3 cups hot cooked and drained spaghetti or fettuccine noodles
- Salt and freshly grated pepper to taste
- Pinch or two of nutmeg *(add more to taste if desired)*
- ¼ cup shredded Parmesan cheese *(add more at the table if desired)*

Preparation:

1. Boil fettuccine noodles.

2. Combine cream cheese, ¼-cup fat-free half-and-half, and flour in a small mixing bowl or food processor. Beat or pulse until well blended. Slowly pour in remaining half-and-half or milk and beat until smooth.

3. Melt 1 tablespoon butter in large, nonstick frying pan or saucepan over medium heat. Add the milk mixture and continue to heat, stirring constantly, until the sauce is just the right thickness *(about 3-4 minutes)*. Turn the heat to low and add the hot noodles and turkey strips. Toss to coat noodles and turkey well with sauce. Add salt, pepper, and nutmeg to taste if desired. Stir in grated Parmesan and serve.

Yield: 4 servings

Nutritional Information: Per serving: 419 calories, 37 g protein, 44 g carbohydrate, 9 g fat *(3.8 g saturated fat, 2.8 g monounsaturated fat, 1.6 g polyunsaturated fat)*, 79 mg cholesterol, 2 g fiber, 332 mg sodium. Calories from fat: 23%.

Recipe Source: medicinenet.com

Turkey Meatloaf

Prep Time: 20 minutes

Cook Time: 50 minutes

Ingredients:

	Per slice:
Calories	108
Calories from Fat	32g
Total Fat	3.7g *(sat1g)*
Cholesterol	28mg
Sodium	193mg
Carbohydrate	10g
Fiber	0.8g
Protein	8.9g

- 1 ½ cups plain breadcrumbs
- ⅓ cup nonfat milk
- 1 medium onion, cut into large pieces
- 1 medium carrot, cut into fourths
- 1 8 oz. pack sliced mushrooms, finely chopped
- 2 cloves garlic
- 1 ¼ pounds 93 percent lean ground turkey
- ½ cup egg substitute
- 1 tbsp Worcestershire Sauce
- ¼ cup tomato ketchup

Preparation:

1. Preheat oven to 400 degrees. Line a large rimmed baking sheet with parchment paper or foil wrap.

2. Place breadcrumbs and milk in a small bowl, and allow to soak for a few minutes.

3. Place onion, carrots, and garlic cloves in a food processor with a grater attachment, or grate by hand. Transfer grated vegetables to a large bowl; add mushrooms.

4. Crumble ground turkey in with the grated vegetables. Add breadcrumb/milk mixture to the vegetable and turkey mixture. Stir well with a fork.

5. Add egg substitute, Worcestershire sauce and ketchup. Mix well with light fingers.

6. Divide mixture into two and form two loaves on the baking sheet, each about 7 x 4 inches.

7. Bake for 50 minutes to an hour. Remove from oven and check the internal temperature has reached 160 degrees F. Allow meatloaves to rest for 10 minutes before slicing. Each loaf makes about 8 slices.

Recipe Source: lowfatcooking.about.com

Seafood/Fish

Asian Glazed Salmon

	Per Serving
Calories	237
Calories from Fat	76
Total Fat	8.4g *(sat 1.8g)*
Cholesterol	64mg
Sodium	587mg
Carbohydrate	8.7g
Fiber	0.2g
Protein	31.5g

Prep Time: 30 minutes

Cook Time: 10 minutes

Ingredients:

- 2 tbsp maple syrup
- 1 tbsp freshly grated ginger
- ¼ cup reduced-sodium soy sauce
- 2 tbsp chopped scallions
- 1 tbsp lime juice
- 4 5-oz. salmon fillets

Preparation:

1. Combine maple syrup, ginger, soy sauce, lime juice and scallions in a large resealable plastic bag. Add salmon fillets. Seal, pressing out

excess air, and refrigerate for 20 minutes.

2. Preheat broiler or grill. Coat broiler pan with nonstick cooking spray. If grilling, spray grill before preheating.

3. Remove salmon from plastic bag, reserving marinade, and place on broiler rack or grill. Cook for 10 minutes until fish flakes easily. Brush with marinade once or twice during cooking. Serves 4

Recipe Source: lowfatcooking.about.com

Easy Herb Butter Scallops

The less you fuss with scallops, the better they tend to taste. Serve these scallops on a bed of whole-wheat pasta or steamed brown rice and with a side of steamed vegetables and/or a green or fruit salad.

Ingredients:

- 1 pound large sea scallops, rinsed in cold water then patted dry with paper towels
- 2 teaspoons olive oil or canola oil
- 1 tablespoon whipped butter
- 2 tablespoons finely diced shallot
- ¼ cup dry white wine or champagne
- 1 tablespoon finely chopped parsley
- 1 tablespoon finely chopped chives
- Salt and freshly ground black pepper *(optional)*

Preparation:

1. Heat a large nonstick frying pan over medium-high heat for a minute or so. Add 1 tablespoon of olive oil and let it heat up about 30 seconds. Place scallops in the pan with plenty of room between them so they will sizzle instead of steam.

2. Let the scallops sizzle until the bottom side is browned and crisp *(2 to 4 minutes)*. Gently turn over and cook the other side until well browned *(2 to 4 minutes)*. When you cut into a scallop, it should be barely firm to the touch and a more solid white color throughout.

3. Take the pan off the heat. Move the scallops to a plate and cover with a sheet of foil to keep them warm.

4. Return pan to the stove over medium heat. Add a tablespoon of whipped butter and the shallots and saute for about a minute. Add the

wine and simmer until it is reduced by about half *(1-2 minutes)*. Reduce heat to low, stir in the parsley and chives, and continue to simmer for only a minute. Turn off the heat and add the scallops. Let sit about a minute to warm the scallops and meld flavors. Add salt and pepper to taste, if desired.

Yield: 4 servings

Nutritional Information: Per serving: 141 calories, 19 g protein, 4 g carbohydrate, 5 g fat, 1.6 g saturated fat, 2.3 g monounsaturated fat, 0.6 g polyunsaturated fat, 43 mg cholesterol, 0 g fiber, 203 mg sodium. Calories from fat: 33%.

Recipe Source: medicinenet.com

Low Fat Breaded Fish

	Per Serving
Calories	195
Calories from Fat	29
Total Fat	3.2g *(sat 0.7g)*
Cholesterol	106mg
Sodium	248mg
Carbohydrate	12.1g
Fiber	2g
Protein	29.4g

Prep Time: 10 minutes

Cook Time: 10 minutes

Ingredients:

- 1 ¼ pounds firm white fish, such as cod or halibut
- 1 egg lightly beaten
- 1 ½ cups breadcrumbs
- 1 tsp dried mixed herbs
- 1 tsp paprika
- Freshly ground black pepper

Preparation:

1. Preheat oven to 450 degrees. Place a large cookie sheet coated with nonstick cooking spray in the oven.

2. Meanwhile cut fish into chunks. Put beaten egg into a small bowl, and combine breadcrumbs, herbs, paprika and pepper in a large shallow bowl.

3. Remove cookie sheet from oven.

Recipe Source: lowfatcooking.about.com

Sea Bass with Dried Fruit Salsa

Ingredients:

- 4 *(5 to 6 oz.)* sea bass fillets, about 1-inch thick
- 2 teaspoons olive oil
- 2 teaspoons ground coriander
- 1 teaspoon ground cumin
- ¼ teaspoon cinnamon
- ¼ teaspoon cayenne pepper
- ¾ teaspoon salt
- ¼ cup of each dried fruit, mango, papaya, cherry and pineapple
- ⅓ cup apple juice or cider
- 2 tablespoons cider vinegar
- 2 tablespoons apricot jam
- 2 tablespoons chopped cilantro

Preparation:

1. Rub fish with olive oil.
2. Combine coriander, cumin, cinnamon and cayenne pepper; mix well. Set aside ½ teaspoon of the mixture for the fruit salsa. Add salt to remaining mixture.
3. Rub seasonings over both sides of fish.
4. Heat a large nonstick skillet over high heat until hot.
5. Add fish. Reduce heat to medium, cook 3-5 minutes or until fish is browned and seared. Turn fish over; cook about 5 minutes or until fish is slightly firm and flaky.
6. Combine dried fruit, juice, vinegar and ½ teaspoon reserved seasoning mixture in a small saucepan or microwave-safe dish. Bring to a boil. Stir in jam. Let stand 5 minutes.
7. Transfer fish to serving plates. Top with fruit salsa and sprinkle with cilantro.

Yield: 4 servings

Nutritional Information: Per serving: Calories 337, Fat 6 g, Calories from Fat 16%, Protein 28 g, Carbohydrates 43 g, Fiber 3 g, Cholesterol 58 mg, Sodium 241 mg.

Recipe Source: medicinenet.com

Seasoned Salmon with Lemon Caper Sauce

When I want to fix salmon fast, this is one of the recipes I tend to grab. It takes five minutes to put together and 10 minutes to broil the salmon! And it tastes terrific—can't get much better than that.

Ingredients:

- 1 pound salmon fillet
- Canola cooking spray
- ⅛ teaspoon salt
- ⅛-¼ teaspoon freshly ground pepper *(depending on preference)*
- ¼-½ teaspoon garlic powder *(depending on preference)*
- ½ teaspoon dill weed

Lemon Caper Sauce

- ½ cup fat-free or light sour cream
- 1 tablespoon drained capers
- 2 teaspoons lemon juice
- ½ teaspoon finely chopped lemon zest or peel *(optional)*

Preparation:

1. Preheat broiler. Line a 9-inch round pan or dish with foil. Coat the foil with canola cooking spray.
2. Rinse and dry salmon fillet well. Place the salmon skin-side down in the prepared pan.
3. Coat the top of the salmon fillet *(flesh side)* with canola cooking spray.
4. Sprinkle salt and pepper evenly over the top of salmon. Then sprinkle garlic powder and dill weed evenly over the top of salmon. Place under broiler *(about 6 inches from the heat)* for five minutes. Flip salmon over *(skin-side up now)* and broil five minutes longer. Check the thickest part of the salmon to test if it is done.
5. Peel off the skin *(it comes off easily)* and throw away. Serve the salmon seasoned-side up *(spoon any juices and seasoning in the bottom of the pan over the top of the salmon)*.
6. While the salmon is broiling, add sour cream, capers and lemon juice *(lemon zest if desired)* in small food processor and pulse about five seconds to blend well. If you don't have a food processor finely chop the capers and blend the capers, lemon juice and sour cream together well in a small serving bowl.

Yield: 4 servings

Nutritional Information: Per serving: 191 calories, 24 g protein, 5 g carbohydrate, 7.5 g fat *(1.4 g saturated fat)*, 65 mg cholesterol, 0.1 g fiber, 206 mg sodium. Calories from fat: 36%.

Recipe Source: medicinenet.com

Spicy Shrimp Kebabs

Cook Time: 5 minutes

	Per Serving
Calories	140
Calories from Fat	28
Total Fat	3.1g *(sat 0.6g)*
Cholesterol	170mg
Sodium	699mg
Carbohydrate	4g
Fiber	0.2g
Protein	23.9g

Ingredients:

- ¼ cup reduced-sodium soy sauce
- 1 tsp sesame oil
- 1 tsp brown sugar
- 1 garlic clove, minced
- 2 tsp freshly grated ginger
- 1 tsp chopped jalapeno pepper
- 4 scallions, finely chopped
- 1 pound medium shrimp, peeled, deveined

Preparation:

1. Combine soy sauce, sesame oil, sugar, garlic, ginger, jalapeno and scallions together in a glass bowl. Add shrimp and stir well. Cover and marinate for up to an hour.
2. Pre-soak bamboo skewers in cold water. Preheat broiler or grill. Thread marinated shrimp on to skewers—4 or 5 per skewer, and broil or grill for 4-5 minutes, turning once. Serve as an appetizer or as an entree with whole grain rice and steamed vegetables.

Yield: Serves 4.

Recipe Source: lowfatcooking.about.com

Beef, Lamb and Pork

Apple-Spiced Pork Roast

This dish works well with steamed yams or sweet potatoes. Any leftover sliced pork works well for sandwiches the next day, too.

Ingredients:

- 2 teaspoons finely chopped fresh rosemary
- 2 teaspoons finely chopped fresh thyme
- 1 teaspoon dried marjoram *(you can also substitute dried sage)*
- ½ teaspoon salt
- ½ teaspoon white or black pepper
- 2 ⅓ to 2 ½ pound pork sirloin tri-tip roast
- 1 cup spiced apple cider *(bottled)*
- 2 Fuji or Granny Smith apples, cored and cut into ¾- inch pieces
- 1 large red onion, cut into ¾-inch pieces
- ¼ cup dark brown sugar, loosely packed
- ½ teaspoon ground cinnamon
- 2 tablespoons maple butter *(you can substitute maple syrup)*
- 2 tablespoons quick-mixing flour

Preparation:

1. In a small bowl, mix together rosemary, thyme, marjoram, salt, and pepper. Rub the herb mixture all over the outside of the pork roast. Place in the slow cooker. Pour apple cider around the roast. Cover roast with apple pieces, then top apples with onion pieces. Sprinkle brown sugar and cinnamon over the top of the apples and onions.
2. Cover slow cooker and cook on low about 4-5 hours *(a meat thermometer inserted into the center of roast should register at 165 degrees)*. When cooked throughout, remove roast to serving platter.
3. Turn slow cooker to HIGH. Add maple butter to a microwave-safe custard cup and microwave on HIGH for about 5 seconds to soften. Stir in flour *(add a tablespoon of juice from slow cooker, if needed)*. Stir maple paste into the apple-onion-cider mixture in slow cooker. Cook for 30 minutes longer, or until thickened nicely. Meanwhile, after pork has cooled slightly *(about 10 minutes)*, cover with foil to keep warm.
4. Serve sliced pork roast with apple-onion sauce, and steamed yams if desired.

Yield: 6 servings

Nutritional Information: Per serving: 365 calories, 26 g protein, 27 g carbohydrate, 12 g fat, 4 g saturated fat, 107 mg cholesterol, 2 g fiber, 250 mg sodium. Calories from fat: 30%.

Recipe Source: medicinenet.com

Barbecue Boneless Ribs

Who doesn't love the taste of barbecue ribs? These ribs have the taste and fall-off-the-bone texture of restaurant ribs—but without all the grease!

Ingredients:

- 2 ½ pounds boneless, very lean beef short ribs, trimmed of visible fat *(my butcher makes it from the center brisket)*
- Black pepper
- Garlic powder
- Canola no-stick cooking spray
- 1 onion, sliced
- 16 oz. of the best barbecue sauce you can get your hands on

Preparation:

1. Sprinkle ribs lightly with pepper and garlic powder.
2. Start heating large nonstick frying pan or skillet over medium-high heat. Spray pan generously with canola no-stick cooking spray. Place ribs in pan and brown ribs on all sides if possible *(about 6-8 minutes altogether)*.
3. Put sliced onion in Crock-Pot. Cut ribs into serving size pieces and put in Crock-Pot. Pour in barbecue sauce. Cover and cook on LOW about 8-9 hours *(HIGH about 5 hours)*.

Yield: Makes about 8 servings

Nutritional Information: Per serving *(if half of the BBQ sauce is consumed)*: 221 calories, 28 g protein, 12.5 g carbohydrate, 5.6 g fat *(1.8 g saturated fat)*, 83 mg cholesterol, 1.3 g fiber, 404 mg sodium. Calories from fat: 23 percent.

Recipe Source: medicinenet.com

Beef Stroganoff

Ingredients:

- About 2 pounds top sirloin steak, trimmed of visible fat, cut into ⅓-inch strips
- Salt and pepper *(optional)*
- 1 tablespoon canola oil
- ½ cup finely chopped shallots
- ¾ pound thickly sliced mushrooms
- 10 ½-oz. can beef consomme
- 2 tablespoons Cognac *(vodka can be substituted)*
- ¾ cup fat-free half-and-half
- 1 tablespoon Dijon mustard
- 1 tablespoon chopped fresh dill
- 8 cups cooked whole-wheat blend pasta of your choice
- Paprika, as desired

Preparation:

1. Pat meat strips well with paper towels, and sprinkle lightly with salt and pepper if desired. Heat oil in heavy nonstick frying pan over high heat. Add meat in single layer and cook just until brown on both sides *(about 1 minute per side)*. Remove meat to a holding plate.
2. Add shallots and mushrooms to the same frying pan and heat over medium-high heat. Pour ⅛ cup consomme over the top and simmer until mushrooms are tender, scraping up browned bits as it cooks *(about 6 minutes)*.
3. Pour in the remaining consomme and cognac and continue to cook until liquid thickens *(about 10 minutes)*. Stir in the fat-free half-and-half and the Dijon mustard. Add the meat strips and any juices from the holding plate. Simmer over medium-low heat until the meat is heated through and cooked to your desired doneness *(about 2 minutes)*. Stir in chopped dill. Add salt and pepper to taste if desired.
4. Serve stroganoff over cooked noodles and sprinkle paprika over the top as desired.

Yield: 6-8 servings

Nutritional Information: Per serving *(if 8 per serving)*: 410 calories, 38 g protein, 43 g carbohydrate, 9.5 g fat, 3 g saturated fat, 76 mg cholesterol, 6 g fiber, 331 mg sodium. Calories from fat: 21%.

Recipe Source: medicinenet.com

Low Fat Beef and Black Bean Chili

Prep Time: 10 minutes
Cook Time: 40 minutes

	Per Serving:
Calories	279
Calories	from Fat 53
Total Fat	5.7g *(sat 1.8g)*
Cholesterol	35mg,
Sodium	304mg
Carbohydrate	37mg
Fiber	9.3g
Protein	19.4g

Ingredients:

- 2 tsp canola oil
- 1 medium yellow onion
- 1 large red pepper, deseeded and chopped
- 1 jalapeno chile pepper, deseeded and chopped
- 1 large carrot, chopped
- 2 tbsp chili powder
- 1 tbsp cumin
- ¾ pound extra-lean ground beef
- 1 15-oz. can crushed tomatoes
- 1 15-oz. can low sodium black beans, drained
- 2 cups frozen sweet corn

Preparation:

1. Heat oil in a large Dutch oven on medium heat. Add onion, red pepper, jalapeno pepper and carrot. Saute for 5 minutes, until onion has softened. Sprinkle chili powder and cumin over the vegetables and stir for 1 minute. Crumble in ground beef; cook on medium-high until no longer pink. Add canned tomatoes and black beans. Turn down heat and simmer for 15 minutes. Add sweet corn and cook for a further 5 minutes.

2. Serve with a dollop of fat free sour cream or a light sprinkling *(1-2 tbsp)* of reduced fat Jack cheese.

3. Serves 6-8.

Recipe Source: lowfatcooking.about.com

Low Fat Spaghetti and Meatballs

	Per Serving:
Calories	404
Calories from Fat	60
Total Fat	6.9g *(sat 2.4g)*
Cholesterol	52mg
Sodium	242mg
Carbohydrate	58.4g
Fiber	3.4g
Protein	27.7g

Prep Time: 25 minutes
Cook Time: 30 minutes

Ingredients:

- ¾ pound extra-lean ground beef
- ⅓ cup breadcrumbs *(about 1 slice)*
- 1 tsp dried oregano
- ½ cup finely chopped onion
- ¼ cup canned no-salt-added tomato sauce
- 1 garlic clove, crushed
- ¼ cup fresh parsley, finely chopped
- 2 ½ cups low fat, low sodium marinara sauce *(such as Amy's or Trader Joe's)*
- 8-oz. spaghetti or angel hair pasta

Preparation:

1. Preheat oven to 400 degrees, and spray a cookie sheet with nonstick cooking spray. Crumble ground beef into a large mixing bowl. Add breadcrumbs, oregano, onion, tomato sauce, garlic and parsley. Combine ingredients thoroughly, either with fingers or with a fork.

2. Roll meatball mixture into 1-inch balls and place on cookie sheet. You should have about 20 meatballs. Bake in the oven for 16-18 minutes, turning once in the middle of cooking.

3. Cook spaghetti in a large pot according to package directions, without added salt or oil. In a large pan, heat marinara sauce; add cooked meatballs to the sauce and simmer until the pasta is ready.

   Serves 4.

Recipe Source: lowfatcooking.about.com

Lemon and Herb Lamb Chops

	Per Serving *(1 chop)*
Calories	165
Calories from Fat	61
Total Fat	6.7g *(sat 2.4g)*
Cholesterol	76mg
Sodium	77mg
Carbohydrate	2g
Fiber	0.5g
Protein	23.9g

Prep Time: 15 minutes

Cook Time: 10 minutes

Ingredients:

- 4 lamb loin chops *(4 oz. each)*
- ¼ cup fresh lemon juice
- 1 tsp dried oregano
- 1 tsp dried thyme
- 1 tsp freshly ground black pepper

Preparation:

1. Trim chops of all visible fat. Place in a glass baking dish with the lemon, oregano, thyme and black pepper. Turn to coat and marinate for 15 minutes.

2. Coat a heavy nonstick skillet with olive oil cooking spray. On a medium-high heat, cook chops 4-5 minutes each side depending on thickness and desired doneness.

3. Serve with minted new potatoes, baby carrots and asparagus. Serves 4

Recipe Source: lowfatcooking.about.com

Slow Cooker Pulled Pork

If you like pulled pork sandwiches, this is a recipe that will make sure your BBQ sauce-soaked pork will be ready for you when you step in the door after work.

Ingredients:

- 2 pork tenderloins *(about 1.5 pounds)*
- ¼ teaspoon garlic powder *(or ½ teaspoon garlic seasoning blend like Mrs. Dash Garlic & Herb)*
- ½ teaspoon salt
- ¼ teaspoon pepper
- 1 large sweet or yellow onion, chopped
- ¾ cup bottled barbecue sauce *(your choice)*
- ½ cup non-alcoholic amber beer or light beer

Preparation:

1. Coat the inside of the slow cooker with canola cooking spray. Place the pork tenderloins in the bottom of the slow cooker and sprinkle the garlic, salt, and pepper evenly over the top.

2. Sprinkle chopped onions over the pork and top that with the barbecue sauce and beer. Add the cover and cook on LOW for 8 hours. Shred the pork with a fork and stir to combine all of the ingredients.

3. Serve the pork filling on a whole grain bun or roll.

Yield: Makes about 6 servings of pork filling

Nutritional Information: Per serving: 150 calories, 23 g protein, 6 g carbohydrate, 3.5 g fat, 1.2 g saturated fat, 55 mg cholesterol, .5 g fiber, 780 mg sodium. Calories from fat: 21 percent.

Recipe Source: medicinenet.com

Spice-Rubbed Pork Chops

	Per Serving
Calories	231
Calories from Fat	74
Total Fat	8.2g *(sat 2.6g)*
Cholesterol	89mg
Sodium	137mg
Carbohydrate	7g
Fiber	1.9g
Protein	32.3g

Cook Time: 10 minutes

Ingredients:

- 2 tbsp chili powder
- 1 tbsp paprika
- 1 tbsp brown sugar
- 1 tbsp cumin
- Freshly ground black pepper
- 4 4-5 oz. ½-¾ inch boneless pork loin chops, trimmed of all visible fat

Preparation:

1. Combine spices in a small bowl using a small whisk. Rub spice mixture on both sides of each pork chop. Transfer chops to a dish large enough to accommodate chops in one layer, and cover; or place pork chops in a gallon-size resealable storage bag and lay flat on a plate. Refrigerate and allow spices to penetrate the chops for 6-8 hours.

2. Preheat broiler. Place chops on a lightly oiled broiler rack and broil 5 minutes each side until

done. These work equally well on the grill. Serves 4.

Recipe Source: lowfatcooking.about.com

• •

Vegetarian Dishes

Goat Cheese, Fig and Basil Pizza

Ingredients:

- 4-oz package dried figs, chopped
- 1 tbsp aged balsamic vinegar
- 3 tbsp water
- 1 large pizza crust or 4 round pita breads
- 1 cup crumbled soft goat cheese *(a 4-oz package will yield 1 cup)*
- 3 tbsp chopped fresh basil
- 1 tbsp pine nuts
- ½-1 tbsp olive oil

Preparation:

1. Preheat oven to 400 degrees.
2. Combine the figs, balsamic vinegar, and water in a small saucepan over medium heat. Cook 5 minutes, stirring frequently.
3. Place the figs in a small bowl. Season with salt and freshly ground pepper.
4. Top the pizza with the goat cheese and figs, and sprinkle with the basil and pine nuts. Drizzle the olive oil over the top. Bake for 12-15 minutes or until the cheese melts.

Yield: 8 servings

Nutritional Information: Per serving: 168 calories, 6 g protein, 26 g carbohydrate, 5 g fat, 2.3 g saturated fat, 7 mg cholesterol, 2 g fiber, 215 mg sodium. Calories from fat: 25%.

Recipe Source: Kathleen Zelman, MPH, RD/LD

Vegetarian Enchilada Crock Pot Casserole

Ingredients:

- 8 corn tortillas
- Canola cooking spray
- 12-oz. package Morning Star Meal Starters Grillers Recipe Crumbles *(Veggie Crumbles)* or similar soy product that mimics cooked ground beef, thawed
- 24 oz. bottled or canned enchilada sauce
- 2 cups shredded reduced fat cheddar and jack cheese blend

- 2-4-oz. can sliced black olives, drained *(optional)*

Garnish:

- 1 cup fat free sour cream
- 6 green onions, white and part green, chopped
- 1 avocado, thinly sliced *(optional)*

Preparation:

1. Begin heating a medium nonstick frying pan over medium-high heat.
2. Coat both sides of a corn tortilla with canola cooking spray and place it in the pan. When both sides are lightly browned, remove it from the pan and repeat this step with the remaining tortillas. Cut each of the tortillas into 4 wedges.
3. In medium bowl, combine veggie crumbles with enchilada sauce.
4. Layer wedges from two tortillas *(8 wedges)* in the slow cooker pan and spread one-fourth of the enchilada mixture over the top. Sprinkle ½ cup of the shredded cheese over the top and some of the black olives if desired.
5. Repeat step No. 4 until you have made 4 layers and used up all of the ingredients. Cook on HIGH for 1-2 hours or LOW for 2-4 hours.
6. Right before serving, spread fat-free sour cream over the top of the enchilada casserole and sprinkle with chopped green onions and avocado slices if desired.

Yield: Makes about 6 servings

Nutritional Information: Per serving: 316 calories, 22 g protein, 30 g carbohydrate, 12 g fat, 4.5 g saturated fat, 22 mg cholesterol, 5.5 g fiber, 998 mg sodium. Calories from fat: 34 percent.

Recipe Source: medicinenet.com

Tomato and Bean Burritos

Ingredients:

- 3 tomatoes *(large)*, approx. 2 ½ lbs.
- 1 tablespoon Vegetable oil
- ½ cup onion, chopped
- 1 teaspoon garlic, minced
- 1-2 tablespoons chili powder
- 1 teaspoon ground cumin
- 1 ¼ cups cooked red kidney beans or 1 *(10 ½ oz)* can red kidney beans, drained and rinsed
- 2 tablespoons cilantro or parsley, chopped

- 8 6-inch flour tortillas, warmed

Preparation:

1. Use tomatoes held at room temperature until fully ripe. Core tomatoes; coarsely chop *(makes about 4 cups)*; set aside.

2. In a medium saucepan heat oil until hot.

3. Add onion and garlic; cook and stir until softened, 3 to 4 minutes.

4. Add chili powder and cumin; cook and stir for 1 minute.

5. Add kidney beans, ¼ cup water, and reserved tomatoes; bring to a boil; reduce heat and simmer, uncovered, until mixture is thickened, about 20 minutes.

6. Stir in cilantro; remove from heat.

7. To serve: Spoon about ⅓ cup bean mixture in the center of each tortilla; roll up tortilla. Repeat with remaining tortillas.

Yield: 4 servings

Nutritional Information: Per serving:Calories 372, Fat 9 g, Calories from Fat 21%, Cholesterol 0 mg, Fiber 11 g, Sodium 620 mg, Protein 12 g.

Recipe Source: Frieda's, Inc./ Official 5 A Day recipe.

Tricolor Stuffed Peppers Recipe

Ingredients:

- 6 colored peppers *(red, green and yellow)*- washed and cored
- ½ cup brown rice
- 6-8 dried apricots, sliced
- 2 Tablespoons dried cranberries
- 6-8 pre-roasted and peeled jarred chestnuts- thinly sliced *(optional)*—may substitute
- pecans or almonds
- ½ cup silken tofu
- ¼ teaspoon nutmeg
- salt and pepper to taste
- 6-basil leaves- for garnish

Preparation:

1. Cook ½ cup brown rice per directions on package.

2. While rice is cooking, wash and core peppers.

3. Pre-heat oven to 350ºF. Lightly spray Pam on a baking dish.

4. In a large bowl, mix cooked rice, apricots,

cranberries, chestnuts, silken tofu, nutmeg, salt, and pepper.

5. Evenly divide the brown rice mixture among the 6 peppers.

6. Place peppers on baking dish and bake at 350ºF until outside of peppers are soft *(about 30-40 minutes)*.

7. Garnish with basil leaves.

Yield: 6 servings

Nutritional Information: Per Serving *(one pepper)*: 124 calories, 4.6 grams protein, 26.6 grams carbohydrates, 1.1 grams fat and 7% calories from fat.

Recipe Source: The Art Institute of New York City

Vegetable and Tofu Noodle Stir-fry

Ingredients:

- 2 *(3-oz.)* packages chicken or pork ramen noodles and 1 of the seasoning packets
- 1 ½ tablespoons canola oil
- ½ medium cauliflower head *(cut away the core and cut the rest into florets)*
- 3 carrots, thinly sliced
- 1 block firm tofu, diced
- 2 medium onions, peeled and quartered, then sliced
- ½ small head cabbage, thinly sliced
- 2 tablespoons light soy sauce
- 1 teaspoon sesame oil

Preparation:

1. Cook ramen noodles in medium saucepan according to the package directions, then drain well. Add back to saucepan and sprinkle the seasoning over the top of noodles and stir to blend; set aside.

2. Heat canola oil in heavy, large nonstick skillet over medium heat. Add cauliflower, carrots, tofu, and onions. Cover skillet and cook, stirring frequently until crisp-tender *(about 6-8 minutes)*.

3. Spread cabbage over the top of vegetables, stir into vegetables, cover pan, and continue to cook, stirring frequently, until cabbage is softened *(about 3 minutes)*. Remove from heat. Mix in cooked noodles, soy sauce, and sesame oil and serve!

Yield: Makes 4 large servings

Nutritional Information: per serving: 337

calories, 21 g protein, 37 g carbohydrate, 14 g fat *(1.7 g saturated fat)*, 0 mg cholesterol, 8 g fiber, 560 mg sodium. Calories from fat: 37 percent.

Recipe Source: medicinenet.com

Yule Manicotti with Roasted Red Pepper Sauce

If you're feeding a crowd, double the recipe. Set each manicotti on top of a small pool of red pepper sauce on the dinner plate, or serve them with an ample drizzle of the red pepper sauce on top. If you want to skip roasting the peppers, substitute 1 cup of bottled roasted red peppers for the 2 sweet red peppers.

Ingredients:

- 8 large dried manicotti pasta shells *(or similar)*
- 2 sweet red peppers
- 2 teaspoons olive oil
- ½ cup 1% milk
- 1 teaspoon minced garlic
- Pepper to taste
- Salt to taste *(optional)*
- 1 ½ cups low-fat or part-skim ricotta cheese
- ¾ cup firmly packed, frozen, chopped spinach *(thawed, with excess water gently squeezed out)*
- 6 tablespoons shredded Parmesan cheese
- ¼ cup prepared pesto sauce *(like Armanino®, found in the frozen pasta section)*
- 4 green onions, white and part of green, chopped
- 1 teaspoon Italian seasoning

Preparation:

1. Preheat oven to 375 degrees. Coat a 9x13-inch baking dish with canola cooking spray.
2. Boil manicotti shells according to directions on package until tender. Drain, rinse with cold water, and carefully set aside.
3. While manicotti is boiling, turn on the broiler. Cut each red pepper into quarters and remove inside flesh and seeds. Cut each quarter in half to make eight strips total. Lay strips, skin side down, on a nonstick baking sheet *(line with foil for easy cleanup, if desired)*. Brush the tops of pepper strips with olive oil. Broil until the top sides are nicely brown, watching carefully. Flip and broil until brown. Let peppers cool slightly. Preheat oven to 350 degrees.
4. In a food processor, puree pepper strips with milk, garlic, and pepper to taste. Add salt to taste if desired. Keep sauce at a low simmer in a small, covered, nonstick saucepan while you bake the manicotti.
5. Mix filling ingredients *(ricotta, spinach, Parmesan cheese, pesto, green onions, and Italian seasonings)* in a bowl with spoon or fork. Stuff shells with the cheese mixture. Arrange in a baking dish. Cover with foil and bake for 15 minutes, then uncover and bake 10 minutes more.
6. Serve one or two manicotti shells per person; decorate each shell with ample red pepper sauce.

Yield: 8 manicotti

Nutritional Information: Per serving: Per manicotti: 218 calories, 10 g protein, 26 g carbohydrate, 8 g fat, 14 mg cholesterol, 1.5 g fiber, 164 mg sodium. Calories from fat: 33%.

Recipe Source: 2003 Vegetarian Resource Group

Beverages/Drinks

Light and Minty Hot Chocolate

Ingredients:

- 3 tablespoons Splenda
- 3 tablespoons cocoa *(preferably Dutch processed)*
- 2 cups 1% milk or skim milk or fat-free half-and-half
- ¼ teaspoon peppermint extract

Preparation:

1. Add Splenda and cocoa to small saucepan and blend with whisk. Gradually add milk to cocoa mixture and whisk until blended.
2. Cook over medium-low heat until thoroughly heated. Stir in the peppermint extract and serve immediately.

Yield: 2 servings

Nutritional Information: Per serving: 120 calories, 10 g protein, 16 g carbohydrate, 3.7 g fat, 2.3 g saturated fat, 10 mg cholesterol, 3 g fiber, 125 mg sodium. Calories from fat: 25%.

Recipe Source: www.medicinenet.com

Lemon-Ginger Iced Tea with Berry Cubes

Cook Time: 6 min

Level: Easy

	Per Serving: *(1 serving equals 1 ½ cups iced tea plus ice cubes)*
Calories	80
Total Fat	0 g *(Sat Fat 0 g, Mono Fat 0 g, Poly Fat 0 g)*
Protein	0 g
Carb	21 g
Fiber	2 g
Cholesterol	0 mg
Sodium	15 mg

Yield: 6 servings

Ingredients

- 1 cup *(4 oz.)* raspberries, rinsed
- Water for ice cube trays, plus 8 cups water, divided
- ⅓ cup honey
- ½ cup *(2 oz.)* coarsely chopped fresh ginger
- 6 white tea bags
- 3 lemons, juiced *(about ½ cup)*
- Lemon slices
- Mint sprigs, for garnish

Preparation:

1. Place about 4 raspberries in each compartment of an ice cube tray, 6 hours before serving iced tea. Fill with water and freeze.

2. Place honey, 2 cups water and ginger in a saucepan and bring to a boil. Reduce heat and simmer over low heat for 5 minutes. Remove from heat and add tea bags. Let mixture steep for at least 30 minutes and up to 1 hour, then strain out solids.

3. In a pitcher combine strained liquid with 6 cups water and lemon juice. Chill in refrigerator.

4. To serve, place 3 ice cubes in a tall glass and pour iced tea over cubes. Garnish with lemon slices and mint sprigs.

Recipe Source: foodnetwork.com

Mint Iced Tea *(0 calories)*

Ingredients:

- ½ tablespoon tea
- Several fresh mint leaves
- No-calorie powdered sweetener *(aspartame, etc.)*

Preparation:

1. Pour boiling water over the tea and mint leaves. Steep for a few minutes and strain.

2. Add sweetener *(optional)* and serve chilled with ice.

Yield: 1 serving

Recipe Source: www.medicinenet.com

Peach Pie Smoothie

Prep Time: 10 min

	Per Serving:
Calories	240
Total Fat	0 g; *(Sat Fat 0 g, Mono Fat 0 g, Poly Fat 0 g)*
Protein	12 g
Carbs	49 g
Fiber	3
Cholesterol	5 mg
Sodium	150 mg

Level: Easy

Yield: 1 serving, serving size: 2 cups

Ingredients:

- ½ cup nonfat or 1 percent lowfat milk
- ½ cup nonfat plain yogurt
- 1 cup unsweetened frozen peaches
- 1 tablespoon honey, plus more to taste
- ¼ teaspoon vanilla extract
- ⅛ teaspoon ground cinnamon
- Pinch ground nutmeg
- Pinch ground ginger

Preparation

Put all ingredients into a blender and blend until smooth.

Recipe Source: foodnetwork.com

Spiced Apple Cider

Ingredients:

- 62-oz. bottle apple cider
- 1 large apple *(green or red)*
- About 30 cloves
- About 3 cinnamon sticks

Preparation:

1. Add the apple cider to a slow cooker and begin heating it on HIGH.

2. Cut the top and bottom off of the apple and cut what's left into ½-inch slices widthwise. Use a dinner knife to carve out the center portion of each slice *(the part with the seeds)*. Poke the sharp end of the cloves into the apple slices *(about 8 per slice)*. Add the spiced apple slices to the apple cider.

3. Add the cinnamon sticks.

4. After the cider is nice and hot, you can turn the slow cooker to LOW and let simmer for hours or until needed.

Yield: 8 servings of 8 oz. each.

Nutritional Information: Per serving: 104 calories, 0.1 g protein, 25 g carbohydrate, 0.2 g fat, 0 g saturated fat, 0 mg cholesterol, 0.2 fiber, 6 mg sodium. Calories from fat: 2%.

Recipe Source: Medicinenet.com

Strawberry Light Lemonade

Add more or less Splenda® and sugar depending on your taste preference.

Ingredients:

- 2 cups sliced or halved strawberries
- 5 tablespoons superfine sugar *(regular sugar will work, too)*
- 8 tablespoons Splenda®
- 12 tablespoons freshly squeezed lemon juice
- Ice cubes as desired
- ⅔ cup club soda, mineral water or seltzer water per glass

Preparation:

1. Puree strawberries and 1 tablespoon sugar in blender or small food processor.

2. Spoon 3 tablespoons of strawberry puree into each glass, then add 2 tablespoons Splenda® and 1 tablespoon sugar to each glass.

3. Add 3 tablespoons lemon juice to each glass;

stir to blend well. Stir in ⅔ cup of club soda (or similar) into each glass, add some ice and serve.

Yield: 4 glasses

Nutritional Information: Per serving: 97 calories, 1 g protein, 25 g carbohydrate, 0.3 g fat, 0 g saturated fat, 0 mg cholesterol, 1.5 g fiber, 1 mg sodium. Calories from fat: 3%

Recipe Source: www.medicinenet.com

Vanilla Iced Mochaccino

Prep time: 20 minutes

Cook time: 5 minutes

Ingredients:

- 2 coffee cups of strong French roast coffee
- 2 cups of fat-free milk
- 1 tablespoon of unsweetened cocoa powder
- 1 tablespoon sugar
- 1 teaspoon vanilla extract

Preparation:

1. Brew 2 cups of French roast or espresso-style coffee and pour into a small saucepan with fat-free milk, cocoa powder, sugar, and vanilla extract; simmer for 5 minutes.

2. Let cool for 5 minutes; pour over ice in 2 large lidded cups and shake well before serving.

Note: This beverage can also be prepared warm. After simmering ingredients, blend with a handheld electric mixer to create a frothy top and carefully pour into coffee mugs.

Yield: 2 servings

Nutritional Information: Per serving: 130 calories, 9 g protein, 20 g carbohydrate, 2 g fat *(1 g saturated fat)*, 5 mg cholesterol, 30% Daily Value of calcium, 1 g fiber, 130 mg sodium.

Recipe Source: National Dairy Council

• •

Desserts

The 100-Calorie Chocolate Cupcake

Ingredients:

- 18.25-oz. box Devil's Food Cake Mix
- 1 ⅓ cups water
- ½ cup fat free sour cream
- 5 large egg whites *(or ¾ cup egg substitute)*
- ¼ cup powdered sugar

Preparation:

1. Preheat oven to 350 degrees. Line cupcake pans with paper baking cups.

2. Beat cake mix, water, fat free sour cream, and egg whites or egg substitute in large bowl on low speed for 30 seconds. Increase speed to medium speed and continue beating for 2 minutes, scraping bowl occasionally. Divide batter between the 24 cupcake cups.

3. Bake for about 17 minutes or until toothpick inserted in center comes out clean. Cool completely.

4. Dust the tops of the cupcakes with powdered sugar using a sifter, sugar shaker, or wire mesh strainer.

Yield: Makes 24 cupcakes

Nutritional Information Per serving: 98 calories, 2 g protein, 18.5 g carbohydrate, 1.8 g fat, .5 g saturated fat, .5 mg cholesterol, .5 g fiber, 200 mg sodium. Calories from fat: 16 percent.

Recipe Source: medicinenet.com

Apple Pie Crisp

With the wonderful crumb topping, you'll hardly notice there isn't any crust.

Ingredients:

Crisp Topping:

- ½ cup walnuts
- ½ cup unbleached white flour
- ½ cup whole-wheat flour
- 3 tablespoons brown sugar
- ¼ teaspoon ground cinnamon
- 3 tablespoons no-trans-fat margarine with 8 g fat per tablespoon, melted
- 3 tablespoons maple syrup, pancake syrup, or light pancake syrup

Filling:

- 4 cups cored and thinly sliced apples *(pippin and Granny Smith work well)*, firmly packed
- ¼ cup sugar *(or substitute 2 tablespoons Splenda)*
- 1 teaspoon apple pie spice
- 2 tablespoons unbleached flour

Preparation:

1. Preheat oven to 375 degrees. Coat a 9x9-inch baking dish, 9-inch cake pan, or deep-dish pie plate with canola cooking spray.

2. Toast the walnuts by spreading on a pie plate and heating in oven until fragrant *(about 7 minutes)*. Chop the nuts medium-fine.

3. Combine the flours, brown sugar, and cinnamon in a mixing bowl. Drizzle the melted margarine and maple syrup over the top and blend on LOW speed until crumbly. Add the chopped nuts and mix well. *(The topping can be prepared up to a week ahead and refrigerated)*.

4. Put the sliced apples in a large bowl. Add the sugar and apple pie spice to a 1-cup measure, then pour over the apples and toss. Sprinkle 2 tablespoons of flour over the apples and mix gently. Pour the mixture evenly into the prepared baking dish.

5. Spoon the topping over the apples, pressing down lightly. Place the dish on a baking sheet *(if necessary)* to catch any overflow. Bake on the center rack of oven until the topping is golden brown and the juices have thickened slightly, about 35-45 minutes.

Yield: 8 servings

Nutritional Information: Per serving: *(using no trans fat margarine)*: 227 calories, 4 g protein, 37 g carbohydrate, 7.5 g fat *(0.7 g saturated fat, 2.7 g monounsaturated fat, 3.8 g polyunsaturated fat)*, 0 mg cholesterol, 3 g fiber, 35 mg sodium, 1 g omega-3 fatty acids, 4 g omega-6 fatty acids. Calories from fat: 35%

Recipe Source: medicinenet.com

Apple Sweet Potato Bake

Sweet potatoes have all three of these antioxidants: Vitamin A, C and E! And they are the star ingredient in this side dish. You can make this recipe without peeling the sweet potatoes or the apples. Peel or don't peel, it's up to you.

Ingredients:

- 5 cups thinly sliced sweet potatoes *(or yams)*, about 1 ½ sweet potatoes
- 2 cups thinly sliced apples, such as Pippin or Granny Smith *(about two small)*
- ¼ cup dark brown sugar, packed
- 2 tablespoons reduced-calorie pancake syrup
- ½ teaspoon ground cinnamon
- ½ cup apple juice or orange juice
- ¼ cup walnut pieces or chopped walnuts

Preparation:

1. Preheat oven to 375°F.

2. In a large bowl, toss the sweet potatoes, apple slices, and brown sugar together. Spoon into a 9x9-inch or similar-sized baking dish.

3. In a small bowl, blend syrup with cinnamon, then stir in the apple juice. Pour evenly over sweet potato mixture. Sprinkle walnuts over the top.

4. Cover baking dish with lid or foil and bake 30 minutes. Remove foil and bake about 15 minutes longer *(or until apple and sweet potatoes are cooked throughout)*.

Yield: 6 servings

Nutritional Information: Per serving: 128 calories, 2 g protein, 24 g carbohydrate, 3 g fat *(0.2 g saturated fat, 0.7 g monounsaturated fat, 2 g polyunsaturated fat)*, 0 mg cholesterol, 2.2 g fiber, 24 mg sodium. Calories from fat: 21%.

Recipe Source: medicinenet.com

Balsamic Strawberries with Ricotta Cream

Per Serving: *(serving size: about ⅓ cup cream and ½ cup berries)*	
Calories	180
Total	Fat 5 g
Protein	8 g
Carbs	27 g
Fiber	2 g
Cholesterol	20 mg
Sodium	80 mg

Cook Time: 2 min

Level: Easy

Yield: 4 servings

Ingredients

- 1 cup part-skim ricotta cheese
- 2 tablespoons honey
- ½ teaspoon vanilla extract
- 3 tablespoons balsamic vinegar
- 2 tablespoons sugar
- 1 *(16-oz.)* container strawberries, hulled
- and quartered
- 2 tablespoons fresh basil leaves, cut into ribbons

Preparation:

1. Put the ricotta cheese, honey and vanilla extract into the small bowl of a food processor and process until smooth, about 1 minute.

Transfer to a small bowl and refrigerate for at least 2 hours.

2. In a small saucepan combine the vinegar and sugar and bring to a boil. Simmer over medium heat for 2 minutes, stirring occasionally. Allow to cool completely.

3. In a medium bowl, toss the berries with the basil and the balsamic syrup.

4. Divide the cream among 4 cocktail glasses, top with the berry mixture and serve.

Recipe Source: foodnetwork.com

Berry Yogurt Frozen Pie

Ingredients:

Graham cracker crust: Filling:

- ½ cups finely ground low-fat *(or regular)* graham crackers
- 2 tablespoons white sugar
- 3 tablespoons honey
- 3 tablespoons whipped butter or less-fat margarine *(with 8 grams fat per tablespoon)*, melted
- 1 ½ tablespoons fat-free half-and-half or low-fat milk
- ½ teaspoon ground cinnamon *(optional)*
- 16-18 oz. of berry-flavored low-fat yogurt
- 3 3-½ cups light whipped topping *(like Cool Whip Lite®)*
- 1 ½ cups finely chopped strawberries, or unchopped raspberries or blackberries
- 10 whole strawberries, or 10 tablespoons of other berries for garnish *(optional)*

Preparation:

1. Mix graham cracker crumbs, sugar, honey, melted butter, and cinnamon *(if desired)* until well blended. Press mixture into 9-inch pie plate; set aside.

2. Mix yogurt, by hand, with the light whipped topping in a large mixing bowl. Gently stir in the berries by hand.

3. Spoon the yogurt mixture into the graham cracker crust. Freeze until firm *(overnight, or at least 4 hours)*.

4. Remove from the freezer and top each serving with a fresh strawberry *(or small spoonful of berries)* if desired.

Yield: 10 servings

Nutritional Information: Per serving: 225

calories, 3.5 g protein, 39 g carbohydrate, 7 g fat, 4.6 g saturated fat, 8 mg cholesterol, 1.5 g fiber, 159 mg sodium. Calories from fat: 28%.

Recipe Source: medicinenet.com

Buncha Banana Pudding

Prep time: 15 minutes

Ingredients:

- 2 *(3 oz.)* packages vanilla cook & serve pudding mix
- 4 cups 1% milk
- About 20 vanilla wafer cookies
- 3 bananas, sliced

Optional garnish:

- whipped cream
- graham cracker crumbs

Preparation:

1. Prepare pudding with 1% milk as directed on package.
2. Spoon one cup of pudding into 2-qt serving bowl and top with 10 cookies and half the banana slices.
3. Continue layering with 2 cups of pudding, remaining cookies, and bananas.
4. Top with remaining pudding; cover and refrigerate 3 hours or overnight.
5. Garnish with whipped cream, graham cracker crumbs, or banana slices if desired.

Yield: 6 servings

Nutritional Information: Per serving: 290 calories, 6 g protein, 60 g carbohydrate, 4 g fat *(2 g saturated fat)*, 10 mg cholesterol, 3 g fiber, 20% Daily Value calcium, 350 mg sodium.

Recipe Source: National Dairy Council.

Chardonnay Spice Cake Recipe

Ingredients:

- 1 box *(18.25 oz)* white cake mix
- 1 package *(5 oz)* instant vanilla pudding mix
- 1 teaspoon ground nutmeg
- ¾ cup fat-free sour cream
- ¾ cup Chardonnay *(or other white wine)*
- 2 large eggs
- ½ cup egg substitute

Preparation:

1. Preheat oven to 350 degrees. Spray the inside of a Bundt pan with canola cooking spray, then dust with about 2 tablespoons of flour.
2. Add cake mix, vanilla pudding mix and nutmeg to mixing bowl and beat with electric mixer on LOW speed to blend well.
3. Add the sour cream, wine, eggs and egg substitute to mixing bowl and beat with mixer on medium speed for 5 minutes *(scraping sides and bottom of bowl after a minute)*.
4. Pour into prepared Bundt pan and bake for 50 minutes or until a toothpick inserted in the center comes out clean. Let cake cool on rack in pan for 10 minutes. Invert pan on serving plate carefully to release the cake. Serve.

Yield: 12 servings

Nutritional Information: Per serving: 259 calories, 5 g protein, 48 g carbohydrate, 5.5 g fat, 1 g saturated fat, 2.3 g monounsaturated fat, 1.9 g polyunsaturated fat, 35 mg cholesterol, 0.6 g fiber, 440 mg sodium. Calories from fat: 23%.

Recipe Source: medicinenet.com

Chocolate Covered Candy Cane Peppermint Sandwich Cookies

Ingredients:

- 11.5-oz. bag semi sweet chocolate chips *(milk can be substituted)*
- 2 boxes of peppermint sandwich cookies, about 66 cookies total *(I buy mine at Trader Joe's—they look like Oreos but the vanilla filling has crushed candy cane in it—but if you can't find them, just use Reduced Fat or regular Oreos)*
- Holiday sprinkles or if you are using regular chocolate sandwich cookies, crushed candy cane works well

Preparation:

1. Pour chocolate chips into a 2-cup glass measure *(or similar)* and microwave on LOW for about 1 minute. Stir gently and if not melted, microwave in 30-second intervals until almost completely melted. Stir with spoon to distribute the heat evenly and finish melting the chips.
2. Line two jellyroll pans with wax paper. Dunk one of the cookies halfway into the melted chocolate and scrape away some of the excess chocolate with the flat side of a dinner knife or use the edge of the glass measure. Lay dipped cookie on the wax paper.

3. Repeat with remaining cookies until all the melted chocolate has been used *(about 33 cookies per cup of chocolate cups)*. Sprinkle holiday cookie decorations/sprinkles or crushed candy canes over the chocolate of each of the cookies. Place jellyroll pans in the refrigerator to harden the melted chocolate.

4. Place cookies in holiday gift bowls, bags or boxes, or on cookie plates. If you use about 11 decorated cookies for each gift, this recipe will make about 6 gifts!

Yield: makes about 66 halfway dipped cookies

Nutritional Information:

77 calories, .6 g protein, 11 g carbohydrate, 3.8 g fat, 1.4 g saturated fat, 0 mg cholesterol, .6 g fiber, 60 mg sodium. Calories from fat: 44 percent.

Recipe Source: medicinenet.com

Chocolate Sherbet

	Per Serving
Calories	151
Total Fat	(g) 6
Saturated	(g) 0
Cholesterol	(mg) 2
Sodium	(mg) 6
Carbohydrate	(g) 23
Fiber	(g) 1
Protein	(g) 1

Makes: 12 to 16 servings

Prep: 25 minutes

Chill: overnight

Freeze: according to manufacturer & directions plus 4 hours

Ingredients:

- 8 oz. 70%-or-greater-cacao chocolate or bittersweet chocolate, chopped
- 2 cups of water
- ⅔ cup sugar
- ½ cup whole milk
- teaspoon vanilla
- oz. 70%-or-greater-cacao chocolate or bittersweet chocolate *(optional)*

Preparation:

Reserve ½ cup of the 8 oz. chopped chocolate; cover and set aside. In a medium saucepan, stir together remaining chopped chocolate, the water, sugar, and whole milk. Bring to boiling, whisking constantly. Boil gently for 1 minute. Remove from heat; stir in vanilla. Cover and chill overnight.

Stir the reserved ½ cup chopped chocolate into the chilled chocolate mixture. Freeze mixture in a 1-quart ice cream freezer according to manufacturer's directions. Allow to firm up in freezer for 4 hours before serving.

To serve, scoop into small glasses or dishes. If desired, chop the 1 oz. chocolate; sprinkle over individual servings.

Recipe Sourcemy.hearthealthyonline.com

Chocolate Raspberry Pound Cake

Dust this cake with powdered sugar and serve with fresh raspberries and a dollop of Light Cool Whip, if desired.

Ingredients:

- ¾ cup less-sugar raspberry preserves
- 1 cup whole-wheat flour
- 1 cup unbleached white flour
- 1 cup granulated sugar
- ½ cup Splenda
- ¾ cup baking cocoa
- 1 ½ teaspoons baking soda
- 1 teaspoon salt
- ½ cup less-fat margarine *(with 8 g fat per tablespoon)*, preferably with plant sterols added
- 3 tablespoons raspberry-flavored liqueur *(fat-free half-and-half can be substituted)*
- 16 oz. fat-free sour cream
- 2 large eggs *(use higher omega-3 type, if available)*
- 1 ½ teaspoons vanilla extract
- Powdered sugar *(for dusting)*

Preparation:

1. Preheat oven to 350 degrees. Coat a tube pan with canola cooking spray and dust lightly with flour. Place the raspberry preserves in a small microwave-safe bowl and heat on HIGH for 15 seconds or until softened.

2. Add whole-wheat and white flours, sugar, Splenda, cocoa, baking soda, and salt to large mixing bowl and beat on low to blend well. Stop mixer and add margarine, liqueur, sour cream, eggs, vanilla, and softened preserves all at once. Beat on medium speed for two minutes, scraping sides of mixing bowl after a minute.

3. Pour batter into prepared pan and bake for 50-60 minutes, or until cake tester inserted

in center comes out clean. Cool in pan 10 minutes, then remove cake from pan and place on serving plate to cool completely. When ready to serve, dust powdered sugar over the top. Serve with fresh raspberries and a dollop of whipped topping or whipping cream. if desired.

Yield: 16 servings

Nutritional Information: Per serving: 195 calories, 5 g protein, 36 g carbohydrate, 4 g fat, 1 g saturated fat, 3 g fiber, 311 mg sodium. Calories from fat: 18%.

Recipe Source: medicinenet.com

Crock Pot Chocolate Kahlua Cake

This moist cake is absolutely amazing straight from the warm slow cooker, served with a small scoop of light vanilla bean ice cream.

Ingredients:

- 1 box *(18.25 oz.)* Devil's Food Cake Mix
- 1 cup fat free sour cream
- 1 cup 1% lowfat milk *(nonfat milk or 2% milk can be substituted)*
- 2 large eggs, higher omega-3 if available
- 2 egg whites or ¼ cup egg substitute
- ¾ cup kahlua liqueur *(or similar)*

Preparation:

1. Coat the inside of the slow cooker dish with canola cooking spray.

2. In large mixing bowl, combine cake mix, sour cream, milk, eggs, egg whites, and kahlua by beating on medium for about a minute.

3. Pour cake batter into prepared slow cooker dish. Cover slow cooker and cook on LOW for 6-8 hours or on HIGH for 3-4 hours.

4. Cut cake into about 16 wedges and using a cookie dough scoop, serve each slice with a small scoop of light vanilla bean ice cream if desired.

Yield: Makes 16 servings

Nutritional Information: Per serving: 210 calories, 4 g protein, 33 g carbohydrate, 5.5 g fat, 1.4 g saturated fat, 29 mg cholesterol, 1 g fiber, 314 mg sodium. Calories from fat: 23%.

Recipe Source: medicinenet.com

Frozen S'Mores

Ingredients:

- 1-½ cups cold 1% milk
- 1 pkg. *(4 serving size)* Jell-O Chocolate Flavor Instant Pudding
- 1 cup thawed light or fat-free whipped topping
- ¾ cup miniature marshmallows
- 7 whole low fat graham crackers, broken in half

Preparation:

1. In mixing bowl, combine milk and pudding mix, beating with electric mixer or wire whisk about 2 minutes. Scrape sides of bowl halfway to incorporate all of the pudding mix.

2. Stir in whipped topping and marshmallows.

3. Spoon about ¼ cup of the mixture on top of each graham cracker half. Place them on a freezer-safe tray. Freeze about 2 hours or until firm. Serve straight from the freezer.

Yield: 14 frozen S'more halves

Nutritional Information: Per serving: 61 calories, 1 g protein, 13 g carbohydrate, 0.5 g fat, 0.2 g saturated fat, 1 mg cholesterol, 0.4 g fiber, 53 mg sodium. Calories from fat: 7 percent.

Recipe Source: medicinenet.com

Healthy Brownies

	Per Serving
Calories	**95**
Total Fat	3g
Saturated Fat	1g
Cholesterol	--
Sodium	75mg
Total Carbohydrate	17g
Dietary Fiber	1g
Sugars	--
Protein	2g
Calcium	--

Yield: 16 brownies

Total Time: 50 min

Cook Time: 35 min

Ingredients:

- 1 teaspoon(s) instant coffee powder or granules
- 2 teaspoon(s) vanilla extract
- ½ cup(s) all-purpose flour
- ½ cup(s) unsweetened cocoa

- ¼ teaspoon(s) baking powder
- ¼ teaspoon(s) salt
- 1 cup(s) sugar
- ¼ cup(s) trans-fat free vegetable oil spread
- 3 large egg whites

Preparation:

1. Preheat oven to 350°F. Grease 8" x 8" metal baking pan. In cup, dissolve coffee in vanilla extract.

2. On waxed paper, combine flour, cocoa, baking powder, and salt.

3. In medium bowl, whisk sugar, vegetable oil spread, egg whites, and coffee mixture until well mixed; then blend in flour mixture. Spread in prepared pan

4. Bake 22 to 24 minutes or until toothpick inserted in brownies 2 inches from edge comes out almost clean. Cool in pan on wire rack, about 2 hours

5. When cool, cut brownies into 4 strips, and then cut each strip crosswise into 4 squares. If brownies are difficult to cut, dip knife in hot water; wipe dry, and cut. Repeat dipping and drying as necessary.

Recipe Source: Good Housekeeping

Holiday Angel Cake

What a beautiful cake to behold! And so tasty with so few calories.

Ingredients:

- 1 cup cake flour
- 1 cup granulated sugar
- ½ cup Splenda®
- 12 egg whites
- 1 ½ teaspoons vanilla extract
- 1 ½ teaspoons cream of tartar
- ½ teaspoon salt
- 1 cup fresh cranberries or ½ cup dried cranberries
- 1 tablespoon finely chopped orange zest *(or substitute lemon zest)*

Preparation:

1. Preheat oven to 375 degrees. Double check that your tube pan is clean and dry. *(Any trace amounts of oil could cause your whipped egg whites to deflate)*.

2. Stir flour, ¼ cup of the sugar, and Splenda® together in medium bowl and set aside.

3. In a large mixing bowl, whip the egg whites with the vanilla, cream of tartar, and salt together with mixer until medium-stiff peaks form. Gradually add the remaining sugar *(¾ cup)* while continuing to whip to stiff peaks. When you think the egg whites have reached maximum volume, gradually fold in the flour mixture, one third at a time.

4. Stir in 1 cup fresh cranberries or ½ cup dried cranberries and orange zest. Be careful not to overmix.

5. Pour the batter in the prepared tube pan and bake 40-45 minutes or until cake springs back when touched. Balance the tube pan upside down on the top of a bottle to prevent decompression while cooling. When completely cool, run a knife around the edge of the pan and invert onto a serving plate.

Yield: 8 large servings

Nutritional Information: Per serving: 171 calories, 7.5 g protein, 36 g carbohydrate, 0.1 g fat, 0 g saturated fat, 0 mg cholesterol, 0.8 g fiber, 216 mg sodium. Calories from fat: 1%.

Recipe Source: medicinenet.com

Old-Fashioned Tapioca Pudding

Enjoy some fresh fruit along with this pudding. It will add flavor and color, along with fiber.

Ingredients:

- 3 tablespoons Minute Tapioca
- 3 tablespoons Splenda
- 1 tablespoon granulated sugar
- 2 tablespoons light pancake syrup *(or honey)*
- ¼ teaspoon salt
- 1 large egg *(use higher omega-3 egg, if available)*
- ¼ cup egg substitute
- 2 cups 1% low fat or skim milk
- ½ teaspoon vanilla extract
- Pinch of ground cinnamon *(optional)*

Preparation:

1. Add tapioca, Splenda, sugar, pancake syrup, salt, egg, egg substitute and milk to a medium nonstick saucepan and whisk until smooth. Let stand *(don't stir)*, for exactly 5 minutes.

2. Cook over medium heat, stirring often, just until mixture comes to a full boil. Stir in vanilla extract and ground cinnamon, if desired. Transfer pudding to a medium bowl

that is sitting in a larger bowl partly filled with ice. Let stand, stirring occasionally, for about 12 minutes.

3. Spoon into 4 serving dishes or cups and eat immediately, or cover dishes with plastic wrap and store in refrigerator *(serve within 2 days)*.

Yield: 4 servings

Nutritional Information: Per serving: 131 calories, 8 g protein, 19 g carbohydrate, 2.5 g fat *(1.1 g saturated fat)*, 60 mg cholesterol, 0 g fiber, 268 mg sodium. Calories from fat: 17%.

Recipe Source: medicinenet.com

Strawberry Shortcake

This recipe was inspired by the outrageously delicious and popular dessert served at the Club level of SBC Park in Northern California.

Ingredients:

Biscuits:

- 1 ¼ cup unbleached flour
- ¾ cup whole-wheat flour
- ½ teaspoon salt
- 4 teaspoons baking powder
- ½ teaspoon cream of tartar
- 2 tablespoons sugar
- ½ cup Take Control® margarine *(keep in freezer)*
- ½ cup plus 1 to 2 tablespoons fat-free half-and-half

Topping:

- 2 cups sliced strawberries
- 2 tablespoons brown sugar
- 1 teaspoon vanilla extract
- 5 cups sliced strawberries
- 10 dollops of light whipped cream *(about 2 cups)* or Light Cool Whip®

Preparation:

1. Preheat oven to 425°F. In large food processor bowl, thoroughly combine flours, salt, baking powder, cream of tartar, and sugar.

2. Add margarine in pieces and briefly pulse just until mixture is coarse and crumbly.

3. Add the fat free half-and-half and briefly pulse just until blended *(do not overmix)*.

4. Turn onto a lightly floured surface and knead gently 4 or so times.

5. Pat dough until about ⅓- to ½-inch thick.

Using a 2 ½- to 3-inch round cutter, cut out biscuits and place them on a baking sheet coated with canola cooking spray.

6. Bake until nicely brown, about 12-14 minutes. Let cool.

7. Meanwhile, add 2 cups sliced strawberries, brown sugar, and vanilla to food processor and pulse until a strawberry puree is created *(about 5 seconds)*.

8. Split a biscuit in half and place both halves, cut side up, on a dessert plate. Drizzle about 1 tablespoon of the strawberry puree mixture over the top of each half. Top both halves with a total of ½ cup of strawberry slices and a dollop of light whipping cream or Light Cool Whip®.

Yield: 10 large biscuits

Nutritional Information: Per serving: 275 calories, 5 g protein, 31 g carbohydrate, 13 g fat *(5 g saturated fat, 5.9 g monounsaturated fat, 2.2 g polyunsaturated fat)*, 25 mg cholesterol, 3.5 g fiber, 390 mg sodium. Calories from fat: 42%.

Recipe Source: medicinenet.com

Sweet Potato Praline Pie Recipe

Ingredients:

- 1 cup All-Bran® Cereal, finely crushed
- ¼ cup pecans, finely chopped
- 1 egg white, slightly beaten
- 2 cups sweet potatoes, mashed
- ¼ cup brown sugar
- ¼ cup granulated sugar
- 1 teaspoon cinnamon
- ½ teaspoon nutmeg
- ½ teaspoon ginger
- pinch cloves
- 1 egg, plus 1 egg yolk, slightly beaten
- 1 scant cup milk, 2% low-fat

Praline Sauce

- ½ cup brown sugar
- 1 tablespoon cornstarch
- ¾ cup coffee
- 1 teaspoon butter
- ¼ cup pecans, finely chopped

Preparation:

1. Combine first three ingredients, press into bottom and sides of 9-inch pie tin lightly

sprayed with nonstick spray *(easiest to do with dampened hands)*.

2. Bake in 400-degree oven for 10 minutes.

3. Mix sweet potatoes in electric mixer for 5 minutes until smooth.

4. Add sugars, spices and eggs, mix to blend.

5. At low speed add milk until well blended.

6. Pour into prepared shell and bake at 400 degrees for 45 to 55 minutes or until knife inserted into filling comes out clean *(center may be soft but will set when cool)*.

7. Refrigerate until ready to serve. Cut into 10 wedges per pie. Serve with Praline sauce, below.

Praline Sauce

1. In saucepan combine brown sugar and cornstarch.

2. Stir in coffee. Cook and stir until bubbly. Cook and stir for 2 minutes more.

3. Stir in 1 teaspoon butter until melted.

4. Stir in pecans.

5. Serve warm with Sweet Potato Praline Pie, approximately 5 teaspoons per serving.

Yield: 10 servings

Nutritional Information: Per serving: Calories 198, fat 6g, protein 3g, carbohydrates 35g, cholesterol 47 mg, sodium 43mg.

Recipe Source: medicinenet.com

Thumbprint Cookies

You can fill these fun, festive cookies with an assortment of jam or preserves.

Ingredients:

- ½ cup no- or low-trans fat margarine with 8 g fat per tablespoon *(such as Land O' Lakes® Fresh Buttery Taste Spread or Take Control®)*
- ¼ cup granulated sugar
- ¼ cup Splenda®
- 1 large egg yolk *(or substitute 2 tablespoons egg substitute)*
- ½ teaspoon vanilla extract
- ½ teaspoon almond extract
- ¾ cup unbleached white flour
- ½ cup whole-wheat flour
- ¼ teaspoon salt
- ½ cup whole blanched almonds
- ⅓ cup less-sugar preserves *(or lemon curd)*

Preparation:

1. Preheat oven to 350 degrees. In large mixing bowl, beat the margarine with sugar and Splenda® on medium speed until light and fluffy *(about 3 minutes)*.

2. Add egg yolk or egg substitute and vanilla and almond extracts; beat well.

3. In a 4-cup measure, whisk the flours and salt together. Beat flour mixture into the margarine mixture gradually on low speed, just until combined.

4. Put almonds in a small food processor and process until nicely ground. Beat into cookie dough mixture on low speed, just to combine.

5. Use a cookie scoop *(⅛ cup)* to put dough on nonstick cookie sheet or jellyroll pan, about 2 inches apart *(line with parchment paper if desired)*. Make a deep indentation in the center of each ball with your thumb.

6. Bake for 8 minutes, then remove from oven. Fill center of each cookie with a slightly heaping 1-teaspoon measure of jam *(if necessary, press down center of cookies again before filling with jam)*. Bake about 8 minutes more or until golden brown. Place cookies on wire rack to cool.

Yield: About 15 large *(bakery size)* cookies

Nutritional Information: Per cookie: 136 calories, 2.5 g protein, 15 g carbohydrate, 7 g fat *(1.2 g saturated fat, 3 g monounsaturated fat, 2.5 g polyunsaturated fat)*, 14 mg cholesterol, 1.3 g fiber, 78 mg sodium. Calories from fat: 49%.

Recipe Source: medicinenet.com

White Chocolate-Cranberry Coffee Cake Recipe

Ingredients:

- ½ cup less-fat margarine *(with 8 grams fat per tablespoon)*
- ½ cup light cream cheese
- 1 cup firmly packed brown sugar
- ½ cup Splenda or Equal for baking *(or ¼ cup granulated sugar)*
- 2 large eggs
- ½ cup egg substitute
- 2 tablespoons grated orange zest *(or 1 tablespoon orange zest + ½ teaspoon orange extract)*
- 3 tablespoons orange juice
- 1 cup whole-wheat flour

- 1 cup unbleached white flour
- 2 teaspoon baking powder
- 1 ½ cups fresh or frozen cranberries
- ¾ cup white chocolate chips *(or white baking chocolate chopped into pieces)*

Preparation:

1. Preheat oven to 350 degrees. Coat a 9-inch tube pan or bundt pan with canola cooking spray.

2. Add margarine, light cream cheese, brown sugar, and granulated sugar *(or sugar substitute)* to large mixing bowl and beat with electric mixer on medium speed until fluffy. Add eggs one at a time, then egg substitute *(¼ cup at a time)*, orange zest and orange juice, mixing well and scraping sides of bowl at least once.

3. Measure a cup of whole-wheat flour and stir in the baking powder. Slowly add the whole-wheat flour mixture to the mixture in the mixing bowl, beating on low speed. Slowly beat in the white flour. Stir in the cranberries and white chocolate chips with a spoon.

4. Pour into the prepared pan and bake for about 1 hour or until toothpick inserted in the center comes out clean. Cool completely and serve.

Yield: 14 servings

Nutritional Information: Per serving: 200 calories, 5.5 g protein, 30 g carbohydrate, 7 g fat, 3 g saturated fat, 36 mg cholesterol, 2 g fiber, 177 mg sodium. Calories from fat: 32%.

Recipe Source: medicinenet.com

Meet *Dr. Sharon*
Sharon Allison-Ottey, MD
www.drsharononline.com

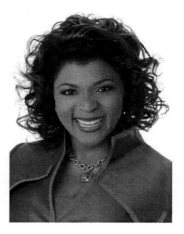

Sharon Denise Allison-Ottey, MD is an energetic and engaging speaker, author, health educator/physician and health strategist/consultant. Dr. Allison-Ottey serves as Executive Director of The COSHAR Foundation, a national nonprofit organization that educates and empowers communities to increase health awareness and outreach. Dr. Allison-Ottey completed a three year residency program in Internal Medicine (Adult Medicine) and two year fellowship in Geriatric Medicine (Adults over 65). She received her medical degree from East Carolina University School of Medicine. Dr. Allison-Ottey is a proud alumna of North Carolina Central University where she earned dual degrees in Biology and Chemistry with minors in Physics, African American History and English with honors.

Dr. Allison-Ottey is an avid medical researcher with numerous publications and presentations. She was named the American Geriatric Society's 1999 Investigator of the Year in recognition of her pioneering work in AIDS in the Elderly and was one of the first in the world to publish on this topic. *Her current research interests include Health Literacy, Patient/Physician Communication, the Role of Spirituality in Medical Outcomes, Direct to Consumer Marketing's effect on Physicians and Patients and Patient Adherence/ Compliance with Medical Treatment.* She provides invaluable insight and guidance to the numerous commissions, advisory boards and committees on which she serves. She is a consultant for several Fortune 500 companies and is also frequently invited to give expert testimony/advice to government and other organizations.

Dr. Allison-Ottey has appeared on Black Entertainment Television (BET) as well as other local and national television programs. She co-hosted a popular radio program for several years and is a frequent guest on nationally syndicated as well as regional/local radio programs across the country. She's been quoted and interviewed by several print publications including Redbook, Essence, Heart and Soul, Jet, Ebony, USA Today, Black Enterprise, The Wall Street Journal and numerous other media outlets. Because of the colorful and down to earth manner in which she addresses health, relationships and offers motivation; Dr. Allison-Ottey is a well-recognized and requested speaker for conferences, universities/schools, churches, corporations, community groups and a host of other outlets.

One of Dr. Allison-Ottey's passions is writing and in 2006 she introduced a new genre to the world of fiction, "fiction with a purpose". This genre marries an engaging fictional storyline with health education that leaves the reader enriched and empowered. Her first novel, *All I Ever Did Was Love a Man*, received much acclaim and continues to make an impact on the lives of her readers. Not one to rest on her laurels, the sequel, *My Breaking Heart* will be released in 2010. In light of her creation of "fiction with a purpose", in 2009 she launched an innovative greeting card line, *Cards by Dr. Sharon* which are "cards with a purpose." This full greeting card line mixes beautiful graphics, artsy and creative words with the unique *Moment of Health & Wellness* which appears on the back of each of the cards. The line was greeted with overwhelming success and continues to expand and make an impact. Dr. Allison-Ottey released a non fiction/self-help book entitled; *Is That Fried Chicken Wing Worth It?*

Contact Information:
Sharon D. Allison-Ottey, MD
www.drsharononline.com
Phone: 301.773.4811
Email: drsharon@sharondeniseallisonottey.com